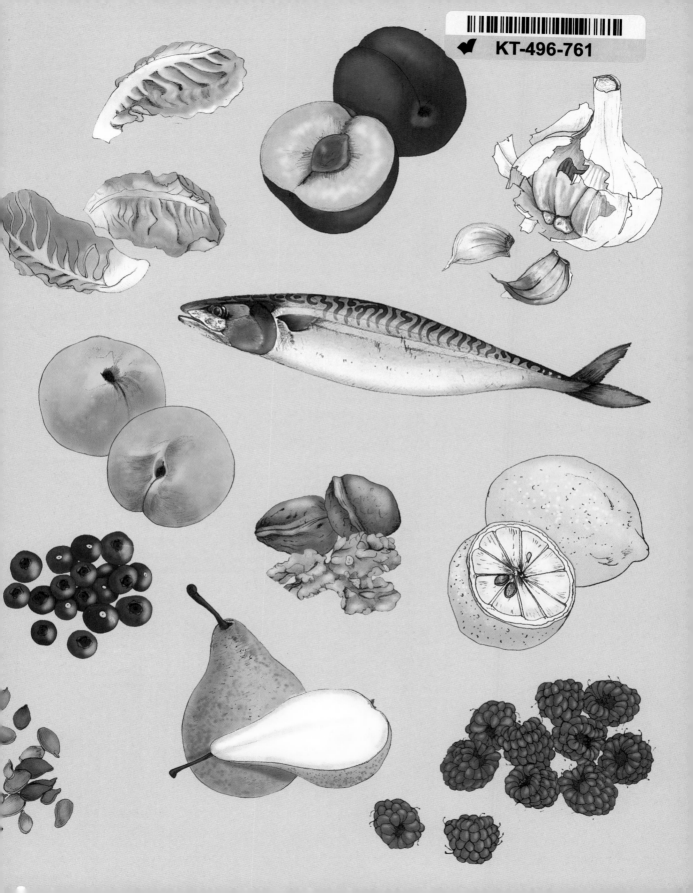

Gillian McKeith's FOOD BIBLE

THE COMPLETE A–Z GUIDE TO A HEALTHY LIFE

MICHAEL JOSEPH
an imprint of Penguin Books

This book is dedicated to my lovely daughters

MICHAEL JOSEPH

Published by the Penguin Group
Penguin Books Ltd, 80 Strand, London WC2R 0RL, England
Penguin Group (USA) Inc., 375 Hudson Street, New York, New York 10014, USA
Penguin Group (Canada), 90 Eglinton Avenue East, Suite 700, Toronto, Ontario, Canada M4P 2Y3
(a division of Pearson Penguin Canada Inc.)
Penguin Ireland, 25 St Stephen's Green, Dublin 2, Ireland (a division of Penguin Books Ltd)
Penguin Group (Australia), 250 Camberwell Road, Camberwell, Victoria 3124, Australia
(a division of Pearson Australia Group Pty Ltd)
Penguin Books India Pvt Ltd, 11 Community Centre, Panchsheel Park, New Delhi – 110 017, India
Penguin Group (NZ), 67 Apollo Drive, Rosedale, North Shore 0632, New Zealand
(a division of Pearson New Zealand Ltd)
Penguin Books (South Africa) (Pty) Ltd, 24 Sturdee Avenue, Rosebank, Johannesburg 2196,
South Africa

Penguin Books Ltd, Registered Offices: 80 Strand, London WC2R 0RL, England

www.penguin.com

First published 2008
1

Text copyright © Gillian McKeith, 2008
Photography copyright © Jonathan Buckley, pages 17, 24, 29, 60, 97, 107; Dan Jones, page 9;
David Loftus, pages 37, 73, 78, 128, 139, 144, 165; Noel Murphy, pages 42, 50, 55, 153
Illustrations copyright © Samara Bryan, 2008

The moral right of the author has been asserted

Designed and typeset by Smith & Gilmour, London
Printed in Great Britain by Butler and Tanner, Frome, Somerset.

A CIP catalogue record for this book is available from the British Library

ISBN: 978–0–718–14890–4

Every effort has been made to ensure that the information in this book is accurate. The
information in this book will be relevant to the majority of people but may not be applicable
in each individual case, so it is advised that professional medical advice is obtained for specific
information on personal health matters. Neither the publisher nor the author accepts any legal
responsibility for any personal injury or other damage or loss arising from the use or misuse
of the information and advice in this book. All vitamin, mineral and herbal supplements are
sold in varying strengths, so always check the dosage on the packaging.

Contents

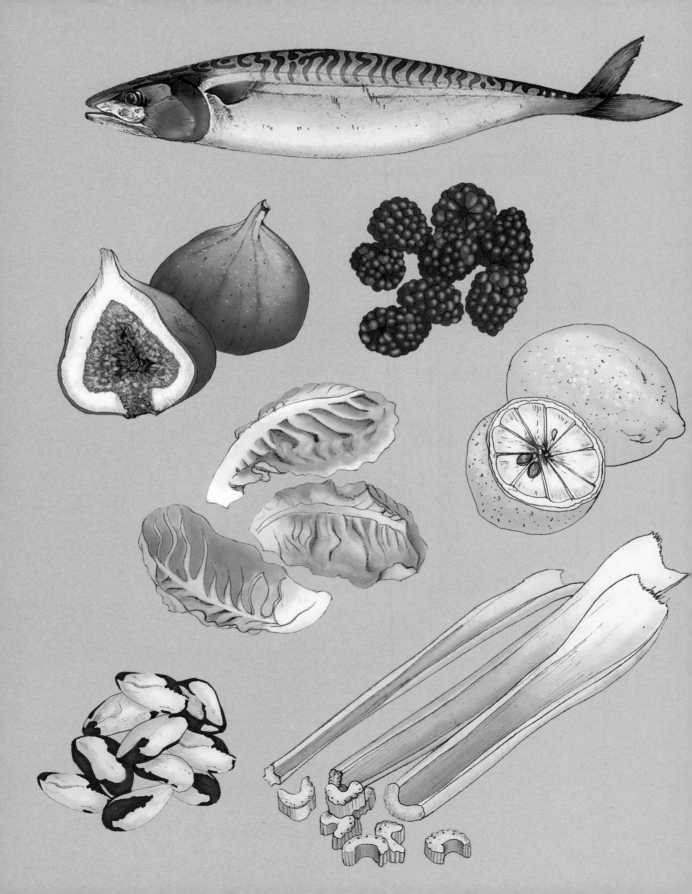

Introduction

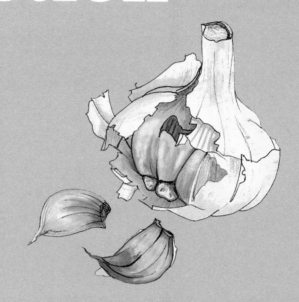

I know I'm a tough talker – my style has always been more bootcamp than health spa – after all, you wouldn't expect me to sugarcoat the message! The reason is, I truly care about empowering people to be healthier, and the best way you can do this is with food.

Your health really is in your hands, and your kitchen. Know that you have the power to heal and revitalize your body, mind and soul. But you need to be ready and willing to take up the reins. From the moment of conception, and even before, food gives us life. It has the power to heal, provides energy, lifts your moods and even boosts your chances of conception to start the life cycle all over again. That's why it breaks my heart to see people making themselves unwell, or even shortening their precious lives, through food ignorance and poor food choices.

But I'm not here to nag you, I'm here to help. I've decided to put my life's work into one must-have food bible. It's a book you can dip in and out of or read cover to cover. You can search for specific foods or ailments, or learn just how foods affect your wellbeing, from head to toe, birth to old age. Whether you want to learn what to eat to help protect you from winter colds, sail through the menopause or banish your IBS, my book provides the answers at your fingertips. Think of me as your personal food oracle. No need to struggle alone – just ask Gillian!

After working in the field of food and nutrition for more than 15 years, I've observed hundreds of clients, attended seminars and workshops all over the world and quizzed more boffins than you could shake a mango smoothie at. While it's absolutely fascinating, the sheer amount of information can be overwhelming. That's why I've made it my passion to absorb, understand and distil it all for you. As I've found so often with my clients, simplicity is the key to success. And success equals a healthier, sexier, more radiant, happier you.

I believe there are three crucial elements when it comes to your general health. They are each very simple, and very powerful:

1. Open up
2. Be the real you
3. Think of food as energy: positive and negative

The first two might not seem very relevant in a book about nutrition, but to get an overweight, beer-guzzling, burger-munching man to swap over to aduki beans, he needs to open up his mind, body and spirit. The same goes for all of us who want to change. We need to open up to who we really are, what we want and go for it. Shed your baggage and reach your core. Become open-minded to all the new and exciting foods that you will discover and the possibilities for health, energy and lifestyle are endless.

The following exercise will help you do it:
1) Upon waking, listen to your breath for a couple of minutes. Then give a soft-spoken command to your body: 'My body is free to be totally open.' (If you have a partner snoring next to you, you may want to say it silently) Repeat the command three times.
2) Get out of bed and stand up with your bare feet firmly planted on the ground. Raise both arms above your head. Just notice your body and how it feels.

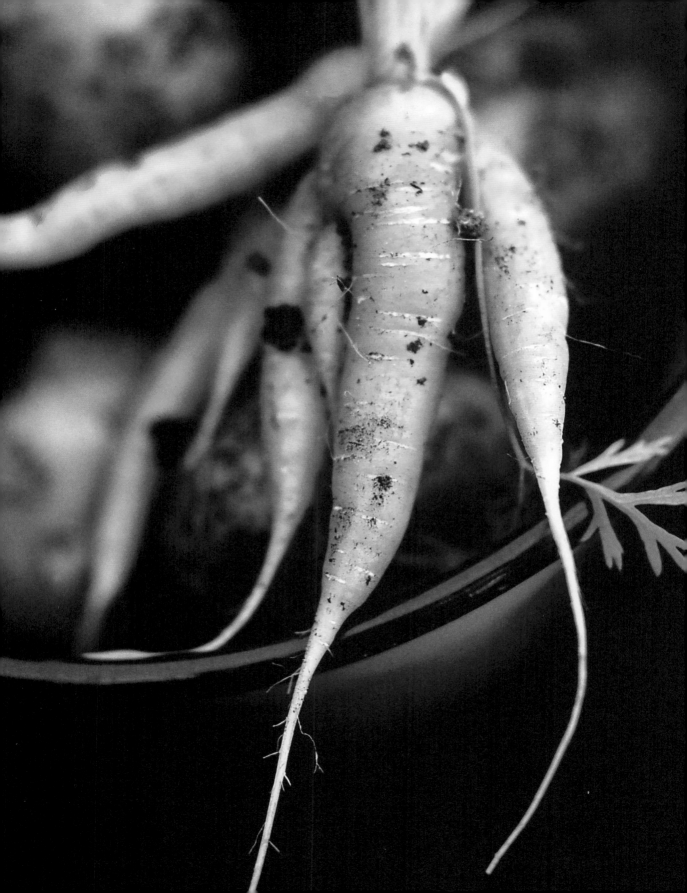

The key is to stay out of your head and be in your body. *Just be*. Stop thinking and don't ask so many questions of yourself. The end result is that you process your emotions better and you will be more open to everything, new ideas, new philosophies, new directions, new foods – a new you.

Once you've opened up, you need to stay true to your new ideals – be the real you. When you eat healthily, you are going to think differently. You will be stronger in body, clearer in thought, more intuitive and able to make the right decisions in life. But some people around you may feel threatened by the change. They might try to stop you because of what it might mean for them. You may hear the usual snide comments:

► That's bird food.
► It's so expensive.
► You're not feeding me that.
► I won't like it.

Don't be discouraged, don't be drawn in. Take note of comments like these, then let go and move on. In order for you to access your own harmony, you must stand your ground. Be who you really are. It's your journey.

The third element is simple, but incredibly effective when it comes to making a real connection to the food you eat and your health. Once you 'get' the concept, it'll be so obvious – you'll wonder why you haven't always thought this way. I want you always to think of food as energy, which can be positive or negative. Just think of the vibrant energy you can taste as you bite into a ripe yellow peach in the summer, or when you pick and eat blackberries in the autumn. Pure, positive energy. But, on the negative side, think about how your body reacts to a fast-food burger and chips, or a bottle of bright blue pop, full of sweeteners, colourings and chemicals. You feel drained and lethargic once the stimulant wears off, and will be more prone to illness.

Once you master the art of seeing food as energy, then you'll begin to really care about what you're eating, to want to enjoy foods in their natural, pure state rather than altered and packed full of additives. I want you to see healthy foods as delicious, high vibrational energy bytes. Raw foods contain food enzymes – an amazing source of positive food energy. Just think about the colour of vegetables when they are still crunchy and full of flavour, versus the rather unpleasant smell and sad, lifeless look of overcooked cabbage. Simply adding more raw foods to your diet, or lightly steaming your vegetables so they maintain their vibrancy and goodness, will show in how you feel, think and look – I guarantee it!

OK, I appreciate that it's not always so easy in the hustle and bustle of today's world to eat perfectly well. We have so many choices but too little time to make the most of those choices. Food has gradually dropped down our list of priorities – we'll grab a sandwich at our desks for lunch, pop an overprocessed meal in the microwave or speed eat in front of the TV. Too many people are addicted to sugar, caffeine, alcohol and artificial flavourings. How ironic that healthy food, in its natural state, should seem so very inconvenient.

I am here to change all that. In this book, you will discover the convenience factor of healthy food, the tastiness and of course the healthfulness of healing foods. I hope this book will inspire as well as inform. It is in four easy-to-navigate sections: The Key Health Factors, The Foundations of a Healthy Diet, Food and the Stages of Life and the A–Z of Conditions. If there's anything you ever need to know about food and health, it's now at your fingertips. Use it every day for you and your loved ones to be the best you can be. You now have the power to be healthy, vibrant and in charge of your own life.

Wishing you love and light

Gillian

www.gillianmckeith.info

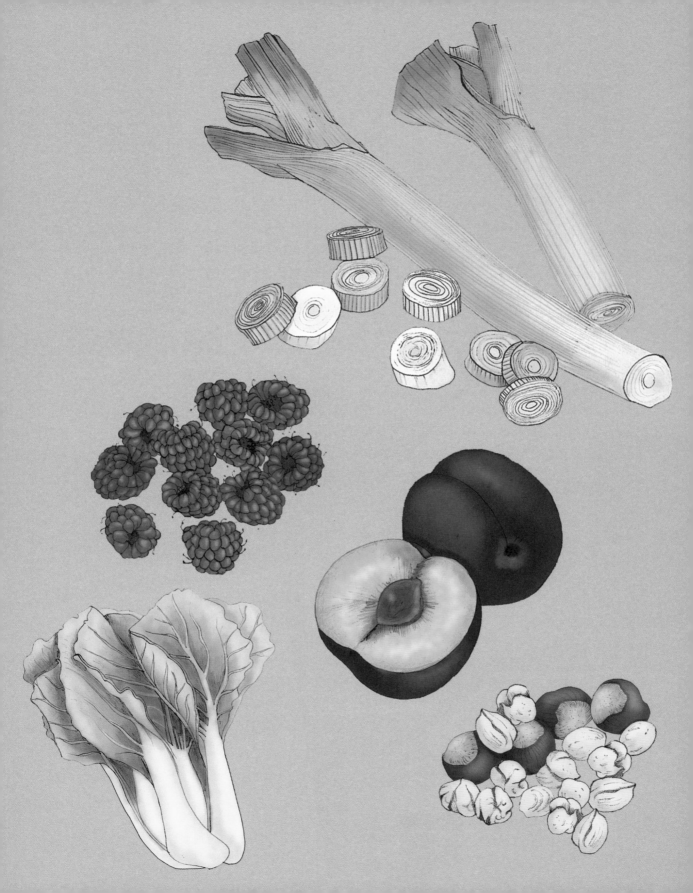

The key health factors

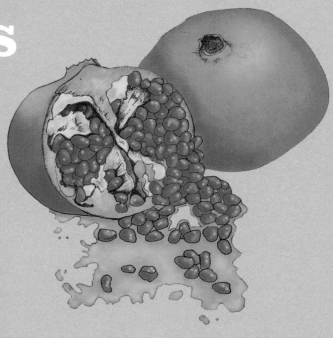

Each of our body systems needs nutrients and natural life-giving energy for constant regeneration. And you can provide that easily with a balanced, varied and vibrant diet. Eat well, follow my suggestions, and you'll work wonders on your wellbeing. Without even knowing it, you'll be empowered by following my key health factors:

► **Digestion**
► **Blood Sugar/Energy**
► **Food Sensitivity**
► **Heart and Circulation**
► **Hormones**
► **Thyroid/Metabolism**
► **Mind and Mood**
► **Detoxification**
► **Stress**
► **Immunity**

The nutrients that influence these health factors include vitamins, minerals, essential fatty acids (EFAs), fibre, water, plant nutrients (phytonutrients) and amino acids. Imbalances in any of these factors and insufficient nourishment will affect how you look and feel. They can contribute to weight gain, skin issues, low energy, mood swings, sexual performance, headaches, irritability and a myriad of aches and pains, not to mention greater susceptibility to degenerative illnesses and diseases.

I lived on pot noodles and cheese on toast, I prided myself on not touching anything green, and the only exercise I got was dancing the weekends away. Then a work colleague recommended your book, I did the questionnaire and it suddenly dawned on me that while I thought I was a healthy 20+ year old, I was actually neglecting and abusing my body. If I didn't do anything about it soon it would only be a matter of time before my body would start letting me down. Small signs were already there – lack of energy, chronic fatigue, bloating, mood swings, irregular bowel movements, etc. and I am convinced that if I hadn't made the necessary changes that these symptoms would have got worse and I probably would have eventually been plagued by potentially more serious illnesses. For me, it was about making small changes and understanding more about food and what the body needs to function at its best. With time I have been able to introduce most types of vegetables to my diet, I'm more conscious of drinking more water, I try and exercise three times a week, and more recently I have started juicing which I'm loving... I'll know I've made it when I start sprouting my own seeds...

Your Key Health Factors

Digestion

Yes, I am always going on about good digestion. I'm not going to apologize for it! Because I see more health problems linked to the way the body digests and absorbs food than anything else. If you've never given your digestion a second thought then it's time to do your body a favour.

Put simply, digestion involves the breakdown of food molecules for absorption into your body, thanks to acid produced in the stomach and digestive enzymes released in your saliva and by the pancreas. Get the process off to the best start by always chewing your food until it becomes liquid. Don't inhale your meals!

Raw foods contain their own enzymes, so eat more of them to give your digestive system a helping hand. My simple rule is every time you eat something cooked, eat some non-cooked food with it (Never tried raw broccoli? You're missing out).

A good gut diet is fibre-rich with plenty of water. Too much processed white sugar, refined foods, red meat, dairy products and processed foods overload and weaken digestion and invite excess yeast and unfriendly bacteria to make themselves at home in your gut. See the A–Z section for detailed entries on Bloating, Indigestion, Irritable Bowel Syndrome, Crohn's Disease.

Blood Sugar/Energy

If you do not balance your blood-sugar levels, then every day you are putting your body and mind on a rollercoaster ride of highs and lows. And you will probably be a bit of a moody so and so to boot. There are many health problems, big and small, that can be traced to a blood-sugar imbalance caused by food choices.

A quick Gillian McKeith masterclass:

Through the day, your body requires a steady supply of glucose in the bloodstream for mental and physical energy. When we eat complex carbohydrates such as fruits and vegetables, beans,

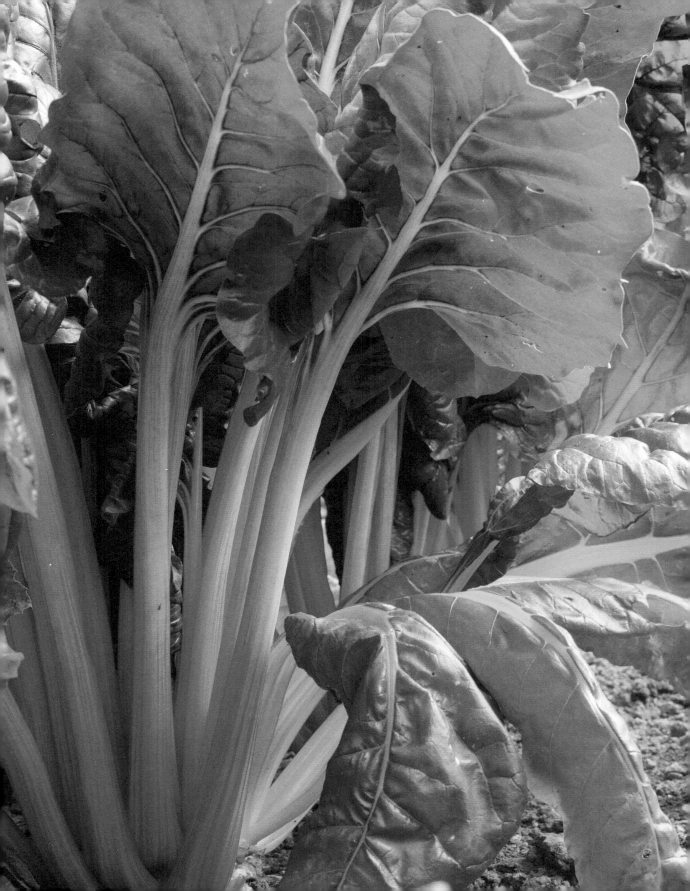

pulses and whole-grains, they release glucose into the bloodstream at a nice steady rate. But refined and sugary foods (such as chocolate, biscuits, cakes, fizzy drinks, sweets or white pasta/rice/bread) break down very quickly and cause an unwanted, rapid rise in blood sugar. This prompts a surge of insulin to remove the sugar, followed by a dramatic drop in blood sugar (hypoglycaemia). That's when you can get the afternoon energy slumps, feel shaky, tired, confused and, surprise surprise, crave more sugar. This yo-yoing causes a host of everyday symptoms and can lead to significant health problems including heart disease and type 2 diabetes.

It sounds complicated, but fortunately the solution is super simple. Just eat regular meals and snacks, never skip breakfast, and avoid refined or sugary foods, caffeine and alcohol. No one who has made this change has ever said to me, 'You know what, Gillian, I think I prefer how I felt before'!

Food Sensitivity

Food sensitivity is a 21st-century epidemic. It has been reported that up to one in three people suffers from unknown food allergies or intolerances. Why unknown? Because symptoms don't always kick in immediately after eating an offending food – they often creep up over a day or two. So you could live for years without realizing a particular food doesn't suit you. Plus, if you've always felt a certain way, you won't know there's anything wrong. When people discover a food intolerance and eliminate it, they feel truly healthy for the first time in their life. It's a joy to see.

Allergies or intolerances of certain foods and chemicals don't just affect your digestive system (although that can take a real bruising). Any number of health factors can be affected, causing all-round illness. Often, it is weakened immunity that is the root cause of a food sensitivity.

The most common food culprits are wheat, dairy and oranges. Others include soy, shellfish, peanuts and yeast. Improving digestive function, enhancing immunity and generally supporting health overall will definitely reduce your chance of suffering a food sensitivity. And rotate foods regularly, in other words don't eat the same thing day in day out. See the A–Z section for detailed entries on Food Allergies.

Heart and Circulation

Made up of your heart and the system of arteries, veins and blood, the cardio-vascular system circulates blood around your body, delivering nutrients and oxygen and carrying away carbon dioxide and waste products.

A few people may have a family history of cardio-vascular problems but for the vast majority (including those with genetic factors) risk can be controlled by lifestyle. Many use family history as an excuse to not even attempt a healthy lifestyle. My father had heart problems and would have been the first to admit that he brought these on himself through 50-odd years of chain smoking. His last message to me was: please tell everyone you possibly can to never ever pick up a cigarette. He would also be first in line to tell you that so many fantastic foods and herbs can make an almighty difference to your quality of life when you have heart issues.

Nourish your heart with foods low in saturated fats, sugar and refined carbohydrates and high in complex carbohydrates, grains, fruits and vegetables. Drink plenty of fresh water but minimize or eliminate alcohol, tea and coffee. See the A–Z section for detailed entries on Heart Disease, Atherosclerosis, High Blood Pressure, High Cholesterol and High Homocysteine.

Hormones

We're all at the mercy of our hormones – and not just women at certain times of the month. So men, this bit's for you, too! Hormones are chemical messengers that travel in the blood to give instructions to certain cells. Their balance affects how you feel, how you age, your sexual performance and how you deal with stress.

Good balance means getting enough essential fatty acids, fibre-rich foods and being well hydrated. Hormone balance can be disturbed by unstable blood sugar, an inability to metabolize fatty acids and malabsorption. Exposure to oestrogenic compounds present in dairy products, red meats, soft plastics (often used to package food) and pesticides which leach into foods are also harmful – another good reason to eat organic foods. Alcohol and caffeine play havoc with hormones, as does deep-fried or burnt food, hydrogenated fat (in margarine and many processed foods) and most saturated fats (in meat, cheese and processed foods). See page 99 for information on male hormones, page 104 for information on female hormones.

Thyroid/Metabolism

The thyroid is one powerful organ. It controls how quickly your body burns calories and uses energy. If you don't have enough thyroid hormones, your body slows down – I'm talking blood pressure, circulation, energy, metabolism and temperature. If you make too many, it speeds up and every system goes into overdrive.

For a healthy thyroid, you need iodine and the amino acid tyrosine. Seaweeds are a good source. And choose foods that include selenium, calcium, zinc and vitamins A, C, E and B-complex. Good old essential fatty acids are also vital, along with making sure you get adequate supplies of complete protein.

Now here's something you never thought you'd hear me say: much as it pains me to utter these words, it is possible for raw cruciferous vegetables to affect an already wobbly thyroid. So, while broccoli, Brussels sprouts, cabbage and kale are fabulous foods, if you have had thyroid problems diagnosed by your GP, eat less of them for a wee while until it's all sorted out. And always make sure you cook them as this will reduce any effects on your thyroid. Invest in a water filter – fluoride and chlorine, both present in tap water, aren't thyroid friends (use a non-fluoride toothpaste, too). And get moving – exercise is brilliant for your thyroid and overall metabolism.

Mind and Mood

Your brain is like a complex chemistry kit, and if the balance isn't quite right, mind and mood problems can result. You may have heard of neurotransmitters, chemicals which the brain uses to communicate with the rest of the body. The main ones are called dopamine, adrenalin, noradrenalin and serotonin, and they're made entirely from molecules derived from food, air and water. Poor nutrition and lifestyle can easily upset your brain-chemical balance.

The brain requires a steady supply of glucose to function properly, so my section on blood-sugar balance is key here, too. In particular, steer clear of caffeine and alcohol. You can argue as much as you like that they perk you up, but in the long term they will mess up your mood – believe me! Swap your cuppa for a thirst-quenching glass of water instead, as good hydration is the best brain booster. See page 156 for brain foods.

Detoxification

Some people might say they don't need to detox, because our bodies do it naturally. But in today's modern world of pollution, radiation, chemicals, pesticides, herbicides, food additives and preservatives (just to get me started!) our bodies are literally under attack. So let me help you detox.

The main detoxification organs are the liver, kidneys, lungs, bowels and skin. Everyone is different, but twice a day for bowel movements is ideal. A congested bowel will exhaust your energy and if your system is clogged up it will soon show in how you look and feel. The bottom line, if you'll excuse the pun, is you need to make sure you're getting all the toxins out, and the best way to do that is through plenty of fibre like brown rice, fruit (yes, prunes are fantastic) and beans (no surprise). Red meat and processed meats contain no fibre; and foods high in sugar or yeast can feed the bad bacteria in your colon, leading to irregular bowel movements. Eggs can also be constipating for some people.

When our toxin load becomes too great, it's our poor liver that takes the brunt. Look after your liver by limiting your exposure to toxins (buy organic, avoid smoking, chemical products, pollution, alcohol) and help your body eliminate those that do get in. To neutralize toxins, especially free radicals, get your antioxidants – vitamins A, C, E, betacarotene, zinc and selenium. Detox your gut by adding beneficial bacteria to overpower the bad. Miso soups, sauerkraut and foods high in B vitamins can help to encourage good bacteria gut growth.

Get into the habit of skin brushing. Use a natural-bristle brush, on dry skin, and sweep it all over your body, towards your heart. This gets your lymph moving and speeds drainage – great if you're prone to water retention or cellulite, too.

Stress

Humans are incredibly adaptable – we're designed to be able
to handle stress. But if a stressful situation gets too much,
or we lose the natural resources needed to cope, it can harm our
health. Most people, when they make better food choices and
modify their lifestyle, find they can handle stress more easily.

It is important if we are stressed or failing to deal well with
stress that we eat nutrient-dense foods. If it doesn't do you good,
don't waste time eating it! Think fresh fruit and veggies (raw
juices, too), raw nuts and seeds and wholegrains. Celery, cabbage
and cucumber are all real stress busters. So next time you're
feeling stressed, don't chew your nails, chew a stick of celery.
A pot of lettuce soup can de-stress in minutes. A stressed body
needs vitamin C, B vits, zinc, potassium and manganese.

Taking regular, gentle exercise is essential, as is finding time
to relax each day. 'I haven't got time' is no excuse. Learn some
deep breathing exercises to restore calm and control. And make
a decent night's sleep – every night – your priority. See page
373 for more detailed nutritional information on combating
and preventing stress.

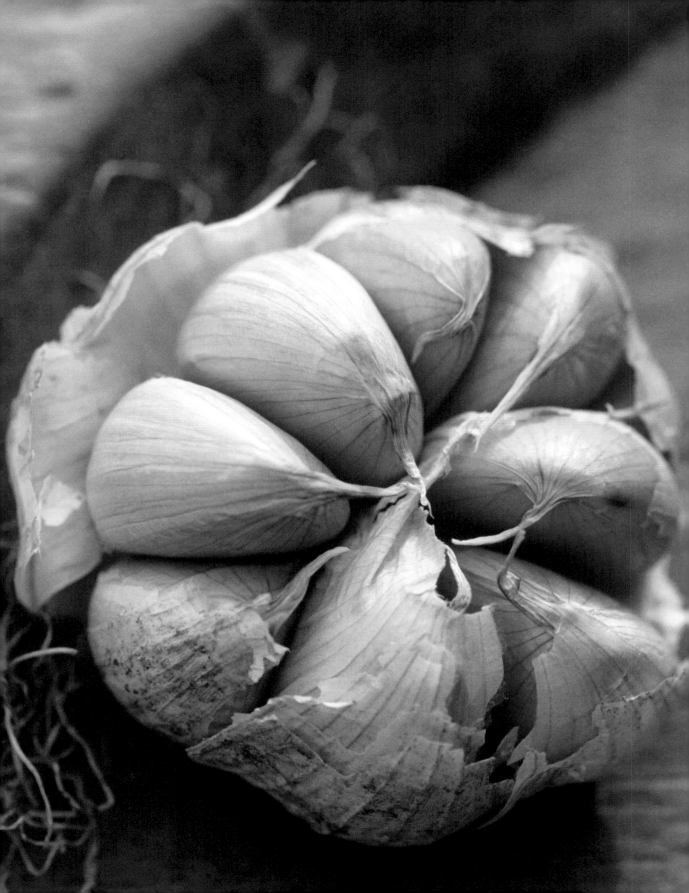

Immunity

You may not have realized it, but every day there's a battle going on. Your body is under constant attack from dangerous free radicals and foreign invaders like bacteria and viruses. What keeps ill health at bay is a strong immune system. Your immune army consists of various antibodies, each with a special protective role, and is dependent on good nutrition and a supportive lifestyle. If your immune system becomes overworked or is not nourished properly, it gives up the fight and surrenders to the bad guys.

The best way to build up your defences is with immune-enhancing antioxidants which disarm free radicals. The key antioxidants are vitamins A, C and E, and the minerals selenium, iron, manganese and zinc. Also ensure an arsenal of B vitamins, for antibody production, and omega-3 and -6 essential fatty acids, to control inflammation. Finally add allicin, an antibacterial, antiviral, antifungal substance in garlic and onions, plus polyphenols, quercetin and rutin – all flavanoids found in plants. Sprouted broccoli seeds and shitake mushrooms are fabulous immune defenders. Give them a go.

If you want to see how these health factors affect you personally, go to www.gillianmckeith.info to take your own unique, individualized, personalized nutritional profile.

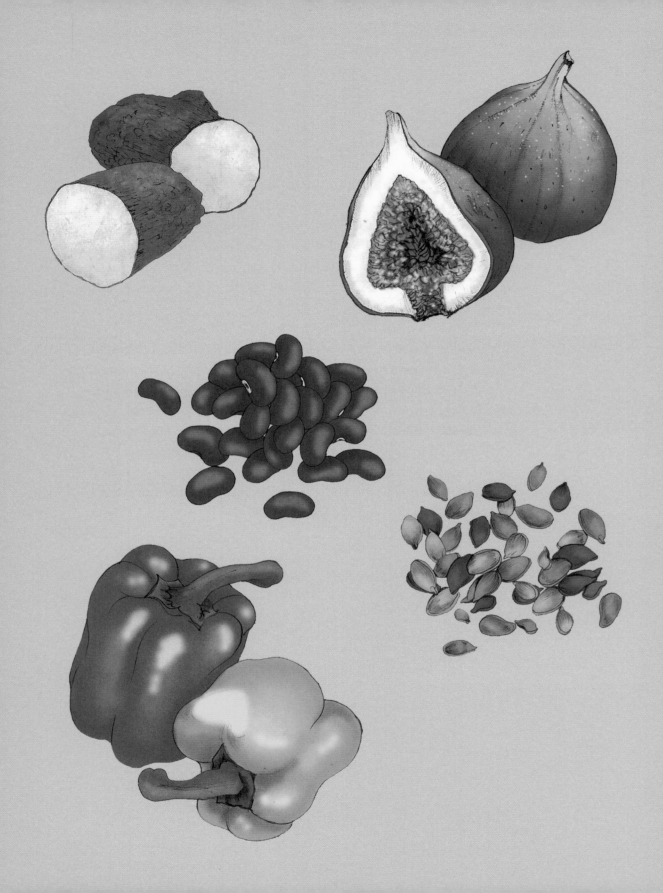

The foundations of a healthy diet

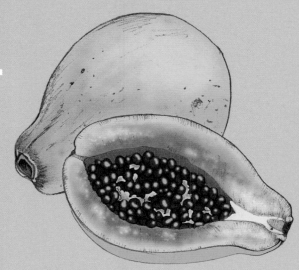

Here is a quick Gillian McKeith masterclass in the essential foundations of a healthy, vital diet. Nutrition is completely personal and individual, so here are the basic principles, from which you will create your own optimum food plan.

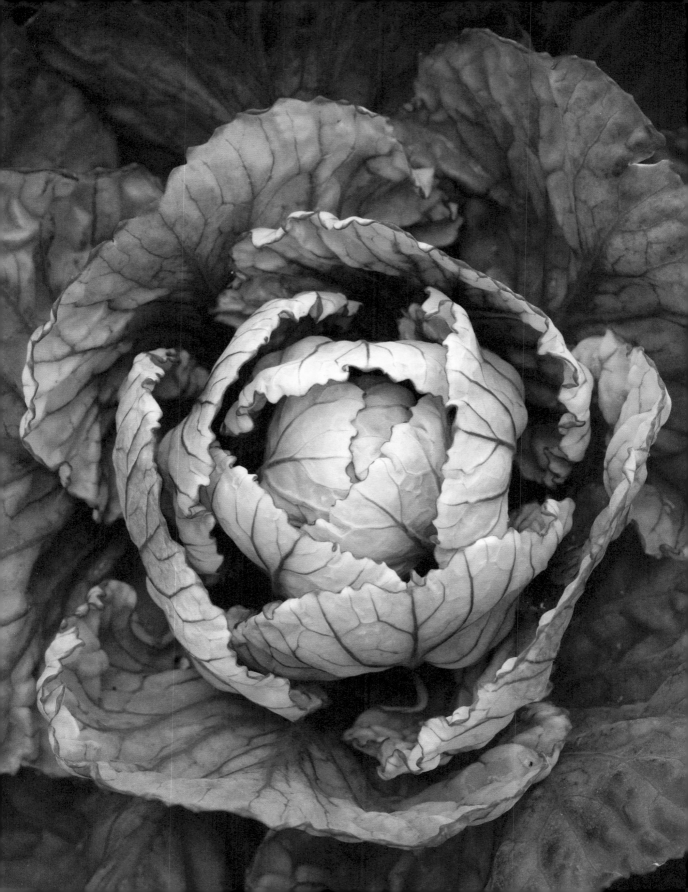

Water

Newborn babies are approximately 77 per cent water. This decreases as we age so that adults are between 45 and 65 per cent water. The muscles and brain are both around 75 per cent water. Even small reductions in body fluids can lead to diminished body function, resulting in digestive problems, lack of energy, poor brain function, slower reaction times and of course dry skin and hair to name but a few.

Water is the major component of every body tissue and fluid. Without it we would be a shrivelled mass unable to function. Digestion, assimilation, elimination, metabolism, respiration and temperature control can only happen in the presence of water. Water dissolves and transports nutrients via body fluids (lymph and blood etc.). Without this transport nothing would be able to happen in the body. The importance of water cannot be over-estimated.

Tap water is the main source of water for most people. It may not, however, be ideal. Undesirable elements it may contain include chlorine, aluminium, fluoride, oestrogens, lead (if the water pipes are lead) and copper (which is needed by the body in moderation but can build up and lead to imbalances if too much is ingested). I highly recommend installing a water filter in your home.

► **Jug filters** – these certainly filter out some impurities from the water. They are relatively inexpensive to buy and maintain, involve no fitting and need little space. Care must taken to change the filter regularly and to keep the jug clean as they can become breeding grounds for bacteria, especially in warm weather.

► **Fitted water filters** – these vary considerably in price, size and how they filter the water. Reverse osmosis water filters usually fit under the sink and attach to the incoming water pipe. There is usually a separate tap from which the filtered water is dispensed. How often the filter needs to be changed varies from 3 months to a service once a year.

There are now also water purifiers that split water into alkaline and acidic water. The alkaline water is for drinking and cooking as this can help to alkalize body tissues and improve health. The acidic water is great for washing up and cleaning purposes as it has an anti-bacterial action.

How much should I drink?

The usual recommendation is to drink 2 litres of water a day. This is a good aim for most people. There is increased water loss when we sweat or breathe heavily so exercise obviously increases our need and this should be taken into account.

Other fluids that can count towards your daily intake include herbal teas and vegetable juices. Vegetable juices can be especially useful to those who find that water just seems to go straight through them. The mineral content of veggie juices means they seem to stay in the body for longer. Thus they can be better for hydrating the body cells.

Tea, coffee, alcohol and soft drinks do not count towards daily fluid intake. These are dehydrating and can lead to nutrient losses.

If you eat foods with high fluid content, then you might get away with drinking slightly less water. Some foods contain a lot of water. But water is like oxygen, it is so very vital to your wellbeing. Fruit can be 90–95 per cent water. Vegetables also have a high water content. Cooked whole-grains can hold some water and this can aid hydration in the body, especially the colon.

Carbohydrates

Foods containing carbohydrates include grains such as wheat, brown rice, oats, and nuts, seeds, pulses, fruit and vegetables. All carbohydrates get broken down into glucose in the digestive tract. This glucose is the body's main source of fuel; in other words it's what gives us energy. Glucose is also what powers the brain; without it we can lose concentration, forget things and feel irritable.

Not all carbohydrates are the same. Although they all get broken down into glucose in the digestive tract, some get broken down more quickly than others. These are called simple carbohydrates and they include white rice, white flour, white bread, white pasta, sugar, pastries, pies, cakes and biscuits, to name a few. During the refining process, the majority of the minerals and vitamins are removed. These foods which also lack fibre behave like sugar in the body causing blood glucose disturbances and cravings; they often contain added sugars too. You may feel angry, tired and irritable. My point is that simple carbohydrates rob your energy levels.

Complex carbohydrates (which I call healthy carbs) break down more slowly. This is partly due to the fibre they contain. Fibre slows down the rate at which the food is broken down and therefore the rate at which glucose is released into the bloodstream. They are also not stripped of their nutrients. End result: sustained energy levels.

Blood sugar levels should remain within very narrow parameters if you are to function optimally. However, because simple carbohydrates break down rapidly into glucose, blood sugar levels rise rapidly. This explains why a person may eat a piece of sponge cake and think they are feeling an upper, but soon after a rapid drop in energy or mood will surely come. Ultimately, simple carbs wear you down.

Complex carbohydrates release their glucose into the bloodstream bit by bit, so tend not to raise blood sugar levels too quickly and a degree of stability is maintained. Complex carbohydrates nourish and enhance energy levels.

Bottom line: simple carbs are bad; healthy carbs are good.

Good sources of complex carbohydrates include:

► **Whole-grains:** brown rice, wild rice, quinoa, millet, buckwheat, amaranth, oats, rye, barley, whole wheat, spelt and kamut.

► **Pulses and legumes:** chickpeas, brown lentils, green lentils, puy lentils, red split lentils, aduki beans, butter beans, borlotti beans, flageolet beans, cannelloni beans.

► **Vegetables:** sweet potatoes, carrots, swede, parsnips, squash, pumpkin, turnips, cauliflower, peas, sweetcorn, broadbeans.

► **Fruit:** apples, pears, cherries, strawberries, blackberries, raspberries, blueberries, plums, papayas, pineapples, mangoes, bananas, peaches, nectarines, apricots.

Simple carbohydrates to avoid or limit include:

► **Refined grains:** white flour, white bread, white pasta, white rice, white cornflour.

► **Sugars:** white sugar, brown sugar.

► Cakes, biscuits, confectionery, sweets, chocolates, pastries, buns, scones, pies.

Fibre

Fibre is basically the term given to indigestible carbohydrates. The walls of plant foods are made up of this indigestible fibre; some animals can digest this fibre but humans do not have the enzymes necessary to break it down. Traditional diets contain lots of unprocessed carbohydrates with fibre intact. In western countries, where more processed foods are eaten with their fibre removed, obesity, diabetes, constipation, haemorrhoids, varicose veins, appendicitis, hernia, heart disease and other degenerative diseases are common. These can all be linked to a low-fibre diet.

In the past, it was thought that fibre had no role as it did not provide any calories or nutrients. That belief led to the removal of fibre and hence all the processed foods we have today.

The fact is that we need fibre – we need food to remain intact, the way nature intended. Fibre can improve:

▶ **Elimination and transit time through the gut:** it can normalize bowel movements in constipation and diarrhoea.

▶ **Blood-sugar control:** fibre slows the breakdown of carbohydrates into glucose. This means glucose is released gradually into the bloodstream and blood-sugar levels will not rise too rapidly.

▶ **Digestion:** pancreatic enzyme (that break down food into its component parts) secretion and activity increase when fibre is eaten.

▶ **Cholesterol and blood-lipid levels:** soluble fibre increases the excretion of these via the bowel and reduces the amount manufactured in the liver.

▶ **Intestinal function:** fibre provides food for the beneficial bacteria in the gut and helps provide an environment in which they can thrive.

Fibre-rich foods

► **Fruit and vegetables:** all of these contain fibre that contributes to their cleansing properties. Juices have their fibre removed in order to free up nutrients for use by the body. These are great for the body, but they should not replace whole fruits and vegetables. Smoothies that are made from blended whole fruits still contain their fibre. I'm a big fan!

► **Whole-grains:** brown rice, wild rice, red rice, oats, barley, rye, millet, buckwheat, quinoa, amaranth.

► **Nuts and seeds:** all contain some fibre. Flax seeds are particularly recommended as they contain a mucilaginous fibre that can aid lubrication and function of the bowel. Ideally, soak the flax seeds overnight, either whole or ground. The seeds and the water can be consumed. Dry-roasted flax seeds are delicious.

► **Pulses and legumes:** all beans and pulses contain useful amounts of fibre. See protein sources for different types.

► **Sprouted grains and pulses:** these are all good sources of fibre.

► **Sea vegetables:** these are a great source of mucilaginous fibre that can help to remove toxins and heavy metals from the body. They include nori, kelp, dulse, arame, kombu, wakame and agar agar.

Protein

Animal proteins are those that come from the body of an animal or are products of an animal. They include meat, fish, eggs and dairy products. Vegetable proteins are those that come from plant foods. Plant foods that contain protein include pulses, nuts, seeds, quinoa, amaranth and green vegetables.

Amino acids are what make up proteins whether they be in plants, animals or ourselves. There are eight amino acids that you need to get from your diet in order for the body to be able to make all the different proteins it needs to function. These are called the essential amino acids. If just one of these is missing or low, protein synthesis in the body will be significantly reduced.

If a food contains all the essential amino acids in the correct ratios, it is called a complete protein. All animal proteins are complete. Vegetable proteins do not necessarily contain all the essential amino acids in sufficient quantities. This is not a problem though as the amino acids that are lacking in some foods can be found in sufficient quantities in other foods.

For example, grains tend to be low in methionine but pulses contain good amounts of this amino acid. Including both grains and pulses together in a vegetarian diet on a daily basis ensures that you get the full range of amino acids in sufficient quantities.

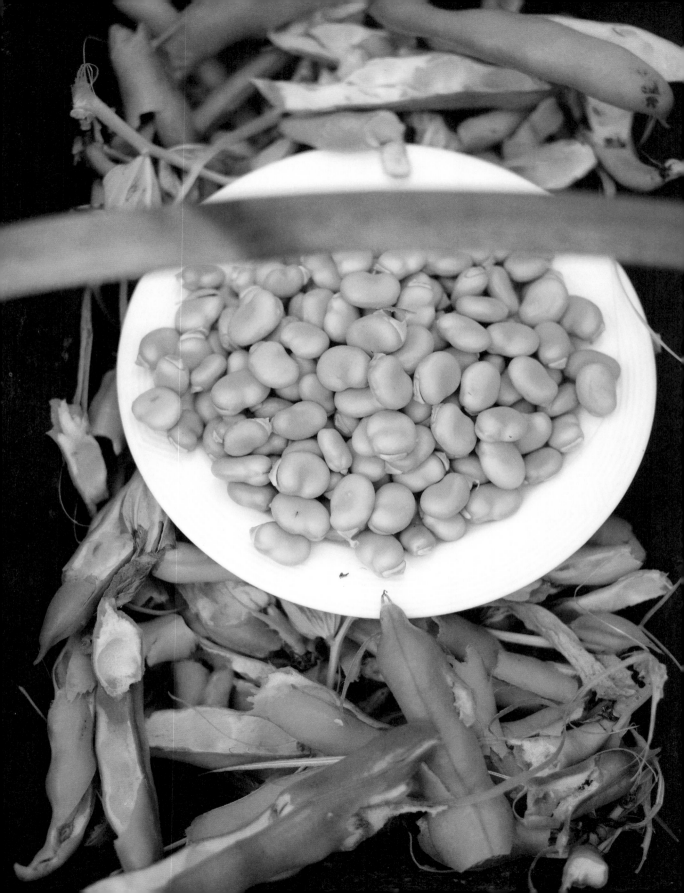

Uses of protein in the body

Protein is vital for the growth and maintenance of all body components. All our tissues, nerves and bones are largely made up of proteins. Muscles, internal organs, blood, skin, hair and nails are also dependent on protein for their structure. Protein is vital for body repair; for example collagen is a protein that makes up scar tissue and strengthens arterial walls.

Body proteins such as muscles can be broken down and converted to energy if there are insufficient carbohydrates and fats available. Excess protein that is not needed for building body tissues or energy can be converted to fat by the liver and stored for future use.

Some hormones are made of proteins. Insulin from the pancreas that helps control blood-sugar levels is made from proteins, as is thyroxine from the thyroid, which helps control metabolism and body temperature.

In addition, enzymes in the body are also made of proteins. Enzymes are what spark all body processes. Without enzymes, no body processes would be able to happen. The main enzymes we talk about are the digestive enzymes that help break down protein, fats and carbohydrates into their component parts. There are many other types of enzymes in the body that are making things happen at all times.

We don't necessarily think of the immune system when we think about protein, but antibodies needed to fight viruses and bacteria are actually made up of proteins, too.

All in all, you can see how vital protein is for life.

Good sources of protein include:

▶ **Lean meats:** chicken, turkey. Get organic where possible as conventionally reared meats may contain antibiotic and hormone residues.

▶ **Fish:** include oily and white fish as they are both good sources of protein – salmon, sardines, mackerel, herrings, sea bass, lemon sole, Dover sole, cod, haddock, trout, red snapper, skate and halibut. Go for wild or organic fish rather than conventionally farmed fish.

▶ **Pulses and legumes:** chickpeas, brown lentils, green lentils, puy lentils, red split lentils, aduki beans, butter beans, borlotti beans, flageolet beans, haricot beans, pinto beans, cannelloni beans, soya beans, mung beans, tempeh, tofu, soya yoghurt, miso.

▶ **Nuts and seeds:** almonds, hazelnuts, cashew nuts, walnuts, pine nuts, Brazil nuts, pecan nuts, macadamia nuts, hemp seeds, sunflower seeds, pumpkin seeds, sesame seeds, flax seeds.

▶ **Quinoa:** this is used as a grain in cooking but is higher in protein than most grains and it contains all the essential amino acids in good ratios, meaning it provides very usable protein.

▶ **Eggs:** there are many different types of eggs around now. The best are often those from small organic farms where the chickens can roam around freely and have plenty of fresh greens and seeds to eat. Other eggs that may be available include quail and duck eggs. Always go for organic and free range.

▶ **Dairy products:** these include milk, cheese, yoghurt, cream and kefir. They are not ideal for many people as they can be allergenic, can upset digestion and be mucus forming. Goat's and sheep's milk products tend to be easier to digest than cow's milk. Fermented dairy products tend to be easier to digest than milk as the beneficial bacteria break down the proteins and sugars to some extent. Natural yoghurt and kefir can be eaten by some people in moderation.

Fats

The body does need good fats. These fats are composed of fatty acids, two families of which are essential (omega-3 and omega-6). The average diet tends to include insufficient essential fatty acids and an excess of the unhealthy saturated and trans-fatty acids.

▶ **Saturated fats** tend to be solid at room temperature and include butter, lard and palm oil. They are very stable and can be heated without becoming damaged. But saturated fats (with the exception of coconut) can contribute to weight gain. If eaten in excess, they can also contribute to high blood cholesterol levels.

▶ **Mono-unsaturated fats** tend to be liquid at room temperature but may start to solidify if refrigerated. Food sources include olive oil and avocados. It is not essential to get mono-unsaturated fats from the diet as they can be made in the body from other fats. However, dietary intake of olive oil and other mono-unsaturated fats seems to lower some types of cholesterol and may be a useful adjunct to a healthy diet. Mono-unsaturated fats can be heated gently, as in gentle frying and roasting, and can also be used in salad dressings.

▶ **Poly-unsaturated fats** tend to be liquid at room temperature and when refrigerated. They should not be heated as this damages them and leads to the formation of trans-fatty acids (see below). Included in the family of poly-unsaturated fats are the two essential fats, omega-3 and omega-6, so called because the body needs them to function but it can't make them. They are needed for brain function and structure, hormonal activity, proper metabolism, cell membranes, and skin, hair and nail health. They are anti-inflammatory so are particularly needed in conditions such as arthritis and inflammatory skin disorders like eczema and psoriasis.

▶ **Trans-fats** are poly-unsaturated fats that have been processed or damaged. Margarines and shortenings that contain hydrogenated fats are examples. Trans-fats have no part to play in a healthy diet. They create free radical damage in the body and block the use of the essential fats.

Effects and uses of fats in the body

Every cell in the body contains fats in the cell membrane. It is important that cell membranes are largely made up of unsaturated fats as these give the cells flexibility and allow nutrients and wastes in and out of the cell.

The essential fats also break down into prostaglandins that control inflammation in the body.

Fats are vital for hormone balance as some hormones are made from fats, particularly the sterols such as cholesterol. Adrenalin, noradrenalin, oestrogen, progesterone and testosterone are all examples of fat-dependent hormones. This is why low-fat diets are not recommended and also why so many women who diet have hormone imbalances.

Essential Fatty Acids (EFAs) are vital for brain structure and function. Skin, hair and nails need oils to be truly healthy. Oils hold moisture in the body tissues and cells. Without sufficient oils, skin, hair and nails will dry out.

Fats in foods also carry fat-soluble nutrients. When fat is removed from food, the vitamins are also removed. Without them, body function can suffer.

In addition, good fats in food carry flavour and provide feelings of satiety for longer. That is why low-fat diets might leave you feeling hungry and unsatisfied.

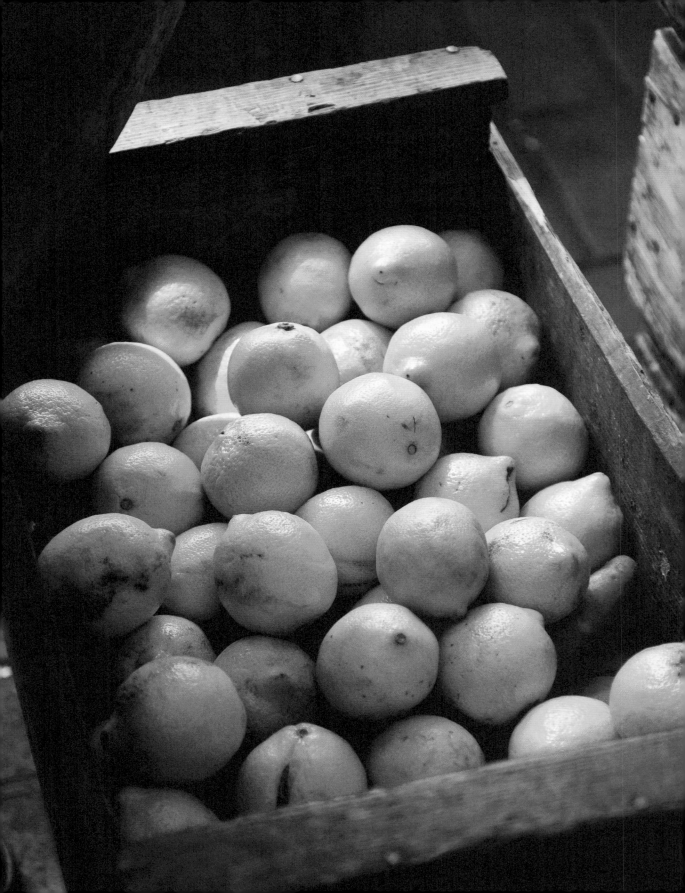

The cholesterol myth

Many people talk about cholesterol as the 'baddie'. We could not function without it. Ninety per cent of the body's cholesterol is found in body tissues and cells, especially those of the brain and nervous system, liver and blood.

When people talk about high or low cholesterol they are talking about measurements taken from the blood. Bad cholesterol refers to low-density lipoproteins (LDL) that carry cholesterol to the cells and can oxidize and damage the arteries. Good cholesterol refers to high-density lipoproteins (HDLs) that carry cholesterol out of the body. Cholesterol is not the problem; it is the ratio of HDL to LDL that is important.

Factors that raise the bad cholesterol in the body include saturated fat, sugar, refined carbohydrates, excess carbohydrates, alcohol, stress and lack of exercise. Factors that raise the good cholesterol ratios include olive oil, garlic, onions, oats, fruit, vegetables, pulses, nuts, seeds, oily fish and exercise. See page 295 for more detailed information on High Cholesterol.

Good fats

Omega-3 fats:

► **Fish:** mackerel, salmon, trout, herrings, sardines, pilchards, halibut.

► **Nuts, seeds and oils:** raw shelled hemp seeds, pumpkin seeds, walnuts, avocados and flax seeds and their cold-pressed oils. Oils must be cold pressed and stored in a cool, dark place as heat, light and air all damage oils and render them harmful to the body.

► **Other animal products:** eggs from chickens that have been fed seeds and greens, some organic meat and dairy products where the animals have had grass freely available and feeds high in essential fats.

Omega-6 fats:

▶ **Seeds and oils:** raw shelled hemp seeds, sunflower seeds, pumpkin seeds, sesame seeds and their cold-pressed oils. Wheatgerm oil is also a good source of omega-6 fats.

▶ **Nuts and oils:** almonds, hazelnuts, pecans, cashews, apricot kernels, pine nuts, macadamia nuts and their cold-pressed oils.

Mono-unsaturated fats:

These are not essential but are useful as they can withstand higher temperatures than the poly-unsaturated fats above and also have health benefits such as improving the ratio of LDL to HDL cholesterol.

▶ **Olives and avocados.** Olive oil can be used in gentle cooking such as stir fries and roasting as long as temperatures do not get too hot.

Saturated fats:

I don't want you to eat foods high in saturated fats. Coconuts are my exception, however.

▶ **Coconuts and coconut oil** are high in saturated fat but much of this is in the form of medium chain triglycerides that do not need to be processed by the liver and have a slight thermogenic effect (meaning they can raise metabolic rate slightly). They are very stable so can be used for sautéing and stir frying.

▶ **Ghee:** this is clarified butter, meaning it is butter that has had all its impurities and milk proteins removed. It may be tolerated by those with dairy intolerances. It is high in saturated fat so should be used only in small quantities. I do not recommend it for those with a tendency to weight gain or high cholesterol.

Fats to avoid

▶ **Processed fats:** hydrogenated or trans-fats should be avoided at all costs. They cause damage in the body and block the use of the essential fats. Their intake has been linked to many disease states including heart disease, obesity, diabetes and strokes. They can be found in margarines, processed foods, crisps, chips, fries, pastries, biscuits, cakes, chocolate and burnt or fried foods.

▶ **Excess saturated fats:** fatty meats, eggs and dairy products. Omega-3-rich eggs are fine in moderation. Goat's and sheep's milk products such as natural yoghurt are OK for those who can tolerate them. But the yoghurt must be sugar and sweetener free and preferably organic.

▶ **Heated or rancid oils:** many oils sold in plastic bottles that are not cold pressed will have lost their beneficial properties. Oils should be stored in a cool, dry place away from heat, light and air. The fridge may be the best place. Those sold in brown or green bottles rather than clear bottles should be chosen when possible as these will be better protected from light.

Vitamins and Minerals

Vitamins and minerals are essential to life. Each has a role to play in our health and they are best provided in what you eat and drink, although supplementation may also be beneficial.

Vitamin A and the carotenoids

► Essential for vision, eye health and skin.
► Enhances immunity.
► Important for bone and teeth formation.
► Acts as an antioxidant to help protect against disease.
Note: taking large amounts of vitamin A can be poisonous, particularly to the liver. And during pregnancy liver-derived vitamin A is best avoided (but you can continue to eat green and orange vegetables and fruits).

Sources of vitamin A:
► Green and orange vegetables and fruits
► Eggs

Sources of betacarotenes (converted into vitamin A in the body):

► Apricots
► Asparagus
► Broccoli
► Carrots
► Dulse
► Kale
► Peaches
► Papaya
► Spinach
► Watercress
► Mango
► Goji berries

The B vitamins

► Essential for the nervous system.

► Helpful for digestion, healthy muscle, skin, eyes, hair, liver and brain function.

► Good for stress and mood.

► Essential for the release of energy from carbohydrate foods.

Sources:

► Eggs
► Whole-grains
► Brewer's yeast
► Brussels sprouts
► Asparagus
► Oats
► Fish

► Chicken
► Nuts
► Shitake mushrooms
► Brown rice
► Quinoa
► Pulses: chickpeas, lentils, aduki beans
► Sunflower seeds

Vitamin C

► Acts as an antioxidant, a protector for the body.

► Necessary for tissue growth and repair, healthy gums and bones.

► Particularly useful for when the body is under stress.

► Helps in the absorption of iron.

Sources:

► Blackcurrants
► Broccoli
► Brussels sprouts
► Red pepper
► Strawberries
► Lemons
► Tomatoes

► Goji berries
► Raspberries
► Rose hips
► Sweet potato
► Peas
► Kiwi fruit

Vitamin D

▸ Required for the absorption and utilization of calcium and phosphorus, so necessary for bone health and development.

▸ Helpful in the prevention and treatment of osteoarthritis and osteoporosis.

▸ Protects against muscle weakness.

Dietary vitamin D is not as easily absorbed as through sunlight, the most important source. Take vitamin D supplements in the winter if you feel you don't get outside enough.

Sources:

▸ Cod liver oil   ▸ Mackerel

▸ Salmon   ▸ Tuna

▸ Herring   ▸ Halibut

▸ Sardines   ▸ Eggs

▸ Trout

Vitamin E

▸ A powerful antioxidant that protects against heart disease, cancer and ageing.

▸ Improves circulation and helps repair tissue damage.

Sources:

▸ Wheatgerm oil

▸ Sunflower, hemp, flax or pumpkin seed oil

▸ Sunflower seeds

▸ Hazelnuts

▸ Almonds

▸ Olives

▸ Avocados

▸ Oatmeal

Vitamin K

► Essential for the normal clotting of blood.

► Promotes healthy liver function.

Sources:

► Dark green leafy vegetables

► Broccoli

► Brussels sprouts

► Cabbage

► Cauliflower

► Asparagus

► Nettles

► Miso

► Alfalfa

Folate

► Essential for healthy cell division and replication.

► Important for regulating homocysteine levels, which are associated with an increased risk of atherosclerosis (see page 193).

► Important in pregnancy and even before conception – helps to regulate embryonic cell formation, vital for healthy development.

Sources:

► Asparagus

► Barley

► Brewer's yeast

► Brown rice

► Split peas

► Lentils

► Broccoli

► Brussels sprouts

► Chickpeas

► Spinach

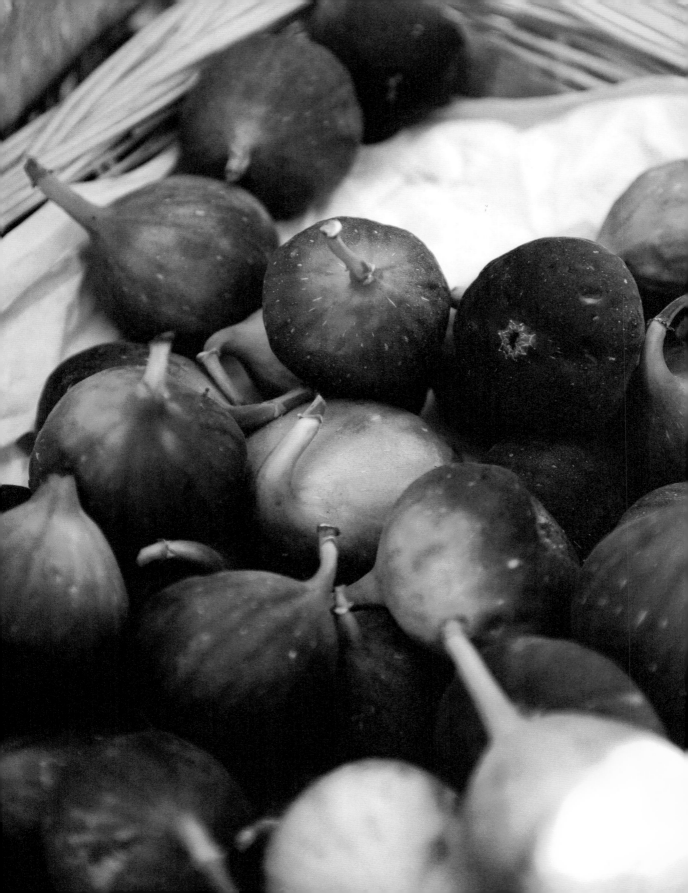

Calcium

► Essential for bone and teeth health.

► Helpful in the prevention of osteoporosis.

► Important for blood clotting and nerve function.

Note: for the optimum absorption of calcium, it is best consumed with magnesium.

Sources:

► Kombu/wakame seaweed	► Nori seaweed
► Broccoli	► Brussels sprouts
► Savoy cabbage	► Cavolo nero
► Kale	► Chicory
► Goat's milk	► Pak choi
► Oats	► Romaine lettuce
► Watercress	► Tahini
► Sesame seeds	► Hazelnuts
► Figs	► Alfalfa

Iron

► Carries oxygen from the lungs to all the cells in the body.

► Required for energy production and a healthy immune system.

Sources:

► Nori seaweed	► Prunes
► Lentils	► Nettles
► Eggs	► Dulse
► Poultry	► Kelp
► Kidney beans	► Parsley
► Watercress	► Amaranth
► Kale	► Quinoa
► Dried apricots	► Fish
► Figs	► Beetroot

Zinc

▸ Essential for fertility and healthy reproductive system.

▸ Good for healthy skin.

▸ Protects the liver.

▸ Protects against free radicals (which promote ageing and disease).

Sources:

▸ Pumpkin seeds
▸ Kelp
▸ Sesame seeds
▸ Wheatgerm
▸ Poppy seeds
▸ Chicken
▸ Nori seaweed
▸ Brown rice
▸ Eggs
▸ Tahini
▸ Fish

Selenium

▸ Acts as an antioxidant, helps protect the body from heart disease, cancer and ageing.

▸ Works with vitamin E to help maintain a healthy heart and liver.

▸ Important for growth, fertility and thyroid.

▸ Good for healthy skin and hair.

Sources:

▸ Brazil nuts
▸ Asparagus
▸ Herring
▸ Dulse
▸ Sardines
▸ Kelp
▸ Broccoli
▸ Wheatgerm
▸ Garlic

Magnesium

- ► Works with calcium to maintain healthy bones.
- ► A vital catalyst in energy release.
- ► Good for heart health.
- ► Has been shown to help relieve PMS (see page 347).

Sources:

- ► Sesame seeds
- ► Raw cacao
- ► Grapes
- ► Avocados
- ► Bananas
- ► Brown rice
- ► Kale
- ► Watercress
- ► Alfalfa sprouts
- ► Dulse
- ► Kelp
- ► Millet
- ► Almonds
- ► Hazelnuts
- ► Rocket

Potassium

- ► Essential for a healthy nervous system and regular heart rhythm.
- ► Helps in promoting healthy blood pressure.
- ► Works with sodium to control the body's water balance.

Sources:

- ► Whole-grains
- ► Apricots
- ► Avocados
- ► Bananas
- ► Brown rice
- ► Dates
- ► Figs
- ► Dulse
- ► Nuts
- ► Butternut squash
- ► Pumpkin
- ► Nettles
- ► Pulses

Phosphorus

► Important in the conversion of food into energy.

► Needed for blood clotting.

► An essential part of all body cells; a deficiency is rare as found in most foods.

Sources:

► Sesame seeds

► Sunflower seeds

► Poultry

► Whole-grains

► Fish

► Oats

Sodium

► Essential for water balance.

► Needed for nerves and muscles.

► Most people consume too much sodium via packaged and processed foods but if you are elderly and take diuretics for high blood pressure (and you follow a low-sodium diet) you may be deficient.

Natural sources (better used by the body):

► Fish

► Sea vegetables

► Celery

► Cabbage

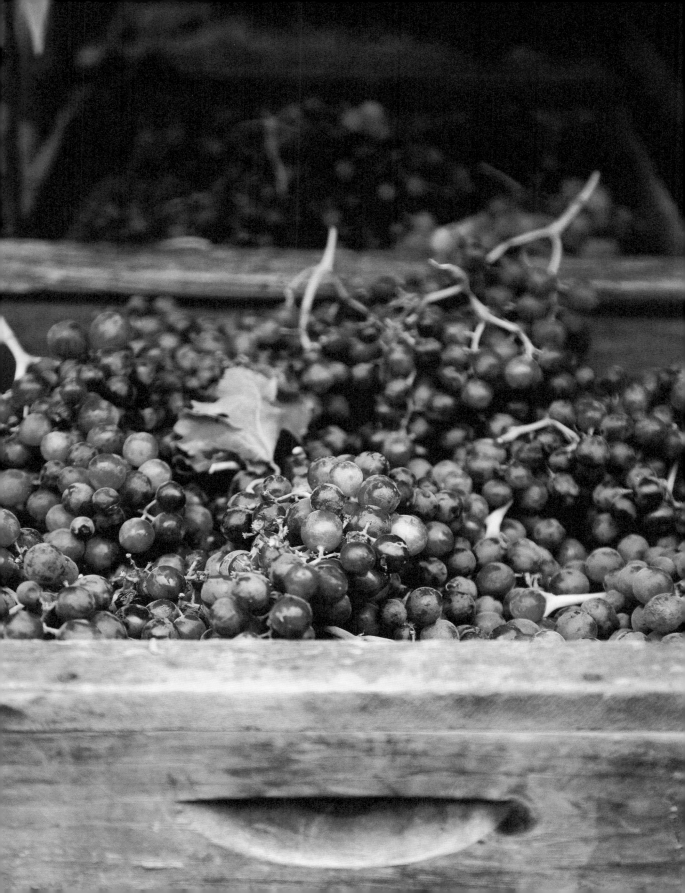

Sources (so avoid if you need to cut down your sodium intake):

- Salt
- Stock cubes
- Salted fish
- Soy sauce
- Bacon
- Ham
- Smoked salmon
- Salami
- Crisps
- Tomato ketchup

Antioxidants and Phytonutrients

These are covered in more detail in Ageing (pages 149–152) but are essential building blocks in a healthy diet. Put simply, researchers have discovered that substances in plants can provide natural resistance to diseases like heart disease and cancer. These foods activate your body's own defences, and have even been shown to slow the growth of tumours. By eating these foods raw or very lightly steamed you will reap many benefits. Almost every whole-grain, legume, vegetable and fruit contains these nutrients.

Sources:

- Onions
- Garlic
- Blueberries
- Raspberries
- Grapefruit
- Tomatoes
- Green tea
- Apples
- Broccoli
- Soya beans
- Spinach
- Carrots

I'm a retired athlete and had fallen into a rut of bad eating habits. To cut a long story short, I have changed my life thanks to Gillian. I no longer eat 'beige'; I eat 'vibrant colours' and feel so good that it's hard to put into words really. My husband is thrilled when I come home with groceries and sees only good things. I wake up excited about breakfast; not because there will be bacon and eggs but because I'm about to have a fruit explosion courtesy of our new juicer! I don't miss anything and the funny thing is I love vegetables – you have no idea how strange that is coming from me... I'd like to say thank you, not for changing my life, because ultimately that is my choice, but rather for providing me with the tools I needed to do so. Oh, and by the way, in five weeks I've lost a stone without even trying...

Putting it all Together – Gillian's Food Pyramid

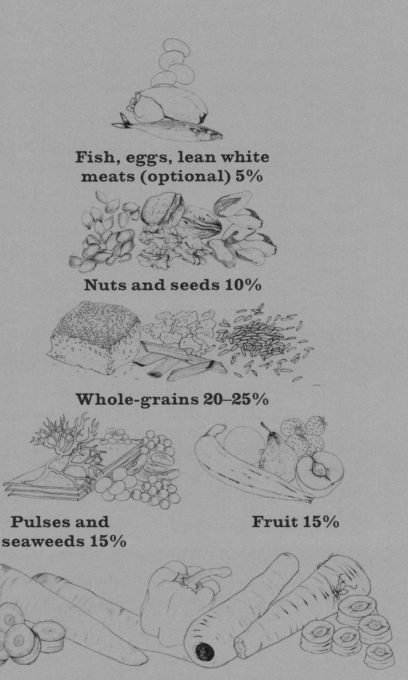

Fish, eggs, lean white
meats (optional) 5%

Nuts and seeds 10%

Whole-grains 20–25%

Pulses and
seaweeds 15%

Fruit 15%

Vegetables raw and/cooked 30–35%

▶ Always drink a cup of warm water with a squeeze of lemon first thing in the morning as the perfect start for your digestion.

▶ Breakfast like queen, lunch like a king, supper like a pauper. Your body gets most of its energy from food eaten early in the day. Foods that provide sustained energy, like complex carbohydrates and protein, are the best choices. Go for variety, so porridge one day, a super smoothie the next.

▶ Eat a variety of whole, natural foods. Expand your possibilities. Buy the basic ingredients and prepare meals from scratch whenever possible.

▶ Slooow down. Eating at a hundred miles an hour on the run causes stress to your body. Savour each morsel and give your body time to digest and absorb the nutrients.

▶ Get to know your body. Really think about how you feel. Are your eyes bright or are there deep circles underneath? Are you feeling full of energy or a little strung out? Choose what you eat accordingly.

▶ Try not to eat big meals in the evening and keep it simple. Eat *more* food in the earlier part of the day. For a restful, vitality-enhancing night's sleep, go easy on red meats and stimulants and opt for soups and salads, veggie stews and herbal teas.

▶ Aim to eat some fruit on an empty stomach each day. This could be first thing in the morning, mid morning as a snack or 30 minutes before lunch or dinner.

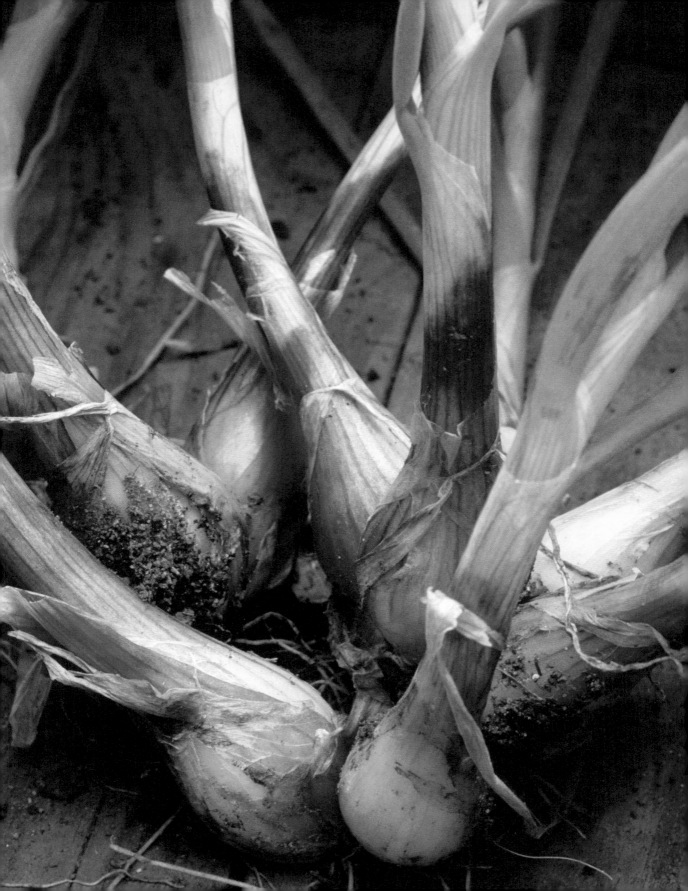

► Have vegetables or salads with lunch and dinner. In the evening they should make up half your plate. They are also useful as snacks with dips or just to munch on. The best ways of cooking vegetables include steaming, water stir frying, baking and roasting. Soups and casseroles are also good ways of incorporating vegetables into your diet.

► Do not eat animal protein more than once a day. If you have fish, chicken or eggs for lunch try to have some vegetable protein in the evening. I prefer fish as it also contains the essential fats and is easier to digest than other animal proteins. Go for wild or organic wherever possible.

► Start experimenting with pulses if you don't already include them regularly. They can be eaten cooked or sprouted in salads, stews, casseroles, soups and stir fries. Cooked pulses can easily be made into dips with just a few other ingredients.

► Include raw nuts and seeds daily. They are a perfect snack and can be sprinkled on salads or cereal. Nut butters are also useful as spreads or mixed with lemon juice and herbs to create dips or sauces. Cold-pressed oils are great in salad dressings; just mix with lemon juice or cider vinegar.

► Eat some raw foods every day.

Let's look at how to put this all into practice with some meal and snack ideas.

Breakfast ideas

▸ Smoothies or fruit salads. These are my favourites, although I often will follow with a porridge about half an hour later.

▸ Soaked muesli: use oat, millet, rice or buckwheat flakes and add nuts, seeds, dried fruit and cinnamon as desired. Soaking overnight makes the muesli more digestible. Soak in rice or oat milk or a mixture of water and natural soya yoghurt.

▸ Natural soya yoghurt with nuts and seeds.

▸ Rye toast with nut or seed butter.

▸ A spinach or mushroom omelette.

▸ Porridge made from oats, millet, quinoa, brown rice or buckwheat. Add cinnamon or ginger for extra flavour.

▸ Cooked grains: if you are having a grain with your evening meal, make extra and re-heat the leftovers in extra water or grain milk for breakfast.

Lunch ideas

Make sure you have some form of vegetable with lunch whether it be as crudités, salads or incorporated into soups or stews.

▸ Soup.

▸ Salad: try fish, chicken, turkey, egg, grain or bean salads.

▸ Sprouted pulses can be incorporated into salads or used as snacks or extras.

▸ Dips and crudités: hummous and other bean or nut dips can be combined and blended with chopped raw vegetables.

▸ Leftovers from previous evening: stews and casseroles can easily be taken for lunch the next day. Just combine with a green salad or blend day-old stew into a soup.

Dinner ideas

Always make sure at least half your plate is made up of vegetables (not potatoes) and/or salad.

► Grilled or baked fish with vegetables or salad. Choose vegetables other than potatoes to avoid putting a strain on the digestive system.

► Grilled chicken with vegetables or salad.

► Bean casseroles and stews: these work well with whole-grains. Good combinations include lentil dahl with brown rice, aduki bean casserole with millet or mung bean stew with quinoa.

► Omelette with salad: spinach, mushroom and tomato omelettes work well with a large green salad.

► Stir fried vegetables with tempeh or chicken. Tempeh is made from fermented soya beans. It is a good source of protein with a meaty texture. Tahini sauce works well with water stir fries; just combine tahini with lemon juice, water, tamari or miso and ginger.

► Nut, seed or grain loaf or bake: various ingredients can be combined to make a loaf. These usually take about ½ hour to bake and are perfect to take for lunch the next day. Works well with steamed vegetables or green salad.

► Risotto: this can be made with brown rice and any combination of vegetable and nut additions. You do not need cheese, cream and butter to make a tasty risotto. Sprouted pulses work well if added near the end of cooking.

► Home-made bean burgers: any beans and cooked grains can be mashed together and shaped into burgers. Herbs and miso can be added for extra flavour. Just brush them with oil and bake them in the oven for 20–30 minutes. Serve with steamed vegetables.

► Chicken, fish or vegetable kebabs: these are great in the summer. They can be cooked on the barbeque or under the grill. Just marinate whatever you choose to use in olive oil, lemon juice and tamari for 30 minutes to several hours in the fridge. Try with courgettes, mushrooms, peppers, aubergines and corn on the cob.

Snack ideas

For blood-sugar balance and stable energy levels and mood, have a snack mid morning, mid afternoon and 30–60 minutes before bed.

► Fresh or dried fruit. Dried fruit is a fairly concentrated source of natural sugar so may be best if soaked for a few hours in water. Look for unsulphured varieties.

► Vegetable crudités: any vegetables can be taken to eat raw as they are or with dips.

► Avocados: transportable and needing minimum preparation.

► Nuts and seeds: raw and unsalted of course (chestnuts too).

► Oat cakes with nut or seed butter.

► Smoothies.

► Vegetable juices.

► Fruit and nut bars (sugar free).

► Crispy seaweed strips (my wee daughters love them instead of crisps!).

Drinks

Start drinking more water. Most of you do not drink nearly enough and you know it. Other options include:

► Herbal teas: nettle, fennel, rose hip, lemon balm, lemon verbena, camomile, liquorice, peppermint, spearmint, dandelion, raspberry leaf, etc.

► Vegetable juices.

► Coffee substitutes: dandelion-root coffee is great (avoid the instant variety as it contains lactose). There are others available containing naturally caffeine-free ingredients such as chicory and barley.

► Warm water with lemon juice: a great way to start the day. This alkalizes the body and kick starts the liver and bowel.

► Freshly pressed fruit juices: have these in moderation because of their sugar content.

Treats

I am definitely not a stick in the mud. I enjoy my treats and you can too. You will find that as your tastes change you no longer want the usual coffee and doughnut. Here are some healthy and delicious ideas instead:

► Carob brownies – see my *You Are What You Eat Cookbook*.

► Soaked dried fruit salad: soak dried apricots, figs, peaches and sultanas in water with a bit of cinnamon or ginger.

► Fruit and nut bites: whiz up dried fruit with soaked almonds, hazelnuts or cashews in the food processor. Shape into balls and roll in raw cacao bean powder, carob powder, coconut or sesame seeds.

► Avocado and date smoothie: blend an avocado with some medjool dates.

► Cashew nut cream: soak cashew nuts and blend with orange juice and zest.

► Cacao bean smoothie: blend two small bananas, half a cup of soya milk, some raw cacao bean nibs and raw cacao bean powder. Add some cinnamon powder or ginger if you fancy. It's a truly delicious pick-me-up!

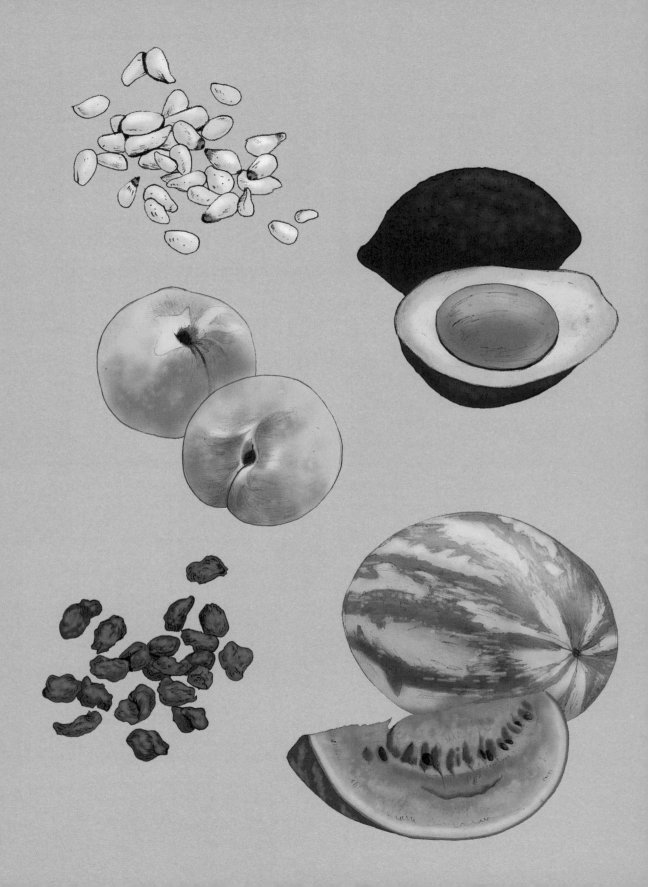

Food and the stages of life

A nutritious diet will go a long way towards meeting your health needs, but these do change throughout life depending on your age and lifestyle. I am passionate about helping you negotiate your life stages and make the most of your health, whatever your age, existing lifestyle or fitness levels.

What's important to remember is that while a healthy diet is a vital foundation throughout life, specific needs change depending on your age and lifestyle. We all need a full complement of nutrients to live well, but, at times, some of us need more than others. A growing baby, for example, must follow a rather different food plan to a teenage boy. A pregnant woman will have different requirements to an elderly lady or gent.

The only people who don't have a say in what they eat are babies and small children. Therefore, parents, please understand the big level of responsibility we owe our wee ones. Everyone else can be empowered to help themselves. If you're a teenager and you're reading this, good on you – the earlier you start to care about your health, the better. It's vital to be empowered with your health and all aspects of your life. Don't let the world and society take control over you. Grasp the real power from within that rests with all of us.

That brings me on to my next topic – ageing. No sooner have we left puberty than some start the feel the pressure to fight the ageing process. It's all about creams, potions and injections to keep us looking young and wrinkle-free. Many people convince themselves that growing older means losing health and vitality. Not at all! I want you to start embracing your age, and your wisdom. I know women in their 50s who are bursting with vitality and sexuality, contrary to all conventional wisdom on the menopause. I have friends in their 80s who are fighting fit and refuse to lead a sedentary life. I knew a man in his 90s who set himself enormous physical challenges to keep active year after year. You don't have to retire at 60 and settle into an armchair. Too many people are programmed to gear themselves into ill health with age. Not moving your body is one of the quickest ways to get old. And the 'not moving' brigade is getting younger and younger.

If you understand your body's requirements through the different stages of life, you can fuel it accordingly and pre-empt any problems. Ageing is not our scrooge but rather the gift of life. You and your family can experience the very best of life at any age, just follow my plan and you will reap the rewards. The following pages will explain how.

Babies

From day one, nutrition plays an essential part in all our lives. Personally and professionally, I am an advocate for breastfeeding, if at all possible. It's good for your baby, and it's good for you, too. For baby, breastfeeding can improve development and growth, immunity, intelligence, organ strength, help prevent allergies and sometimes even promote a calmer disposition. And for mum breastfeeding can be relaxing, calming, bonding, emotionally nurturing, good for your immunity and for more balanced hormones, and thus carries less risk of post-partum blues and other related problems.

I always get a kick out of thinking about when I started to breastfeed my first wee baby. The paediatrician told me that I had the most abundant milk she had ever seen. The funny thing is that my clients often report a similar story: thick milk and milk flow. I know that healthy nutrition is the key.

I must also stress, though, that it is always a mother's choice when it comes to feeding her baby. Don't beat yourself up if you end up not breastfeeding. Occasionally the choice may not be there for you; breastfeeding comes easily to some and not so easily to others. I want you to be happy either way. Acceptance of what you do and who you are is paramount to your physical and spiritual well being.

What's good about breast milk?

Each mammal produces milk that differs in the quantity and type of proteins, fats, minerals, vitamins and trace elements, a biochemical make-up that is unique to that animal. Because breast milk is designed for human babies, it's much easier to digest than formula or cow's milk. Human milk contains at least 100 different compounds not found in formula.

Milk is essential for the development of every organ, bone, cell tissue and physiological system of the new baby. A study published in the *American Journal of Public Health* showed that babies who were exclusively breastfed for the first six months suffered '30 per cent fewer illnesses'. The breastfed babies in the study experienced fewer incidences of diarrhoea, colds, ear infections, vomiting and fever.

Breast milk is especially rich in the nutrients required for brain development, healthy bacteria for baby's digestive system, and iron and zinc, both essential nutrients for growth. The milk you produce in the first few days is ideally suited to the nutritional requirements of your baby at that time. During the first few days of life, it is particularly important that your baby receives a substance from the milk called colostrum, which contains all the maternal antibodies. Since the baby's immune system is not fully developed at birth, these antibodies fight early infections, illness and disease. Colostrum is also extremely high in protein and healthy fats for the development of the brain and nervous system. Easy to digest and loaded with enzymes, colostrum helps establish the foundation of your baby's digestive system for life. As the digestive system matures, the nutritional content of your milk will change accordingly.

It is now thought that babies who are breastfed have less likelihood of developing allergies such as hayfever, asthma and other respiratory problems, and less risk of obesity, heart disease and other conditions later in life.

Advantages for you

Breastfeeding not only promotes bonding in the days after giving birth, but also has many health benefits for mum. It releases the necessary hormones to instruct the uterus to clamp back down to its pre-pregnant size and burns huge amounts of extra calories, helping mum return to pre-pregnant weight more quickly.

Breastfeeding may be the best treatment for post-natal depression because the breastfeeding process itself encourages hormone levels to readjust, slowly settling down from the effects of being pregnant and giving birth. If mothers stop feeding too soon, then the body doesn't have a chance to adapt gradually to these changes in hormone activity; the result is an increased incidence of mood swings and depression. In cases of my own breastfeeding clients, I have noticed that these women tend to be calmer and more balanced.

What's the downside?

To make breastfeeding work, you have to be prepared to feed on demand. Your body knows how much milk to produce only by the frequency of your baby's sucking. The more sucking that occurs, the more milk is produced. If you limit either the amount of time your baby spends on the breast, or how often you allow the sucking, then the amount of milk produced will often not be enough for your baby. In the beginning, until the nipples and surrounding area toughen up, it can be painful. I would urge you not to throw in the towel at the first twinges of discomfort as your nipples will toughen and the breastfeeding will get easier by the day.

Breastfeeding on demand can in turn feel very demanding on your body and your energy. To make it easier, give up trying to be superwoman for a while. Just focus on you and connecting with your new bundle of joy.

The following are the most common problems for breastfeeding mothers and ways to prevent and sort them out. Breastfeeding problems are rare, but armed with this information you run far less risk of ever encountering them.

Let-down reflex

A baby can be positioned perfectly, but if mum feels afraid of feeding, stressed or uninterested, then she may not 'let-down' (release) her milk. The let-down reflex occurs when oxytocin is released from the brain, causing breasts to tingle, tense up

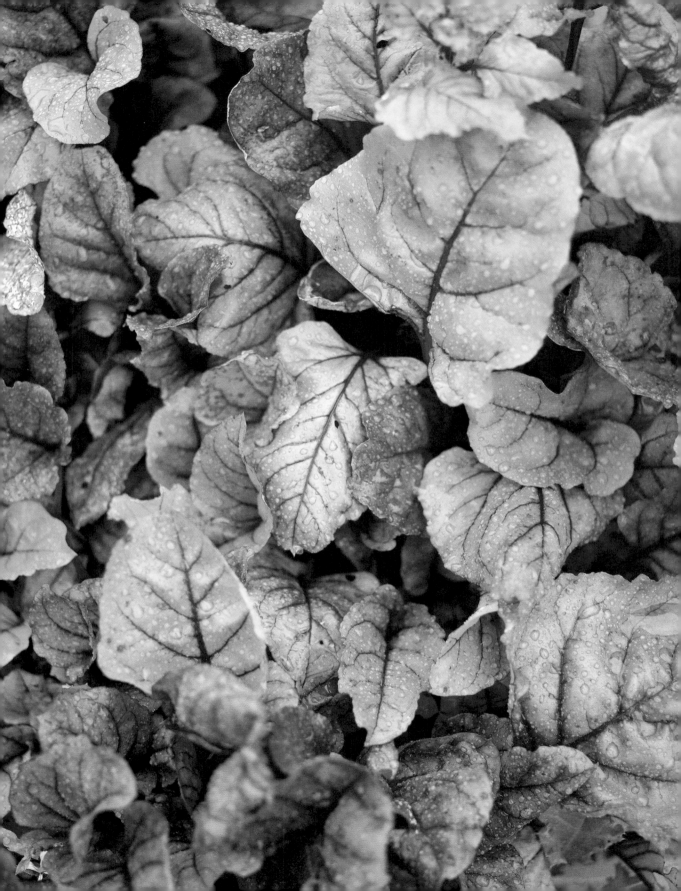

and the nipples stand out; milk will then eject easily. If this reflex does not happen, then the baby will get only a blue-tinged fore-milk or nothing, and certainly not the richer, thicker, more nutritious hind-milk which satisfies hunger. You will know all about it as baby will be fractious and crying a lot. In order to encourage the full release of milk, I always recommend relaxation techniques, breathing exercises and visualization.

Insufficient milk supply

My own mother was told by her GP that she could not breastfeed me when I was a baby, because she had insufficient milk supply. In my experience, most new mothers who are told that they cannot feed their babies actually have poor-quality blood. Many women give up breastfeeding because they think that they do not have a good-enough milk supply. But if you follow my general advice on nutrition and enjoy a diet packed with fresh, natural foods you should produce all the milk your baby needs.

Herbs can help to boost your output

Just take one of these herbs at a time. If you decide to stop breastfeeding, then discontinue the rotation. Herbs can be obtained from the fresh leaves of tea or capsules, tablets or liquid tinctures.

Agnus castus (also called chasteberry or Vitex)

I recommend this for every woman after giving birth. Agnus castus stimulates production of prolactin, helping to ensure a healthy milk supply. It's best to start agnus castus one week before you anticipate giving birth and continue for two weeks. Take for three weeks if you feel that the quantity of your milk is subsiding.

I also recommend:

- Blessed thistle
- Catnip
- Chicory
- Dandelion
- Fennel
- Fenugreek
- Licorice
- Marshmallow root
- Nettle
- Raspberry leaf
- Red clover

Thin Milk

It is common for milk quantity and quality to decrease slightly at around two months after the birth. Some women find their milk has gone thin or watery. You may simply be overtired at this point, so rest whenever you can. Keep putting your baby to the breast as it is the sucking action which will stimulate the milk to flow. Nourish your spleen, liver and blood supply, and the milk will thicken. Use the herbs above in rotation and add one of these superfoods to your daily diet:

- Alfalfa
- Spirulina
- Wheatgrass
- Wild blue-green algae
- Barley grass

Too much milk

Too much milk can result in engorged, uncomfortable breasts. You can buy or rent an express machine to pump out some extra milk and freeze it for a later date. Be cautious of too much expressing, since it gives your body the same message as putting baby to the breast; so your body will continue to produce extra milk. Too much milk usually lasts only for a few days when the milk first comes in and balances itself as your baby becomes more settled. Applying ice bags to the breast can sometimes relieve the pain. If your breasts start getting hard, lumpy and uncomfortable, have a warm shower and gently massage the lumps towards the nipples, while manually expressing out the blocked milk. This will usually relieve the discomfort, while leaving enough milk in the breast to allow your body to naturally regulate milk supply.

Remedies to decrease milk production or reduce engorgement

► Drink an infusion of sage herbal tea three times a day until milk slows down. It's also available in tincture form.
► Parsley contains specific compounds to help slow milk flow.
► Eat generous amounts of lentils, dried figs, basil, mint, papayas and papaya juice.
► It may sound crazy, but place chilled cabbage leaves inside your bra. The anti-inflammatory compounds in cabbage can help reduce swelling. I know first hand as it worked for me!

Blocked milk duct

Blocked ducts are sometimes caused by too much milk, or a bra that is too tight pressing on a duct. You may feel a tiny lump the size of a pea. You need to deal with it quickly, as you do not want it to become infected. First, have your baby suck frequently, changing positions so that every part of the nipple is stimulated. Use a warm compress; after each feed massage breasts down and towards the nipple. My own patients have had great success with the following:

Put 2 drops of phytolacca, plus 6 drops of evening primrose oil, and 10 drops of sage tincture into some water. Drink this every two hours until relief.

Mastitis

Occasionally, if the breasts remain engorged and blocked over a period of time, then the breast tissue can become infected, resulting in a condition called mastitis. The blocked area will appear red and increasingly tender to touch. Your temperature may rise and you might feel ill. It is imperative that you take action at the first signs of mastitis as the symptoms can get worse quite quickly and you can end up with a high fever. Consult your doctor as you may require antibiotic treatment. Encourage baby to feed frequently from that side. While feeding on that side, stroke the hardened part towards the nipple, thus helping the blockage to clear. Manually express the milk by hand in the shower or bath. Take 1,000mg of vitamin C and 6–8 garlic pearls every three hours to combat the infection. You may wish to add two echinacea tablets every three hours. Add 10–15 drops of propolis tincture in warm water twice daily until relief.

You could also try mixing a paste of the herbs marigold, poke root and slippery elm powder with water and spread over the affected breast. If left on for a few hours, this will help the inflammation to reduce. Always carefully wash the breast before feeding.

Sore and cracked nipples

Sore and cracked nipples are usually caused by incorrect positioning of the baby on the nipple. If the baby is allowed to keep sucking incorrectly, then bleeding cracks may quickly appear on the nipple.

Consult a local La Leche League representative (www. gillianmckeith.info/breastfeeding). The league exists to assist breastfeeding mothers.

Add tinctures of marigold and St John's wort to a little boiling water, then allow to cool to air temperature: dabbing on the breast or nipple after each feed may help the delicate breast tissue to heal and harden. Calendula cream can also be helpful as can anaesthetizing the nipple by applying an ice cube before starting to feed.

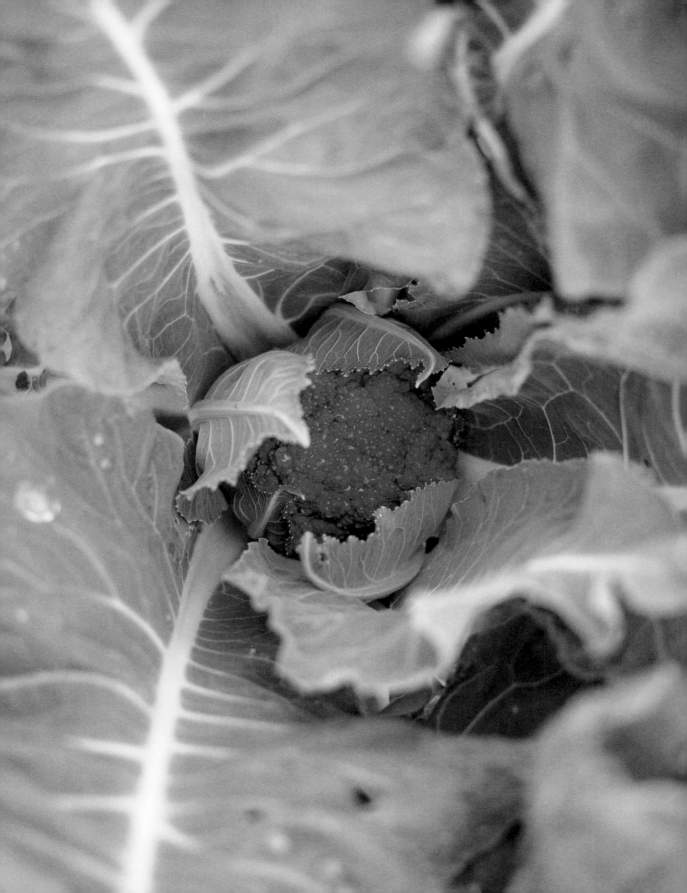

If soreness and bleeding cracks persist, you may have an elevation of the yeast candida. Try submerging your nipples in pure yoghurt (see page 219 for more information on tackling candida).

Baby rejects milk

There are cases where the baby rejects your milk. Babies might scream, grimace, 'pull faces', bring up curdled milk or have green, runny bowel movements. In my experience, this usually indicates a mother's out of balance liver (see page 22) or indigestion (see page 308). You could also try a herbal infusion of the herbs fringe tree, valerian and hawthorn, which are best sought out in a specialist herbal shop.

How long should I breastfeed for?

I generally recommend breastfeeding exclusively for at least the first six months after the birth. After the first six months, you might start to introduce other tastes or fresh juices with some solids. As this process continues after the first six months and your baby begins to eat solid foods or fresh juices, baby should require less breast milk. The length of feeds may shorten; the frequency of breastfeedings may decrease. Allow your child to take the lead. My first child breastfed exclusively for ten months. She had no interest in anything else. Each individual child has different needs and desires as to how long breastfeeding continues. Some babies wean naturally by their first birthday; others are still feeding at two and three years. Ultimately do what feels right for you and your child.

Weaning

Weaning is the process of gradually introducing solid foods to a baby, during the first year or so of its life. Every baby and every mother is different, so let me start by saying that this isn't something to get stressed about – it'll come naturally when the time is right.

Most people begin weaning when their baby is between four and six months old. I wouldn't advise you to start younger than this, because babies' digestive and immune systems probably won't be ready for solid foods and may react badly.

The reason for weaning is a baby's nutritional and calorific requirements increase as they grow. At around six months they are likely to need more than just milk – although it's worth pointing out that this depends on the strength of your milk. My first child didn't fancy solids until she was ten months old; my other daughter was ready at seven months. As some point in their first year, though, your baby will not be able to consume enough milk to meet his or her needs (milk is also low in iron so if weaning is delayed, anaemia can result). Babies usually start to show an interest in food around this time, and chances are they'll demand more frequent feeds.

What foods and when?

Introduce foods to your baby one at a time, leaving three–four days in between each new food so you can monitor any reactions (how's their nappy, their skin, their mood?). I'd suggest keeping a food and symptom diary to help the monitoring process.

Although there's a plethora of baby foods on the market, home-made is always best – and it's pretty darned easy as all you really need to do is blend or mash. Start with a teaspoon of fruit and vegetable purées as these are the easiest to digest. Sweet potatoes, carrots, swede and squash are good vegetables to start the process. For fruits, try pears, apricots and bananas. Go for organic wherever possible to reduce baby's intake of pesticides and maximize nutrient intake. Do not include citrus fruit, berries or tomatoes initially. Soft, well-cooked grains such as rice and millet can be included in the early stages, but avoid gluten grains (wheat, rye, oats, barley) as these can be hard to digest.

By the time your baby is seven–nine months old, they'll be well and truly bored with purées and ready for some new textures. And of course you can continue to introduce new foods, too. Instead of blending to a purée, fruit and veg can be mashed and left lumpier, and babies can be given small amounts of soft food such as bananas or cooked vegetables to encourage chewing. As their food repertoire increases, you'll find they drink less milk. So this is when you start them on a healthy fluid intake for life by making sure baby has water – vegetable juices are a possibility, too. I combined celery, carrot and cucumber juice with a little apple juice and water for my daughters.

When they show an interest, you can start introducing protein – in the form of cooked pulses, fish, and poultry – to replace the protein they were getting from milk. They need to be cooked and puréed.

Of course there are some foods and ingredients your baby definitely won't be ready for. Crucially, you must ensure they don't have any food containing added salt – their kidneys are simply not developed enough to deal with sodium. Sugar, peanuts and stimulants, such as caffeine, must be off limits. And if anyone in your family has a food allergy or intolerance, it's best not to introduce the food in question to your child until they are at least two years old.

By twelve months, your baby should be able to eat three regular meals a day with a milk feed between each, and you can give them finger food to snack on such as slices of avocado, cooked carrots or green beans.

Children

Why is a healthy diet for children important?

There's no way I can soften the message: kids suffer when their diet is poor. Making sure your children eat well is one of the most important and loving things you can do for them.

Studies suggest that a significant number of children today have worryingly low intakes of essential vitamins such as vitamin A, C and D and minerals such as zinc, iron, calcium and magnesium – crucial nutrients for healthy growth and development. A nutrient-poor diet, especially when combined with low activity levels, will significantly affect the future health of your children by increasing the risk of osteoporosis, heart disease and obesity. And, in the short term, unhealthy eating will affect their concentration, energy levels, immunity and cholesterol levels. Add to that something that worries me enormously – the shocking rise of type 2 diabetes in children. It's all down to a sugar-laden, junk-food diet and lack of exercise. In other words, it's completely avoidable, and I'm sorry, mums and dads, but you're accountable.

Given the overwhelming body of evidence of the negative effect of poor diet on the growth, development, intelligence and wellbeing of children, it's never too early to get healthy. The earlier in their lives you start, the easier it will be. Studies have shown that when children are fed healthy nutrient-rich foods like fruit, vegetables and whole grains, not only do they stop overeating and feel more satisfied, but their body weight decreases and they perform better at school. So ditch the family value-pack of crisps and start thinking and shopping healthily, today. Your kids will thank you.

Incorporating healthy foods into your child's diet

I love to watch children play by making food in the kitchen. They have such a great time. Getting kids involved with food preparation as early as possible is one of the best ways to interest them in what they put into their bodies. It's so old-fashioned to think children don't like anything that's 'good for them'. They deserve more credit than that. Allow children to experiment. Healthy habits start young – and, reassuringly, last a lifetime.

By the same token, unfortunately bad habits tend to start young, too. Many kids, if they had their way, would eat the same foods all the time, a habit they usually learn from mum and dad. To get all the nutrients kids need for optimum growth and good health, both now and in the years to come, they need variety, just like you.

► **Grains,** including whole grains, brown rice, porridge oats, rye bread and quinoa (my kids' favourite) should all be on the menu. These foods are high in complex carbohydrates, which are the body's preferred fuel. Give your child the energy to play, pay attention in school and do many other activities. Grains also provide other important nutrients such as vitamin B complex, which helps your child's body to use the protein needed to build muscle. Whole grains contain dietary fibre that can assist in the protection against heart disease and diabetes, and also help control your child's weight and keep their poos moving. I am shocked at how many children suffer from constipation, because they just don't get enough fibre. Always choose whole grains, rather than refined. Refined grains, such as those in white bread and white rice which have been processed, should be avoided because many of the naturally occurring nutrients have been lost.

► **Vegetables** provide many of the essential vitamins and minerals and fibre your child needs for good health. Include a variety of veggies in your child's diet. Green leafy vegetables, such as spinach and broccoli, are a good source of calcium, which helps to build strong bones and teeth and is essential during this stage of rapid growth. Tantalize their taste buds early on with more unusual (but now widely available) vegetables such as pak choi, fennel and butternut squash. Fruits are also wonderful sources of essential vitamins and minerals and give children a natural sweet treat that is also healthy. I notice that my own kids prefer raw veggies over cooked ones.

► **White meats, fish, beans and nuts** provide children with protein to maintain and repair body tissue and build muscle. The proteins from lean meats such as chicken, turkey and fish, as well as eggs and beans, supply essential amino acids that make up our bodies' 'building blocks'. For growth vitamin A helps to build healthy eyes, skin and hair. Vitamin B aids metabolism. Vitamin D helps your child's body to absorb calcium and use it to maintain healthy bones and teeth, along with muscle and nerve functions. Iron also helps to build strong bones, teeth and muscles. Iron is especially important for kids during periods of rapid growth, stress, injury or illness.

► **Fats and oils** contain essential nutrients to maintain brain function, healthy skin and development in children, but trans-fats, found in chips, crisps, pastries and processed foods, have been linked with heart disease and obesity so limit these foods. Foods naturally high in essential fats (particularly omega-6 and omega-3) include nuts (nut and seed butters are great for children), olives, oily fish, soy products and avocados. Omega-3, found in oily fish as well as hemp and flax seeds, has been shown to be particularly important for brain development.

▶ **Water** is the most important drink, and should be encouraged whenever kids are thirsty. Children need water for healthy skin and cell function as much as adults need it when they get older.

▶ **Juicing:** this is far better for your kids than squash or fizzy drinks. Sugary beverages have been linked not just to obesity, but to a host of health problems as well as poor concentration at school. Kids love the juicing and smoothie-making process, so I say let them have a go themselves. This kind of play will build a fabulous foundation for a lifetime love of healthy food.

▶ **Sprouting:** children will eat food they have grown themselves, so buy a sprouter and encourage the kids to sprout their own. Chickpeas when sprouted or soaked overnight are a chewy sweet snack for kiddies. My kids adore these little chewy balls.

Children need regular nibbles to keep their blood-sugar levels steady and to prevent cravings and bingeing on unhealthy food. Temper tantrums are often a direct result of blood-sugar swings. Junk foods will obviously send their levels on a rollercoaster ride and have your kids climbing the walls in no time. Good snack ideas are seeds, sugarless cereal, fruit, raw veggies, hummous sandwiches and natural sugar/sweetener-free yoghurts (yoghurts are only a healthy option when they are free of chemical sweeteners and colourings). My kids love to snack on chestnuts. You can easily find them in the health-food store or supermarket in the winter months for roasting. Replace crisps and snacks with seaweed and nuts. You will be amazed how much children love them. Soak almonds overnight and kids will find them chewy and easy to digest.

What to avoid

Limit the amount of added sugar you feed your child from biscuits, sweets, sugary cereals and other foods. The body stores this extra sugar it doesn't immediately need as fat and this can lead to weight gain and other health problems. You end up addicting your kids to sugar from an early age and that addiction continues into adulthood. It is a vicious cycle, and it's up to parents to take action.

You can help your kids to break the association between sweets and treats. Fruit is sweet and a good treat. Yams, sweet potatoes and squash are sweet and make perfect snacks. Brown rice has a lovely nutty, sweet flavour. Be a good role model and make the healthy choice the norm. You can still include favourite or 'treat' foods now and again. Make them special, not every day. Learn how to prepare all kinds of good healthy options. I make a super healthy carob fudge brownie that is delicious, too. See page 65 for my raw cacao bean smoothie.

Persistence is key

Fussy eaters are a parent's nightmare. I understand just how busy and stressful life can be, and how frustrating it is when you've slaved over a meal only to have it rejected. But please, please, be patient and persevere. Some kids may turn their noses up at new foods and this is entirely normal. Repeated exposure to new foods in an upbeat environment will encourage them to experiment, trust me. As always, lead by example and make sure you are eating the healthy food you want your child to eat. After all, you can't expect your child to snack on seeds while you're scoffing an iced bun, can you?

In my experience, children who help prepare food are more likely to eat it. I have found that most children are very open to trying new things and are eager to get into the kitchen and get involved. So let them! This can be a great time to communicate with your child and discuss healthy eating. Encourage your kids to lay the table and eat with a knife and fork. Take them shopping to the local greengrocer; say that as a special treat they can pick the most unusual fruit or vegetable they can find and you'll try it at home together.

As you try to modify your child's diet for the better, remember that children are natural grazers. They prefer to have several meals and snacks throughout the day rather than big meals. Children have small tummies, so they're not always being fussy when they say they don't want to finish something. Try not to make a big issue of food and eating. Instead, let them stay in tune with their appetite and eat according to it. Just make sure that the meals and snacks you offer them are nutritious and that they sit down to eat and chew slowly rather than snacking on the run (as I happen to know many adults who do!).

AGES 6 TO 11

It's normal at this age for fat to accumulate on the tummy and trunk until adolescence; you should expect children to put on weight before a major growth spurt. They fill out, then shoot up.

⁙ DO
► Start teaching your children the basics of healthy eating.
► Encourage your children to help you with the preparation and selection of food. Allow them to serve themselves and tell them to stop eating when they are full.
► Eat the same food that your children eat and make family meal times fun.
► Set up a healthy snack shelf in your cupboard.
► Encourage your child to eat 3 to 6 servings a day of whole grains and anything made from them; 2 to 4 servings a day of fruit, 3 to 5 servings a day of vegetables and legumes and 2 to 3 servings of healthy protein, such as nuts and seeds, leafy greens and soy or oat milk.
► Enrol them in regular sports activities and take an interest in their progress.
► Set time limits for television and computer time.

⁙ DON'T
► Give children sweet or fizzy drinks. Research shows that children who drink more sweetened beverages tend to have a higher risk of obesity.
► Underestimate the importance of body image if your child is overweight. They may be teased or bullied at school. Take steps to help children feel more positive about their bodies.
► Give unlimited pocket money. Consumption of sweets and crisps on the way to and from school is a major cause of obesity.

THROUGH PUBERTY

We all remember the emotional and physical shift that was puberty. So why not give your teenagers an easier ride? Research shows that a healthy diet can balance overactive hormones and boost physical and emotional health. Stable blood-sugar levels equal a happier, less moody teenager around the house – now that's got to be good news.

This is the age when you might start to see your child's eating habits change. An increased social life can mean fewer family meals and more exposure to fast food, skipped meals or snacking on the run. Girls (and some boys, too) will often develop dieting and body image concerns, and may start to experiment with food fads. Teenagers are further developing their personalities and lifestyles and this is when bad food habits can take root. This is when the kids need your guidance and support the most. Please be there for them.

It's normal during the adolescent growth spurt for boys to gain more fat on their trunks and lose it on their arms and legs. In contrast, girls tend to gain weight everywhere during this period. Don't be overzealous about weight gain, but do be aware of what they're consuming.

Teenage diets are notoriously poor. This is a serious problem because increased nutrition is vital and needed most during growth spurts and the onset of puberty. As a parent, make it your business to know what they are eating outside the home, difficult as that may be. Please be engaged and proactive with them.

Food aside, physical activity levels can be low in teens. I know many adults who were put off exercise for life by badly taught PE at school. Encourage the school to offer more varied, fun activities. Build exercise into your family life – cycle at the weekends, walk the dog, go swimming. If they get into the exercise habit now, they're more likely to stick with it for life.

⠿ DO

▸ Continue to offer healthy meals, even if they are snubbed. Offer fruit when a hungry teenager returns from school and provide healthy snacks for breaks. Ban eating while in front of the television. Do your best to sit down at a table. Make eating a family occasion as much as you possibly can. Teens can seem lazy but I contend they need to be inspired and really listened to. So strike a deal with your teen and encourage them to stay active and get at least an hour of exercise a day. Reward them with an outing, not junk food! Send teens on errands and involve them in household chores – tasks that keep them away from the television and computer.

▸ Encourage your teen to eat breakfast. Eating first thing in the morning benefits thinking power and will help them get really fit.

▸ Banish refined carbohydrates and drinks high in caffeine content. Encourage your teenager to eat plenty of complex carbohydrates, such as fresh vegetables, brown rice, whole grains, sprouted seeds, nuts and seeds. These prevent blood-sugar imbalances, and also serve to spur endorphin production for happy feelings.

▸ Include 'good mood' foods (that contain tryptophan) in your family meals, including oil-rich fish, such as salmon and sardines, avocados, seeds, dried apricots, walnuts, raw cacao beans, turkey, chicken and bananas.

▸ Even if teens don't appear to be listening, you can be sure they will be if you are speaking in a kind and loving manner. Finally, tell your teenager that Gillian wants a word in private without mum or dad around. They just need to go to www.gmk.com for teens only – no adults allowed please! But rest assured, you'll be glad they found me. Just don't tell them that!

::: **DON'T**

► Don't put your child on a fad diet. The teenage years are a period of intense growth and development and teenagers need plenty of nutritious food to grow into their natural body weight.

► Don't force the issue. If your teenager is overweight or obese they will likely feel embarrassed by their size. Please be sensitive, soft and kind. Try to get your teen to open up to talking and recognising issues without further embarrassment. Talk openly with them. Change the whole family's eating habits and choice of leisure activity so that healthier options become a way of life.

Six years ago my partner left me and my son and I had quite a few dark months. I didn't eat properly and smoked like a trooper. I have since found a wonderful man who just loves to cook and we are getting married soon. I have given up smoking and eat all the lovely healthy foods you recommend. Now I am fit, healthy and extremely happy along with my son who has grown into a well-mannered, intelligent boy. My skin has never glowed so much and I have never smiled so much. So thank you Gillian for all your wonderful healthy eating tips.

Girls

Just as girls start to notice their body shape, Mother Nature makes life difficult for them. Girls change shape, gain weight in different places, sprout body hair and between the ages of eleven and fourteen will have to get to grips with periods. You won't be surprised to read that a decent diet and regular exercise will make all these transitions much smoother and easier to deal with. A melting pot of hormones means teens will always be prone to mood swings. But food most definitely affects mood, so help them resist the rubbish.

Good nutrition is critical since a teenage girl grows faster during adolescence than at any other time in her life except for infancy. That requires a mountain of vitamins and minerals best found in food, as well as an average of 2,200 calories a day. But too often teenage girls don't get enough of these crucial micronutrients. I urge all parents to supplement the diets of their teenage children with vitamins – a daily multiple as well as a green superfood such as spirulina, wheat grass or barley grass now and again in a smoothie. Young girls are often deficient in major minerals of the body: magnesium for one, which mobilizes calcium into the bones.

Half a woman's bone mass is formed during adolescence, and low intakes of calcium and magnesium today may lead to osteoporosis tomorrow. Good sources of calcium include natural yoghurt, leafy green vegetables, tofu, soy, sprouted seeds. Magnesium sources include sesame seeds, raw shelled hemp seeds, raw cacao beans, grapes, avocados, bananas, blackstrap molasses, brown rice, kale, broccoli, cavolo nero, savoy cabbage, chicory, romaine lettuce, rocket, watercress, dulse, kelp, millet, almonds, hazelnuts and alfalfa sprouts.

Girls often don't get enough iron. Not only do they lose iron through menstruation, but if their diet isn't varied enough, they won't get enough iron-rich foods. The risk of anaemia is great.

One study found that even a mild iron deficiency resulted in lower test scores in maths. Iron-rich foods include eggs, fish, poultry, almonds, figs, dulse, kelp, kombu, wakame, parsley, watercress, broccoli, cavolo nero, quinoa, amaranth, oats, millet, rye, blackstrap molasses, prunes and nettles.

Boys

There are so many stereotypes about teenage boys that I feel sorry for them, I really do. They're not all spotty, unwashed, rude and moody – especially not the ones whose parents make sure they eat healthily. Girls may have to cope with periods and all their associated woes, but boys have some pretty major life changes going on, too, from hair growth to their voice breaking.

Before puberty, boys and girls have similar muscle-to-fat ratios. But once the growth spurt starts – which in boys lasts from around the ages of twelve to eighteen, a year or so later than girls – they'll gain more muscle than fat. They can also go through periods of looking gangly, as their limbs shoot them skywards, so it's important to reinforce a good body image and keep their self-esteem high.

Teenage boys are going to need more calories a day (2,500–2,800), but this doesn't just give them licence to buy more from the school tuck shop. If you send them to school with a few snack-packs of nuts, seeds, veggie sticks or fruit/dried fruit for breaks, you'll help them get into the habit of healthy grazing.

Having a greater muscle mass, they're going to need plenty of protein for growth and repair. They'll also need iron for energy, especially if they're sporty, as this mineral can be lost through sweat.

And let's not forget those essential fats. They're a must-have for hormone production, brain function, good skin, hair, nails and healthy growth. A fish-oil supplement would be good insurance if getting your growing lad to eat oily fish proves difficult.

An intake of minerals is vital to support the health of growing boys, so as for the girls, I'd strongly recommend a full-spectrum multivitamin and mineral supplement daily. This, alongside a balanced diet, should ensure adequate:

► Calcium – essential for forming a strong skeleton and teeth (with vitamin D, boron, magnesium).
► Zinc – vital for hormone production. Boys need it for healthy sperm production and a deficiency is also a major cause of acne.
► Magnesium – for bone health, hormone balance and energy.

Finally, a word about hormones. Puberty is the time when hormones can start to fluctuate all over the place. Some of this is natural and to be expected, but most of it can be controlled through good diet for a smoother ride through puberty. In boys the chief hormone is testosterone, responsible for the deeper voice, facial hair, broader chest, sex drive and, if you're not careful, aggressive outbursts.

As any parent who's been there will know, convincing teenage boys to eat well takes time, effort and care. Girls often want to be healthy, but boys don't want to be seen munching on what their mates might call 'rabbit food'. You *can* set a good example at home. Explain the 'masculine' benefits of eating well: stronger muscles, more energy, better mental and physical stamina. In other words, he'll be brainier, fitter and better looking.

Tips for parents

▸ Be a good role model; it will help your health and weight, too. Ensure that your child understands how their body changes as it develops, and that healthy lifestyle changes are not about appearance but to help their mood, concentration, skin and health.

▸ Recognize that we're all different shapes and sizes and examine your own feelings and comments about your weight and shape.

▸ Help your child to find something they're good at and enjoy to boost their self-confidence.

▸ Make sure your child has a healthy breakfast as studies show it can significantly improve performance at school.

▸ Don't let your kids eat mindlessly in front of the television. Eat together whenever you can.

▸ Try not to let food become a power struggle, nor a means of reward or punishment.

Health tip: If you have real concerns about your child's diet, weight or eating habits, then see your GP and get a referral to a nutritionist.

I have noticed that our family thrives on the organically grown vegetables and herbs from our allotment. We have spinach, new potatoes, runner beans, beetroot, cabbage, leeks, onions and herbs. Gillian, you have made us all think about our eating habits and how we prepare food.

What if I am a vegetarian?

Lots of teens come home and declare one day that they're vegetarian. It might be a phase or an early lifestyle choice. Either way, it's best to take them seriously and respect their choice. A vegetarian or vegan diet can be a very healthy option as long as you do it well, specifically that it's balanced, nutrient-dense and varied. Vegans and vegetarians need to enjoy an abundance of fruits, vegetables, beans, seeds, nuts, grains, legumes, pulses, seaweeds and veggie juices. Soya products such as tofu, tempeh and miso are tasty proteins. And while vegetarians do eat dairy products, it is worth trying goat and sheep's milk and cheese for a change. They tend to be more easily digested than cow's products.

The acne plague

There is a direct relationship between acne and hormones. Acne usually begins when the body starts to produce androgens. Androgens stimulate the sebaceous glands to enlarge and secrete more sebum (oil). The sebum gets accumulated in the follicle, and moves up the hair shaft to the exterior part of the skin. As the sebum moves up, it mixes with bacteria and the hair follicle gets blocked. This could result in acne, spots, pimples and oily skin.

Hormones regulate every bodily function. Sleep, growth and many other things depend upon your hormones. If your hormones are in balance, then you are less likely to suffer from acne.

In my clinical experience many teenagers with acne have always tested positive for a deficiency in the mineral zinc. A nutritious diet is hormone balancing and a far more effective remedy for acne than topical creams and lotions. See page 171 for my Acne Plan.

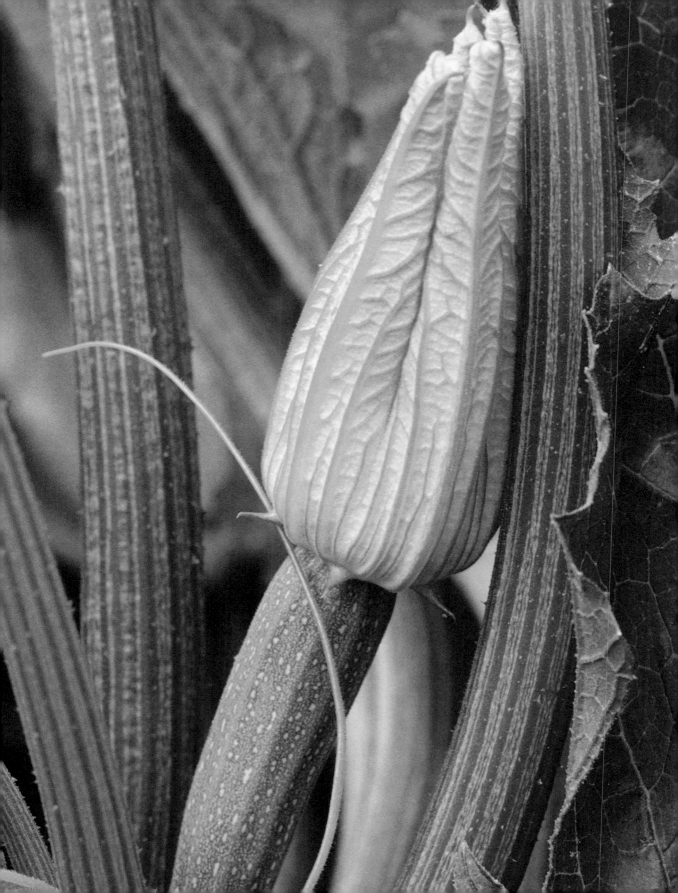

The Fertile Years

Nearly every client who has come to me in the hope of conceiving a baby has been granted their wish. When you think about the purpose of your reproductive organs – creating new life – it's easy to understand how vital it is to nourish them with a vibrant, energy-giving diet. The full spectrum of nutrients is needed for maximum reproductive health.

But you don't just need to think about reproductive health when you're trying for a baby. Far from it. Nutrition plays a crucial role in the development and maturity of male and female reproductive systems, right from childhood. Just take zinc, for example. This mineral is easy to find in food if you follow a healthy diet and it's directly involved in the development of reproductive organs. If your children have white spots on their nails, which is very common, then they are likely deficient in zinc. If this carries right through to adulthood it can put immunity, menstruation, sex life and reproduction at risk.

MEN

Nutrition has a direct impact on the potency of a man's sperm. Research shows that if you eat badly, smoke and drink too much alcohol, the quality and quantity of your sperm will be lowered, and conception more difficult. So here's where I stand on my soapbox. Men, I am talking to you! Don't think that infertility is a purely female problem, and that you can continue drinking, smoking and eating what you like while your partner makes all the lifestyle changes. Did you know nearly half of all fertility problems originate from the man? And in the majority of cases, experts can't even tell which partner has the problem – it might be both of you. The best way to maximize your chance of a healthy, successful conception and pregnancy, whether you've been experiencing problems or not, is for you both to adopt a healthy-eating plan and lifestyle.

Foods to choose

To boost your chances of conceiving a healthy baby, your diet should be balanced, healthy, varied and as organic and free from additives and preservatives as possible. A healthy diet is low in most of the saturated fats, particularly animal fat, sugar, salt and refined and processed foods and high in wholemeal products, fruit and vegetables. In a study of Danish greenhouse workers, an unexpectedly high sperm count was found among organic farmers who grew their products without the use of pesticides or chemicals. Interestingly enough, Danish sperm is one of the most sought after in the world, routinely used to boost up sperm supplies at sperm banks. So, ladies, if you can't find Mr Right, you now know where to go!

The most important nutrients

▶ **Zinc** is vital because it is crucial for the proper development of sperm. Low or no zinc in the man equals no or low sperm count in the penis. Food sources include fish, kelp, brown rice, hulled hemp seeds, wheatgerm, chicken, pulses, pumpkin seeds, sesame seeds, peas, chicken, whole grains and eggs.

▶ **Manganese** is essential for the maintenance of healthy testicles. A lack of the mineral manganese leads to testicular degeneration, sterility and loss of libido. Food sources include avocados, oatmeal, bananas, peas, prunes, kale, raspberries, lettuce, nuts, seeds, sea vegetables, whole grains, pulses and seaweed dulse.

▶ **Selenium** is needed to raise sperm counts. Food sources include Brazil nuts, barley, broccoli, fish, eggs, asparagus, brown rice, chicken, dulse, garlic, kelp and wheatgerm.

▶ Research suggests that the antioxidant activity of **Vitamin E** may make sperm more fertile. An interesting study looked at men with good sperm counts but low fertilization rates during IVF treatments. These men were given vitamin E each day. One month after starting treatment, the fertility rate increased from 19 per cent to 29 per cent. Food sources include nuts, seeds, olives, avocados, oatmeal, wheatgerm and cold-pressed oils.

▶ **Vitamin C** is needed to increase sperm quality. Food sources include berries (strawberries, blueberries, goji berries for example), citrus fruits, kiwi fruits, tomatoes, peppers, blackcurrants, peas and rose hips.

▶ **Essential fatty acids** are crucial because semen is rich in prostaglandins, which require these fatty acids for production. Food sources include flax seeds, shelled hemp seeds, pumpkin seeds, sunflower seeds, sesame seeds, walnuts, avocados, trout, salmon, mackerel, herrings, pilchards, sardines and cold-pressed oils.

▶ **Vitamin B12** is also important for cellular sperm production. Food sources include poultry, eggs, dairy products, herrings, mackerel, salmon and cod.

▶ **Potassium** is another important mineral for increasing male virility. Food sources include pulses, vegetables, apple cider vinegar, whole grains, apricots, avocados, bananas, brown rice, dates, figs, dulse, nuts, squash, pumpkin and nettle.

▶ **Co-enzyme Q10** is a nutrient used in the body for the production of energy, as well as sperm count and motility. Food sources include herring, mackerel, soya, trout and pistachio nuts.

▶ **Deficiency in calcium and vitamin D** can affect a man's fertility. Sources of calcium include yoghurt, kefir, green vegetables, tinned fish with bones, almonds, sesame seeds, tahini, carob, dulse, wakame seaweed, figs, hazelnuts and alfalfa. Sources of vitamin D include eggs, fish and fortified foods – dietary vitamin D is not particularly well absorbed. The most important source of vitamin D is sunlight as the body can make vitamin D by the action of sunlight on the skin.

▶ **Amino acids,** the building blocks for protein, have been proven to be important supplements for men addressing infertility problems and low sperm count. Good food sources include poultry, eggs, lentils, quinoa, amaranth and aduki beans.

Herbal help

Saw palmetto is one of the best herbs for male reproductive health. It acts like a tonic for men and has been used for centuries to help symptoms of an enlarged prostate. Several studies in Europe show that saw palmetto is an effective alternative for many men, especially those in the early stages of enlarged prostate. In Germany, it's sold over the counter as a treatment for enlarged prostate (Benign Prostatic Hyperplasia).

Things to avoid
Alcohol
I know you might think that alcohol gets you in the mood, but I'm here to tell you that it's going to hinder your performance in bed, not help it. And it's certainly not going to help one bit with babymaking. Research clearly indicates that drinking alcohol causes a decrease in sperm count, an increase in abnormal sperm and a lower proportion of mobile sperm. This is because alcohol reduces the level of sperm-making hormones. Men who drink four units of alcohol a day run a risk of lowered sperm count, and as little as one pint of beer (two units) a day could produce abnormal sperm. If you're prone to binge drinking, as so many people in the UK are, know this: experts reckon you can wipe out your sperm count for up to three months after a single bout of heavy drinking. And any sperm that manage to mature while alcohol is still in your system may be less effective and healthy. It's like the sperm are effectively drunk too!

Need any more convincing that alcohol is one of the greatest threats to a man's potency? Well, too much alcohol can alter the way testosterone is produced and then released. Plus, a man who drinks alcohol may accumulate small amounts of female hormones which can lower sperm potency and production. The good news is that all these effects can be reversed in around three to four months by avoiding alcohol and adopting a healthy diet. You might think I'm bossy, but you'll thank me.

Smoking

A man's fertility is adversely affected if he smokes because the chemicals taken in from cigarettes, such as nicotine and carbon monoxide, degrade sperm count.

Drugs

Recreational drugs will compromise a man's fertility:

► Marijuana can lower sperm-producing hormones and reduce libido.

► Cocaine causes lower sperm counts, poorly moving sperm and a high rate of abnormal sperm.

► Heroin can cause a decrease in testosterone levels.

► Some medicines have a direct impact on male fertility and sperm count. These include sulphasalazine (used to treat irritable bowel), nitrofurantoin, tetracyclines, cimetideine, ketoconzole, tricyclic antidepressants, monoamine, oxidase inhibitors, propranol and other medications for conditions such as gout or high blood pressure. Overuse of antibiotics may also pose a problem.

WOMEN

The optimum years for pregnancy are your 20s and early 30s.
Believe me, I know this is easier said than done – you have a job
to hold down, a mortgage to pay, a willing partner to find. Women
certainly get pregnant naturally in their late 30s and 40s but
my advice to you, if at all possible, is to start much earlier to
give yourself the best chance of conceiving.

Age aside, proper nutrition is very important for a healthy
pregnancy and baby. I can help you get your body baby-ready.

Foods to choose for fertility and pregnancy

Choose fresh fruits and vegetables, before and during pregnancy
– women should aim for eight servings daily – grains such as
brown rice, buckwheat, spelt, amaranth and quinoa, high-quality
protein from organic turkey or chicken, nuts, tofu and fish and
a supply of good fats, especially hemp oil, raw shelled hemp seeds,
flax, sunflower and pumpkin seeds, primrose oil and fish oils.
Essential fats, found in nuts, avocados, seeds and oily fish, have
a profound effect on every system of the body, including the
reproductive system, and are crucial for healthy hormone
functioning. Last but by no means least, drink plenty of water.
Water plays a key role in the health of your reproductive organs.

'You are what you eat' is particularly relevant in the case of
reproductive health and fertility. There is no doubt that proper
nutrition is crucial at every stage from the development to the
maturation of the reproductive organs and for healthy hormone
function and the creation of new life.

A spectrum of trace minerals is essential, for example, iron,
calcium, magnesium and zinc. Vitamins C, A, E and the Bs are
also important, as are friendly bacteria.

► **Folic Acid:** found in green beans, spinach, Brussels sprouts, brown rice, peas, asparagus, chickpeas and bananas.

► **Iron:** found in eggs, fish, nettle tea, dark green vegetables, seaweeds and prunes.

► **Calcium:** found in quinoa, seaweeds, natural yoghurts, fish, nuts, tinned fish with bones, broccoli and kale.

► **Selenium:** found in herring, tuna, broccoli, garlic, Brazil nuts, dulse and kelp.

► **Zinc:** found in seafood, pumpkin seeds, raw shelled hemp seeds, squash seeds, whole grains and dried fruit.

► **Manganese:** found in seaweeds, dulse, nuts, whole grains and legumes.

► **Magnesium:** found in dark leafy greens, nuts, vegetables, cooked brown rice, sunflower seeds.

► **Essential fatty acids:** found in pumpkin seeds, hemp seeds, sunflower seeds, linseeds, nuts, avocados, olive oil, flaxseed oil, and fish.

► **B complex vitamins:** found in brown rice, avocados, lentils, quinoa, pulses, sardines, eggs, spirulina and seaweed.

► **Vitamin C:** found in raw fruits, especially berries, broccoli, red peppers and sprouted seeds.

► **Vitamin E:** found in wheatgerm, olives, avocados, nuts and seeds.

► **Vitamin A (betacarotene):** found in carrots, tomatoes, cabbage, spinach, broccoli.

► **Probiotic bacteria:** found in natural (unsweetened) yoghurt, sauerkraut and miso.

► **Prebiotic bacteria:** found in bananas, chicory and artichoke.

Protein

Protein is also vital. Pregnant women need good quality usable protein every day. White meats, eggs, nuts, legumes, green superfoods and whole grains such as quinoa are good forms of protein. Protein builds muscle, tissue, enzymes, hormones and antibodies for you and your baby. These foods also have B vitamins and iron, which is important for red blood cells. Need for protein in the first term is small, but increases in the second and third terms when the baby is growing the fastest and the mother's body is working to meet its needs.

But … excess protein consumption may tax the liver and kidneys. It leaves behind a waste of nitrogen that the body must then eliminate. Fluid imbalances can occur, causing the body to lose calcium and other valuable minerals through the urine. While you definitely need protein, do not overdo it. Moderate protein consumption, preferably from plant food sources, is recommended. These foods contain other vital nutrients.

Nutritious foods containing protein:

▶ Wild blue-green algae
▶ Spirulina
▶ Chlorella
▶ Black beans
▶ Brewer's yeast
▶ Tofu
▶ Soya beans
▶ White meats
▶ Fish
▶ Eggs
▶ Nuts
▶ Quinoa
▶ Tempeh
▶ Sprouted seeds and sprouted legumes
▶ Barley grass

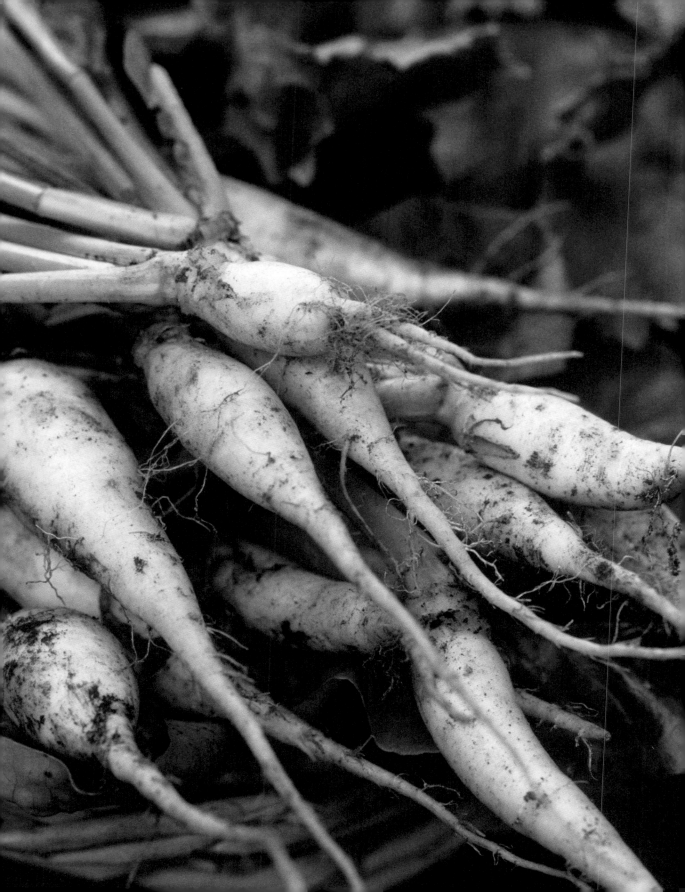

Herbal help for fertility

Herbs can help to improve general health and readiness for conception as well as being generally supportive during infertility treatment.

If you choose one herb for infertility, go for agnus castus. I use the herb agnus castus with my female clients to help balance sex hormones, which will encourage the ovaries to function normally. Agnus castus has been shown to restore hormonal balance and boost reproductive health in women. You can buy it in tincture form in health-food stores.

► **Agnus castus:** Helps regulate periods, balance hormones, stimulate ovulation and significantly enhance fertility.

► **False unicorn root:** Can help to strengthen and normalize the reproductive organs.

► **Dong quai:** A potent blood tonic, it adds important nutrients needed for fertility to the bloodstream and may increase the chance of implantation.

► **Black cohosh:** Useful for women who have an absence of menstruation or irregular cycles.

► **Red raspberry leaf:** Has a long-standing tradition in many tribal cultures as a uterine toner and strengthener.

► **Evening primrose oil:** Rich in essential fatty acids (EFAs) and crucial for fertility.

► **Wild yam:** This is an excellent remedy for progesterone imbalance. Best when taken after ovulation, in the second half of your cycle.

► **Red clover:** Contains isoflavones, which are hormone-like compounds that help to boost oestrogen production.

► **Liquorice root:** This extract is helpful in balancing adrenal gland functions.

► **Unkei-to:** An Asian herbal remedy for fertility.

► **She-oak:** A flower essence that many of my clients swear by.

Please understand that I am not suggesting that you take all of the above herbs at once. My herbal programme is normally in rotation with those plants that are readily available. So you might take agnus castus by itself for one week; then black cohosh for one week; and so on. See how you feel and respond to each herb. This is the best way to approach herbs, on a rotational basis.

Supplements for fertility

Here is the absolute fact: if you want to increase your chances of getting pregnant, you must take your vitamins and minerals. Take a good-quality multivitamin, combined with a wholesome diet.

The fat connection

Fat is essential to fertility. A certain percentage of body fat is vital. Women need body fat in order to ovulate. Studies have shown that 50 per cent of women who have a BMI (Body Mass Index) below 20.7 are infertile. A BMI between 23 and 24 is ideal for conception. The average woman has 27 per cent of her weight as body fat. Being underweight may contribute to infertility in females.

However, you can have too much of a good thing. Being overweight can and does interfere with ovulation, because the extra fat produces extra oestrogen in the system, causing an imbalance in the ratio of the reproductive hormones needed for egg ripening and release. Obesity increases the risk of infertility. The good news is that the effect can be quickly reversed. Just losing a small amount of weight can be enough to stimulate regular ovulation.

Things to avoid

In a nutshell, to boost reproductive health and encourage fertility you need to avoid caffeine, alcohol, smoking and processed or highly refined foods, as research has shown they all have a negative effect on reproductive health in both men and women. You should also avoid xenoestrogens. When you are trying to conceive, one of the most important things you need to do is to balance your hormones. That means avoid anything that might cause an imbalance, and one of the main culprits is xenoestrogens. Xenoestrogens are essentially environmental oestrogens, coming from pesticides, food additives and the plastic industry. One of the best ways to eliminate an excessive intake of xenoestrogens is to buy organic produce.

Smoking

Women who do not smoke are twice as likely to get pregnant as women who do, so don't put it off – give up now! Prior to getting pregnant, cigarettes reduce oestrogen levels. Lowered oestrogen levels cut down the number of fertile years a woman has left to conceive, cause irregular periods, and make eggs and cervical mucus less penetrable to sperm.

Alcohol

The *British Medical Journal* has stated categorically that women should avoid alcohol when trying to conceive and when pregnant. Alcohol may prevent progesterone being produced by the egg capsule, and progesterone is required to maintain a healthy pregnancy. Alcohol and baby making don't go together.

Stress

Like good physical health, emotional health is important for fertility, too. People are of course able to conceive when under stress, but for many it proves very difficult. Stress at work has been identified as a problem for would-be mums. There are studies to show that extreme stress can even stop ovulation. Fertility units such as the Beth Israel Hospital in Boston (USA) and the Harvard University Behavioral Medicine Center have been including stress reduction in their fertility programmes for years.

Caffeine

Drinking just one or more cups of coffee per day has been associated with impaired conception in women trying to get pregnant. Caffeine consumption equivalent to more than two cups of coffee per day has been associated with an increased incidence of infertility due to tubal disease or endometriosis.

Gillian's top fertility foods

- Raw shelled hemp and pumpkin seeds
- Avocados
- Almonds
- Figs
- Berries
- Pomegranates
- Brown rice
- Oats
- Nori seaweed
- Quinoa
- Sprouted clover and sprouted sunflower
- Turtle beans

During Pregnancy

Eat/drink

► At least five portions of fresh fruit and vegetables daily as they are rich in vitamins, minerals and numerous protective antioxidants. When cooking vegetables, steaming and stirfrying are the best methods as they cause minimal nutrient loss. Drinking freshly pressed vegetable juices will help increase your vitamin and mineral intake.

► Whole grains such as rye bread, brown rice, millet, pot barley, buckwheat noodles and sugar-free muesli. These foods are good sources of complex carbohydrates that help sustain energy levels and maintain blood-sugar balance. They also contain plenty of fibre, which is important for preventing constipation – a common problem during pregnancy.

► Your body requires more protein during pregnancy so make sure you include some with every meal. Good sources include organic white meat, fish (see notes in the Avoid section), eggs, tofu, beans, peas, lentils, quinoa and sprouted legumes and seeds. Some plant-based foods contain complete protein similar to animal products (tofu and other soya bean products, quinoa, amaranth and sprouted legumes and seeds) and these are particularly beneficial if you are vegetarian or vegan. In addition, protein absorption from plant-based foods can be increased by combining them in the same meals. So try combining whole grains with legumes or nuts and seeds (for example lentils with brown rice, healthy baked beans on rye toast, bean burgers with millet risotto, tahini on oat cakes).

► Foods rich in essential fatty acids, especially omega-3 fats, which are important in pregnancy for your baby's brain, eye and vision development. Good food sources include oily fish (no more than two portions a week), pumpkin seeds, walnuts, dark leafy green vegetables and unrefined, cold-pressed seed oils such as flaxseed oil or hemp seed oil.

► Calcium needs increase in pregnancy. Include calcium-rich foods such as live natural yoghurt, dark leafy greens, sea vegetables, tofu, chickpeas, sesame seeds, tahini, almonds and dried figs. If you are eating dairy products, always opt for organic dairy products and minimize calcium-containing foods that are high in saturated fat such as whole milk, cream and full-fat cheeses. Vitamin D is needed for proper calcium absorption. Although this vitamin is found only in a small number of foods, the body can produce it naturally from sunlight – so make sure you get outdoors every day.

► During pregnancy, your blood volume increases and iron is a major component of red blood cells. Although red meat is high in iron, it can also be high in saturated fat. Healthier iron-containing foods include beans, lentils, chickpeas, millet, eggs, dark green leafy vegetables, poultry, nettles, raisins and prune juice. There is plenty of choice for vegetarians and vegans. To increase your iron absorption, eat foods rich in vitamin C at the same time.

► In addition to taking a folic acid supplement, include foods high in this vitamin such as broccoli, Brussels sprouts, asparagus, peas, brown rice and chickpeas.

► Healthy snacks to ward off hunger pangs and keep blood-sugar levels balanced: fresh or stewed fruit, dried (unsulphured) fruit with nuts and seeds, rye bread or oat cakes with nut butter, live natural yoghurt, vegetable crudités with hummous or olive tapenade.

► Drink at least eight glasses of bottled or filtered water daily to help control food cravings and to maintain hydration levels.

Avoid

There are various foods that you should avoid during pregnancy, because they might make you ill or harm your unborn baby. These include:

► Foods that may contain bacteria called listeria such as unpasteurized cheeses (Camembert, Brie, chèvre and blue cheeses) and meat-based pâtés.

► Raw or partially cooked eggs as they may contain salmonella, which causes food poisoning. Also foods made using raw eggs such as mayonnaise, salad dressings, some desserts and ice creams.

► Undercooked meats as they may contain salmonella and other bacteria.

► Liver products and supplements containing fish liver oils as they can be excessively high in vitamin A, a build-up of which could be harmful during pregnancy.

► Certain types of fish including shark, swordfish and marlin. In addition, have no more than two portions of oily fish (tuna, mackerel, sardines and trout) a week. This is because these fish contain traces of mercury – a toxic metal.

► Raw shellfish as they sometimes contain harmful bacteria and viruses.

► Alcohol, caffeine and cigarettes.

► Peanuts – if the baby's father, brothers or sisters have a nut allergy. Avoid any foods to which there are allergies in the family.

► Foods that are generally unhealthy such as fried foods; foods high in saturated fats; sugar and all foods that contain sugar; refined grains, white rice and white flour products such as white bread and white pasta; junk foods and table salt.

Supplements

► Folic acid (400mcg) until week 12 of the pregnancy as this B vitamin helps to prevent neural tube defects such as spina bifida. Alternatively take a good multinutrient formula specifically designed for pregnant women as it will contain vital nutrients for this time of life, especially folic acid, calcium, iron and zinc.

► Probiotics to aid regular bowel function and improve nutrient absorption.

► Prenatal multivitamin.

► Taking a superfood supplement containing wheat grass juice or powder or spirulina can also be a useful way of increasing your nutrient intake.

Coping with food cravings

As many as half of all women experience food cravings during pregnancy. The most common are for sweet, salty or spicy foods. Cravings may be because of the increased calorie needs at this time, while another explanation may be that they are signalling nutritional deficiencies. A further reason could be low blood-sugar levels, especially when the cravings are for sweet foods. While it's fine to indulge yourself if the foods you are craving are healthy, try not to give in to them if they are for the wrong types of foods. If you follow my dietary guidelines above, eat a wide variety of foods, include healthy snacks in between main meals and take a prenatal multi-nutrient food supplement, your cravings should begin to subside. Also make sure you drink enough water as this can also help control unhealthy food desires.

MORNING SICKNESS

Morning sickness is common in early pregnancy. It does not often occur before the fourth week of pregnancy and usually does not continue past the sixteenth week. However, it is not limited to the morning and, for some women, continues throughout the pregnancy. Symptoms include nausea and often vomiting. This can make eating a healthy diet difficult at a time when it is most important to do so. With my own clients, I have been able to fully eliminate or at least dramatically reduce nausea during pregnancy through the introduction of B vitamins, mainly B6, zinc and very low-level herbal-source iron. The (B vitamin) nutrients help the liver and gall bladder to unload toxins more effectively so that the reaction to the hormones is lessened or neutralized.

Eat/Drink

► Peppermint and camomile teas, which can be calming to the digestion.
► Oat cakes or rye crackers. Snacking on these can help to stave off the nausea.
► Bland foods rather than heavily flavoured foods. Cooked whole grains such as brown rice and quinoa are ideal.

► Mugs of warm water. It is vital to keep well hydrated, especially if you experience vomiting.
► Freshly pressed organic vegetable juices. These can replace minerals that may be lost through vomiting. They also supply readily available nutrients needed for your health and foetal development.

Avoid sugar and refined carbohydrates, alcohol, spices, caffeine and fatty foods.

Herbs and supplements

► Always consult with your GP before taking any supplements.
► Keep vitamin B6 drops with you and take every four hours. Vitamin B6 has excellent anti-nausea effects.
► Magnesium works well with B6 to reduce nausea and balance hormones.
► Vitamin C and vitamin K taken together may help.

Extra tips

► Although ginger is widely known for its anti-nausea effects, use with caution during pregnancy. Ginger candy or a little bit of grated ginger steeped in hot water every now and then is fine. But do not take ginger capsules while pregnant.

▸ Eat small meals and snacks regularly. Low blood sugar is a common trigger so eat every two to three hours and do not let yourself get really hungry. Have a small snack before you go to bed to reduce the likelihood of waking in the night with nausea.

▸ Get adequate sleep and rest. Having a rest during the day can be helpful.

▸ Avoid wearing clothes that are tight round the middle.

▸ Avoid strong smells such as engine oil, cleaning products, perfumes and strong-smelling foods. Pregnant women have a heightened sense of smell and strong smells can trigger nausea.

▸ Breathe fully. Inhale into the diaphragm and exhale completely.

▸ Acupressure can help. This can be done by wearing a specially designed band that puts pressure on an acupressure point on the underside of your wrist. You can also put pressure on this point yourself. To find the point, measure three finger widths from your wrist crease line. Press on the hollow between the tendons and you will experience a slight tenderness. Press the point firmly with your thumb as you exhale and release the pressure slightly when you inhale. Continue for a few minutes.

▸ If you haven't been able to keep anything down for 24 hours, including fluids, you may have a condition called hyperemesis gravidarum. This refers to excessive vomiting in pregnancy. It is vital that you consult your medical specialist if this is the case in order to avoid complications.

Consult your medical specialist if:
▸ You experience severe, chronic vomiting.
▸ If the sickness persists past the fourteenth week of pregnancy.
▸ If you vomit blood.
▸ If you become dehydrated because you can't keep fluids down.

The labour process itself, lactation, breastfeeding, sleep deprivation, anxiety, fear, worry, malabsorption and the added daily and hourly demands from the new baby – all these deplete nutrients. Supplements, foods, herbs, botanicals, plants and herbal teas can correct the most common nutrient deficiencies of the new mother. By spending a bit of time going through my book, you are taking proactive measures so that you may become a healthier, happier and more nourished mum.

Weight Loss

If you think it's naturally harder to keep the weight off as you age – that it's all down to hormones – then I'm afraid I'm going to have to put you straight. Yes, hormones do play a role, but there's another factor that I contend overrides all that, which is exercise.

I remember one very special visit to my 96-year-old granny. I asked Granny what her secret was – why had she never put on weight? "Cycling my stationary bicycle," she replied. At that moment she insisted I turn on her favourite record and dance together. I have also a friend, Norman, who is 82 years old and never uses a lift. He lives on the 22nd floor of a high rise in New York, looks about 55 and is fitter than most 30-year-olds!

The reason it is so hard to stay trim as we leave our 20s is because we let our activity levels slip. But, as Norman and my granny prove, you don't have to. Just watch a child and you will see perpetual motion in action. They are constantly burning fuel. And of course in school you are required to exercise, albeit some schools encourage it more than others. My eldest daughter attends a high school that does PE four days a week, even double sessions. It's been so good for her stamina and endurance that she's become a great runner. However, PE stops at her school for the year 10 students. The rationale is they have too many academic subjects and not enough time to exercise. What a terrible message to teach our children. PE for kids should never stop.

You can live without studying trigonometry but, frankly, you cannot live life if you don't move your bod. The older you get, the more exercise you need to do. Age is not your cue to slow down. When you exercise, it improves digestion and metabolism; you burn fuel more effectively. And of course what you eat is still crucial. Bad food regimes and poor eating habits catch up with you eventually. In your younger years, some of you might get away with hoovering food down your mouth and living on junk. But you can't do it for years on end and stay looking fit.

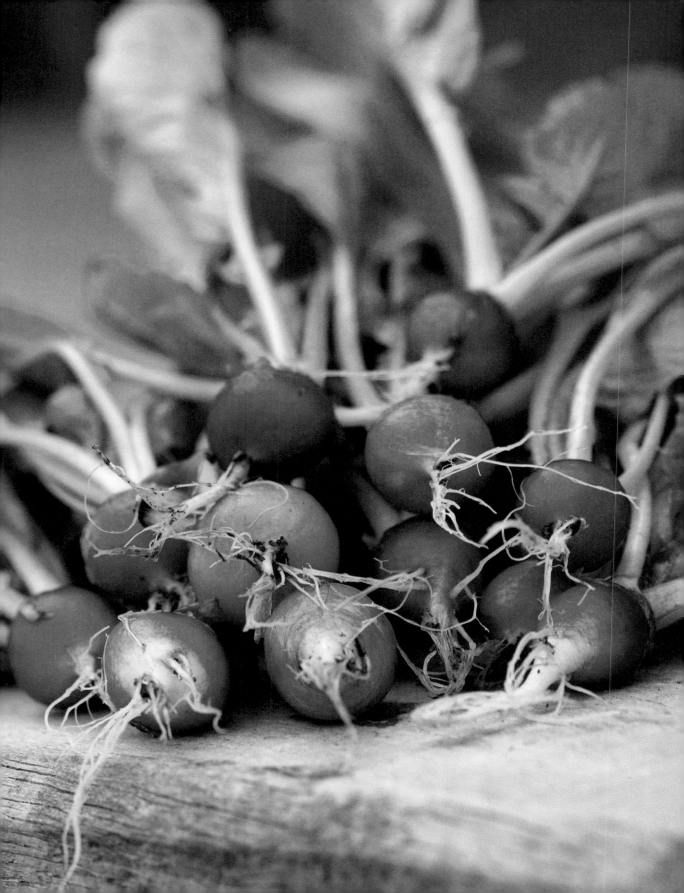

Why do some people seem more prone to putting on weight?

The number one factor is lack of exercise. The number one excuse? 'Gillian, I think there must be something wrong with my thyroid.' Sure, if you really do have an underactive thyroid, it'll trigger weight gain because the thyroid controls your metabolic rate (the rate at which you burn up calories for energy). But I can count on one hand the number of people I have met who fall into the thyroid-malfunctioning category once tested.

The second most common excuse is blaming genetics, and some studies have certainly shown a hereditary factor to body weight. But I believe it is more nurture than nature, where diet and lifestyle habits are inherited.

There is a connection between thoughts, feelings and weight. I am talking about relationships, divorces, marriages, break-ups, disappointments, job losses, bereavement, accidents or illness. I put it all under the heading of 'Stuff'. And Stuff can be a major blockage to weight loss.

Stuff may be big or small, recent or go way back to childhood. Unresolved problems from childhood and our teen years often manifest as comfort eating in adulthood. Anaesthetizing emotional pain with rubbish food is a no-win situation for your health – but you probably don't even know you're doing it. A common result is that you end up yo-yo dieting, which can be a real blow to self-esteem and confidence when the diets don't seem to work in the long run. It's crucial to think of your body and mind when embracing health. Everything is connected. Recognize and acknowledge any negative thoughts; then let them go. Allow your thoughts, words and actions to always be kind, positive and loving. This is my greatest secret to achieving wellness and balance on all levels.

When do you need to start worrying about your weight?

The answer is never. I don't want you to ever be worrying about your weight. Weight balance is a by-product of the work I do, never the focus. Take note of your body, but please do not become obsessed; follow the Gillian McKeith healthy lifestyle and the weight will take care of itself.

The first step is to admit responsibility. Yes, we live in a sedentary, fast-food-loving world. But it's still your choice as to how you live. Remind yourself what your kitchen and your trainers are for. (Clue: they're not for heating up takeaways and looking fashionable.)

There are three main indicators:

1) A BMI of 25 or over

Obesity can be assessed by calculating your BMI (Body Mass Index). This is your weight in kilograms divided by your height in metres squared. In the UK the ideal BMI is 18.5–24.9, while people with a BMI from 25–30 are classed as overweight. Above 30 = obese and over 40 = morbidly obese.

(Note that BMI doesn't take into account body shape or muscle-to-fat ratio, so it's not the best indicator on its own.)

2) A bulging waist that measures over 32in

Carrying fat around your middle is associated with many health problems, including heart disease and diabetes. A waist circumference greater than 80cm or 32in for women and 94cm or 37in for men needs action.

3) A waist-to-hip ratio of over 0.8

The waist-to-hip ratio is also a factor. To calculate it, divide your waist circumference by your hip circumference. If you're a man, a ratio of 1 or more should set alarm bells ringing. Likewise if you're a woman, a ratio of more than 0.8 means you need to get with my plan.

Being overweight puts you at increased risk of developing:

► **Cardio-vascular problems** including high blood pressure, heart disease, heart attacks, strokes and high cholesterol.

► **Diabetes** – being overweight makes you ten times more likely to develop type 2 diabetes. Diabetes is a major cause of kidney failure and adult-onset blindness. It can also lead to diabetic neuropathy and the need for limb amputations.

► **Respiratory problems** – excess weight puts an added strain on the lungs so that even minor activities such as climbing the stairs or carrying shopping become difficult. Sleep apnoea and snoring are also increased in overweight people. These both lead to fitful sleep and tiredness during the day.

► **Musculo-skeletal problems** – carrying extra weight puts a huge strain on the skeleton, joints, muscles and nerves. Being overweight increases the risk and severity of arthritic disorders, gout and backache.

► **Digestive problems** – reflux or heartburn, and gas, are more common in overweight people as the abdominal fat around the stomach increases the pressure on the digestive system, causing stomach acid to rise up into the oesophagus.

► **Urinary incontinence** – can result from the weight of the abdomen weakening the valve in the bladder. This can lead to leakage of urine, especially when laughing, sneezing or coughing.

► **Venal problems** – excess weight can increase the pressure on the veins, leading to varicose veins and skin ulcers.

► **Female hormone imbalances** – being overweight increases the risk of infertility, PMS, menopausal symptoms and problems during pregnancy.

► **Cancer** – being overweight may increase the risk of developing cancers of the uterus, gallbladder, cervix, ovary, prostate, breast and colon.

► **Gallbladder disease** – the risk increases as your weight increases.

Weight-loss inhibitors

▶ Excessive unhealthy food intake

▶ Lack of exercise

▶ Yeast overgrowth

▶ Mineral and vitamin imbalances

▶ Insulin imbalances (caused by too many sugary carbohydrates)

▶ Food intolerances

▶ Poor digestive function

▶ Poor adrenal function

▶ Poor metabolic function

▶ Sluggish liver

▶ Thyroid problems

▶ Water retention

Excessive unhealthy food intake

Eating bad food can inhibit your ability to lose weight. Most junky foods contain unhealthy fat, added white sugars, additives and or artificial sweeteners. So what you are really getting is empty, high calories sludge with little nutritional value. As a result, you never feel truly satisfied. Your body ends up craving and you respond by eating more of the same old rubbish, easily piling on the pounds.

Lack of exercise

Exercise burns calories and also increases muscle mass. Muscle burns more calories when at rest than other body tissue. If you don't move that bahookee, then watch the weight creep on. You might not feel like doing exercise at first but find something that you love, get started and you will be on a natural high as well as trim and slim.

Cravings

Added sugars in food is one of the worst advents of our modern society. You crave sugar if your blood-sugar levels are constantly out of balance by eating sugary foods; if you have nutrient deficiencies, yeast overgrowths; if you eat a diet high in refined, processed carbohydrates. You end up becoming the victim of a rollercoaster of soaring and plummeting sugar levels. This is why if you eat just one chocolate biscuit, you crave more. The sugar gives you the rush, but an energy drop is never far behind. The best way to beat the sugar fix is to go cold turkey: no sugary foods or sweets for a month. The herb astragalus can give you a natural energy lift (500mg daily).

Eat a balanced, nutrient-rich diet to break the cycle of cravings, sugar and weight gain. Eating well not only nourishes your body but regulates your blood-sugar levels so that you don't get those lows.

Certain foods help to regulate blood-sugar levels and tame sugar cravings. Whole grains and fresh veggies are great choices. Yams, sweet potatoes and squash help to curb a sweet tooth, too.

Support your system with live nutrient-dense superfoods like spirulina or liquid algae. A liquid mineral supplement that contains chromium, manganese and magnesium is important, too. Deficiencies of any one of these three minerals cause sugar cravings (more than 80 per cent of chromium is destroyed in the processing of foods). I often ask my clients to take half a teaspoon of L-glutamine powder before meals to inhibit carbohydrate cravings.

Finally, eat smaller, more frequent meals and regular healthy snacks through the day, especially mid morning and mid afternoon, when blood-sugar levels may fluctuate.

Insulin imbalances

When we eat, glucose from the digestion of carbohydrates is absorbed into the blood. At this point, blood-sugar levels are raised. This sends a signal to the pancreas to release insulin. The insulin's job is to carry the glucose from the blood to the cells in order to bring blood-sugar levels back to normal. Once in the cells glucose can be used for energy or stored for later as glycogen.

In a healthy diet this process works perfectly. However, excessive consumption of refined carbohydrates, particularly sugary foods, upsets the balance and everything starts to go haywire. Your body has to produce increasing amounts of insulin to keep blood-sugar levels normal. Eventually you become resistant to the insulin, so more needs to be produced. Once this happens, the glycogen stores become full and glucose is converted to fat.

You are then caught in a vicious cycle where the more unstable your blood-sugar levels, the more prone you will be to craving sweets and unrefined carbohydrates like bread and the easier it is to lay down fat. But this does not need to be the case.

I started going to the gym last year and I started watching Gillian's programmes to lose some weight. I was a dress size 14 weighing 11st 11lbs. Since listening to Gillian's advice I have gone down to a dress size 8–10 and I now weigh 9st 4lbs! I suffered badly with a lack of confidence and losing the weight has really helped. I now have my life back.

Glucose tolerance self-check

If you recognize three or more of the symptoms listed below, you may have a problem with the regulation of insulin and glucose in your body.

► Difficulty in concentrating.
► Excessive consumption of caffeine, chocolate or cigarettes.
► Excessive sweating.
► Excessive thirst.
► Extreme difficulty in getting out of bed.
► Falling asleep in the middle of the day/feeling really drowsy.
► Inability to get going without a caffeine/nicotine fix.
► Irritability without frequent meals.
► Need for more than eight hours' sleep per night.

Breaking the cycle

In order to break this cycle so you don't end up a complete sugar junky on a rollercoaster ride to poor health, you need to eat a diet that keeps insulin levels as low as possible. Over time, this can improve the cellular response to insulin so less is needed to keep blood-sugar levels normal. The less wide the swings of insulin you produce, the less likely you are to store glucose as fat.

► Avoid all foods that cause blood-sugar levels to rise rapidly. These include sugar, white bread, white rice, white pastry, white pasta, white potatoes, crisps, chips, processed foods, alcohol, caffeine, chocolate, cakes, pastries, biscuits, confectionary and soft drinks.

► Eat small, regular meals and snacks rather than large meals.

► Include fibre and protein with each meal as these slow down the release of glucose from carbohydrates. Examples include fish or chicken with vegetables and salad or beans with grains and vegetables.

► Drink herbal teas and water instead of tea, coffee or alcohol. These act as stimulants that raise blood-sugar levels initially followed by a slump, leaving you with cravings for another pick-me-up an hour or so later.

▶ Move that bahookee of yours please. Daily, moderate exercise improves the cellular response to insulin and normalizes appetite.

▶ Stress upsets blood-sugar levels. Learn relaxation techniques such as yoga, tai chi, chi gung or meditation.

▶ Take blood-sugar balancing nutrients such as chromium, amino acid complex, vitamin D, magnesium, zinc and B vitamins. Balancing herbs include nigella, lupin, cloves, cumin, sage, cinnamon and fenugreek.

If you do get a fit of the cravings, the key is not to get flustered. Just take not of it like an observer. Intead, just say, 'Oh, there's that craving,' and allow it to go. A new you is on the way!

If chocolate is your thing, then go for the real thing. Raw cacao bean nibs or powder are from the raw bean that chocolate is made from, but they don't have the added white processed sugar that makes up chocolate. You'll find them in the health-food store.

Food intolerances

We often crave the same foods day in and day out. But if you eat the same foods every day, for years, in many cases you can become sensitive to those very foods, sometimes referred to as food intolerances. And usually the foods that we crave are the same ones that lead to weight gain. It is a vicious cycle.

If you are food intolerant, a delayed immune response may occur in your body. This can happen over several hours or days after the offending food is ingested. Side effects to these foods can be anything from irritable bowel-like symptoms (see page 314) to skin eruptions, ulcerations in the mouth, Crohn's disease (see page 239) or inflammation of the digestive tract, colic, ear problems and tiredness, to name a few. It is not always so obvious.

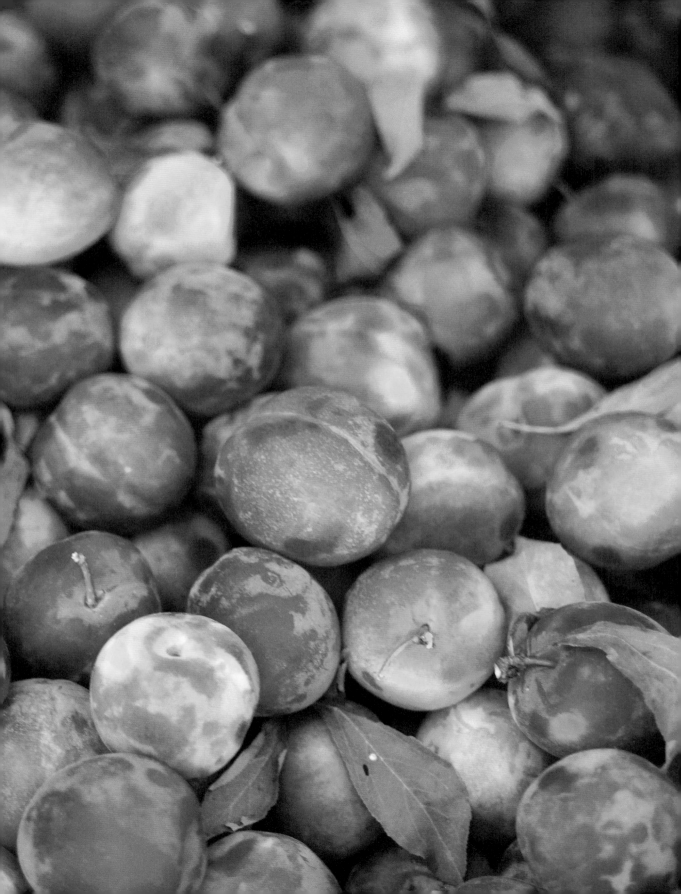

But food intolerances can have a direct effect on the assimilation of nutrients, digestive organ function and weight management. The more common foods such as wheat, dairy, sugar and corn are often implicated as food-intolerance triggers, simply because many of us eat too much of these same foods.

The problem is that when you eat foods to which you are intolerant, every day, you may cause a drastic slowdown of metabolism. Digestive enzyme function might become impaired, which means that your body may not break down fat properly.

Moreover, by eating the same foods every day, you limit your intake of essential nutrients, vitamins, minerals and co-factors. So my best advice here is:

► Always rotate your foods. In other words, if you eat a food today, then try not to eat it again for, say, three or four days. Thus, you may prevent food intolerances.

► It is a good idea to get tested for food intolerances or allergies (www.gillianmckeith.info). In this way, you can know exactly which foods are possibly causing you to gain weight or feel horrible or overly tired and lethargic.

Poor digestive function

Your digestive system is responsible for breaking down food into amino acids, glucose and fats, releasing nutrients from food and the elimination process. If it is not functioning optimally, you will feel unwell and this can lead to overeating as your body starts to crave nutrients. You may well be constipated, too (you should be passing stools twice a day, even once a day is a sign of poor digestion). So improving digestion becomes a serious matter.

Poor adrenal function

When adrenal function is out of balance, then more stress hormones could be released. This hormone release can exacerbate blood-sugar fluctuations, which may cause further weight gain. Your adrenal glands can become compromised from a lack of sleep, a deficiency in B vitamins and a poor diet high in sugary foods. A tell-tale sign of adrenal exhaustion is a beer belly even when you don't drink beer.

Poor metabolic function

If you don't eat food on a regular basis you could actually cause weight problems. Reduced metabolic rate – this can happen if you have yo-yo dieted in the past. Reducing food intake gives a message to the body that food is scarce. In order to ensure your long-term survival, your body reduces the amount of calories you burn on a daily basis. When you start eating more normal amounts again, you will store the extra calories as fat much more easily.

When you starve yourself, your metabolism could slow down to a trickle. I have seen many overweight folks who hardly eat anything. See page 326 of the A–Z for more info.

Sluggish liver

The liver is involved in many different body processes including detoxification, blood-sugar control, the breaking down of old hormones, the manufacture and breakdown of cholesterol and the absorption of protein, fats and carbohydrates.

If the liver is struggling, absorption of nutrients will be compromised and blood-sugar levels will fluctuate. This can lead to cravings for the wrong kinds of foods and reduced energy levels. Boozing on the weekend or at any other time for that matter doesn't help sugar cravings or weight either. Cravings get worse and weight piles on.

Thyroid

The thyroid gland controls the metabolism of your entire body by regulating energy production and oxygen uptake. Continual stress can negatively affect the thyroid gland, depressing its normal function. Overstimulation of the thyroid is caused by the consumption of sugar, coffee and alcohol, sending the thyroid into an exhausted state, which can cause weight gain.

Solutions:

► Kelp supplements can help an underactive thyroid, so can green superfoods. Seaweeds which are high in iodine can help bolster metabolism, too.

► Eat tyrosine-filled food, such as pumpkin seeds, avocados and almonds, to feed your metabolism.

► If you are a compulsive eater, take a tyrosine supplement (500mg, four times a day) along with a zinc supplement (50mg daily).

Thyroid self-check

► Cold hands and/or feet
► Constant headaches
► Constipation
► Exhaustion, even after sleeping for hours
► Feeling cold all the time
► Inability to sweat
► Infertility
► Lethargy in the mornings, while feeling energetic at night
► Loss of outer third of eyebrow hair
► No desire for sex
► Permanent heel cracks
► PMT
► Swollen eyelids, ankles or hands
► Very dry skin and hair
► Yellow tint to skin

If you have three or more of the above symptoms, you may have an underactive thyroid. Ask your GP for a blood test to check it out. Be aware, however, that sometimes if you have a very mild form of thyroid malfunction, it will go undetected in a blood test.

Water retention

If you suffer from water retention, it is somewhat paradoxically, important to drink plenty of water and herbal teas. This is because water retention can be a sign that you are dehydrated meaning the body holds onto water for fear of becoming further dehydrated. It is also a sign that there may be excess sodium in the body. This needs to be flushed out with extra fluids – (not diet/fizzy drinks and coffee). Vegetable juices are perfect due to their high potassium content – potassium is needed to balance sodium in the body. Dandelion and nettle teas both have gentle water balancing effects and contain potassium along with other minerals. B complex, specifically vitamin B6, may also be helpful in relieving water retention.

Good foods for healthy weight loss

► **Aduki beans** – my weight loss bean of choice. High in fibre, low in calories, rich in many nutrients, including potassium, which can help reduce water retention, and magnesium needed for energy.

► **Almonds** – research shows that almonds can assist in weight loss. This may be due to their blood-sugar balancing qualities and rich nutrient content.

► **Apples and pears** – research shows that daily consumption of apples can benefit weight loss. This is partly due to their low glycaemic index meaning they do not cause highs and lows of blood sugar. They thus give you sustained energy while providing very few calories and lots of fibre and nutrients, including chromium needed for blood-sugar regulation and energy.

▸ **Blueberries** – rich in nutrients, fibre and antioxidants.

▸ **Brown rice** – rich in tryptophan, the amino acid that converts to 5HTP and serotonin in the brain, helping reduce appetite and improve mood.

▸ **Cucumbers** – low in calories and have a high water content that can help with internal cleansing and satiety.

▸ **Ginger** – warming spice that can get things moving in the body, particularly the blood and lymph circulation. Good for metabolism generally.

▸ **Leafy greens** – high in fibre and nutrients. They are particularly rich in magnesium, chromium and B vitamins all needed for the conversion of food into energy and blood-sugar stability.

▸ **Miso soup** – whole soy products contain phytoestrogens which have been shown to have a beneficial effect on weight loss. Miso is also rich in bio-available protein needed to keep blood-sugar levels stable and enzymes needed for digestion.

▸ **Oats** – rich in soluble fibre and slow releasing carbohydrates meaning they keep you feeling satisfied.

▸ **Plums** – high in fibre and rich in potassium needed to reduce water retention.

▸ **Quinoa** – highly nutritious grain, high in magnesium, iron, B vitamins, fibre and protein.

▸ **Raw shelled hemp seeds** – my weight loss seed! The essential fats have been found to be beneficial in the treatment and prevention of many diseases including obesity.

▸ **Sea vegetables** – rich in minerals and iodine, a commonly deficient nutrient needed for thyroid function and metabolism.

▸ **Sprouted seeds** – contain bio-available nutrients, protein and fibre needed for blood-sugar control.

Herbs and Supplements for weight loss

▶ **B vitamins** to help metabolize carbs and proteins. Take 50–100mg a day.

▶ **L-tyrosine** to reduce appetite. Take 500mg before all meals.

▶ **Co-enzyme Q10** is a metabolic stimulant that helps facilitate weight loss – especially useful when you're really fatigued. Take 100mg a day.

▶ **Triphala** to clean out your colon.

▶ **Digestive enzyme supplements** to aid nutrient uptake and help suppress appetite. Take one capsule with every meal.

▶ **Gillian McKeith Organic Energy Powder** as a great meal replacement when eating on the run.

▶ **Flax oil supplements** or linseeds to replenish drastically needed EFAs.

▶ **Chromium polynicotinate** to regulate blood-sugar swings. Take 200mcg a day with lunch and dinner.

▶ **Chickweed** to help break down stubborn fat deposits. Drink two cups of chickweed tea a day.

▶ **Kelp** to support the thyroid gland and weight loss. Take three tablets a day or use the seaweed kombu in cooking.

▶ **Lecithin** to utilize body fats. Take a tablespoon of granules twice a day.

▶ **Good-quality fibre** to cleanse your system. Take psyllium husks in between meals – with lots of water.

▶ **Ginseng** to nourish the metabolic system and help the liver to break down fats more effectively. Take two tablets daily (500mg) or drink ginseng tea twice daily.

▶ **Dandelion tea** is cleansing to the liver and a natural diuretic, so helpful in weight loss and fluid retention.

▶ **Nettle tea** is a great weight-loss tea as it supports metabolism and has diuretic properties.

How best to start a new lifestyle and then stick to it

By picking up this food bible, you have already taken a big step towards changing your lifestyle. But when it comes to actually making the change – altering your diet, activity levels, attitude – that's when the self-doubt creeps in. A big worry clients always vocalize to me is that they're not going to be able to stick to it. They have been on every diet known to man and they are still back at square one. To this, I can offer them – and you – absolute reassurance. You will feel so good when you follow the Gillian McKeith way that you will want to stay on the path. The pay off is huge and it's that elusive commodity we all want more of: energy.

Good food not only gives you more energy; it *is* energy. The physical and molecular structure of food itself is energy in its own right. Good food is your fuel that powers you for life.

Years ago, I developed a superfood energy powder from sprouted seeds for my clients. I always remember this story I was told about an old woman who owned a shop in Fulham, London, and how she used dousing to test the vibration of new foods before she would bring them into her shop. It turned out the woman, who also worked with energy healing, was astounded when she discovered the high vibrational charge of my superfood energy powder. She claimed it was the highest level of vibration charge for a new food supplement powder.

My point here is that the food you eat is either of a high vibration or of a low vibration. Food can either heal you or hurt you. For example, fizzy soda drinks, sugary cakes, processed luncheon meats and the like are of the lowest vibrational energy charge. Therefore, they are hurtful and unhelpful. Conversely, sprouted millet or sprouted broccoli seeds are of the highest vibrational energy charge. Feed yourselves with foods of the highest vibrational charge in the most natural state – in other words, all the foods I recommend to you in my food bible – and you'll be living a happy, healthy and loving life.

Top tips for initial weight loss

► Eat more, not less. Eating less than is required to support your basal metabolism will slow your metabolism down. My clients raise metabolism and keep blood-sugar levels stable with regular healthy eating. It also helps to prevent bingeing because you never feel famished.

► Drink more water. Drink eight glasses of water a day between meals. Have a large glass of water 20 to 30 minutes before meals, not during meals as this is a recipe for gas. Dehydration, because it causes headaches, lack of concentration and fatigue, is also often mistaken for hunger. Please drink enough water.

► Slow down. Eating slowly is one method that can help take off pounds. That's because from the time that you begin eating, it takes the brain 20 minutes to signal feelings of fullness. Fast eaters often eat beyond their true level of fullness before the 20-minute signal has had a chance to set in. Put your knife and fork down between each bite, take smaller bites and enjoy and savour every tasty morsel. Nutrient uptake is more effective, too.

► Go through your cupboards, fridge and freezer and throw out salty convenience foods, fatty foods, sugary drinks, chemical snacks, foods with unpronounceable ingredients you can't decipher, hydrogenated oils and processed foods.

► Change your snack mindset. Stop thinking of quick snacks as sugary flapjacks, biscuits, chocolates, crisps and other nasties. Start associating fast, on-the-run snacks with easy, healthy alternatives like your favourite fruits, freshly squeezed juices, nuts and seeds or carrot sticks and sugar snap peas.

► Don't shop when you're hungry. You'll end up buying all kinds of things you know you don't need.

► Cook in the raw. I always advise my clients to include raw foods in the same meal when they prepare cooked foods. This is because raw foods contain food enzymes that are essential for optimum digestion and general wellbeing.

► Keep moving. Walking to the shops, mowing the lawn and taking the stairs at work all count and keep you moving throughout the day.

► Drink warm water in the morning. A warm cup of water first thing in the morning (and even better with a squeeze of lemon) goes right through the bowels and cleans out mucus. Drink another cup of warm water in the evening, too.

► Break the fast. Always eat something healthy and substantial for breakfast. This is the time period when your stomach energies are at their strongest, and your digestive enzyme juices are rearing to go. You will gradually weaken your stomach and digestive function if you skip breakfast. No matter how little it is, eat something decent. Fresh fruit, oatmeal, millet or quinoa porridge are all good morning choices.

► Eat when calm. You physically can't digest food properly if you are upset or have just had an argument.

► Nimble at night. Eat your last meal of the day at least a couple of hours before bedtime and a snack later if you need it. When you eat too late, you stress and wear out your body. You cannot digest a late meal effectively if you go to sleep on a full stomach. It's bad for your digestive organs, heart and liver, not to mention your libido! A light snack is OK.

► Early to bed. The earlier you get to bed, the better you will feel. The liver and gallbladder conduct their detox work generally between the hours of 11pm and 2am. Being tired slows your metabolism and can affect your food choices, making you go for high-calorie, fatty foods for a fast, brief energy burst.

► Go to www.gillianmckeith.info for advice and support especially the Club and Gillian's Boot Camp.

The Menopause

The average age women experience the menopause is 50.
But, like puberty, it's not an overnight experience. The months
and years leading up to menopause (the peri-menopause) and
menopause itself (the very end of your menstrual cycle) last
between five and ten years. During which time, the production
of oestrogen and progesterone by your ovaries gradually wanes.

The decline in hormone production and the associated
symptoms can start as early as 40, although a premature
menopause occurs in only a small minority of women. Common
symptoms can include hot flushes, vaginal dryness, night sweats,
depression, insomnia, headaches, mood swings, lack of energy,
low libido in a few and weight gain that feels harder and harder
to shift. Osteoporosis (page 337) and heart disease (page 283) can
also increase as the protective effects of female hormones lessen.
But notice I said all these symptoms can occur – I didn't say they
will, so don't go looking for them. The menopause is portrayed as
such a negative time for women when often it can be a liberating,
joyous, sensual time, too. And even if you do experience some of
these symptoms, there's plenty of advice I can give you on how
to minimize and even eliminate them.

Raging hormones

You may have heard reports that women reach their sexual
peak later in life than men. Well it's all true. By your late thirties
or early forties you're likely to experience an increase (sometimes
quite intense) in libido. This is down to fluctuating hormone
levels and changes in your menstrual cycle. In the build-up to
menopause, production of the sex hormones – testosterone,
oestrogen and progesterone – can become unpredictable. This
affects different women in different ways, but it will most
probably have some effect on your sex life.

Now, as oestrogen production falls, this triggers your brain
to release higher quantities of other hormones in an attempt

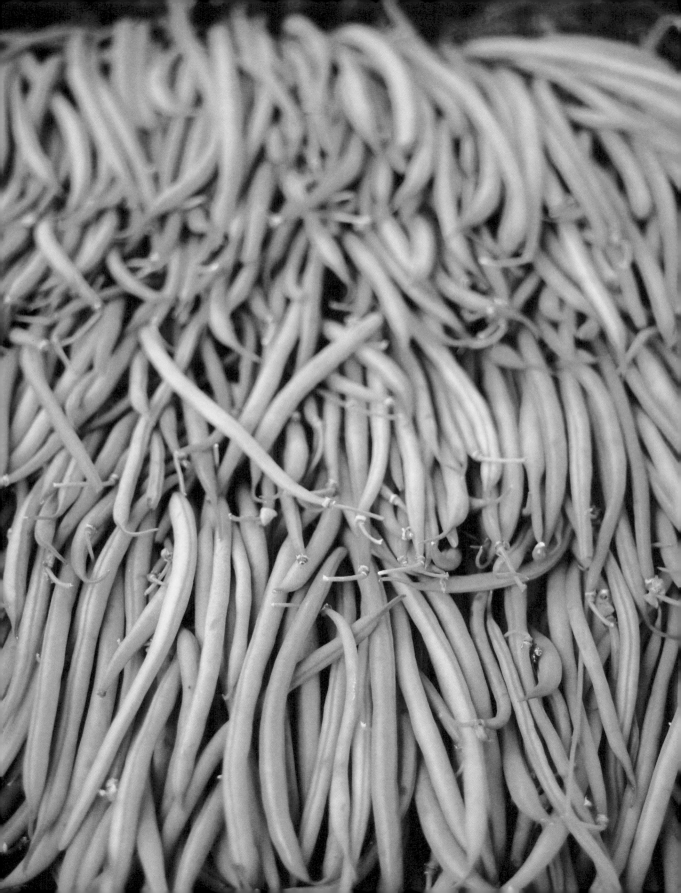

to make your ovaries work harder. Nonetheless the number and quality of the eggs released from your ovaries inevitably falls and your fertility decreases.

As the debate rages in the media about the rights and wrongs of Hormone Replacement Therapy (HRT), I try my best to convince people that the easiest way to ensure a smooth transition is through healthy living. At the risk of sounding like a broken record (again!), eating healthily is absolutely essential during menopause. It enables your body to adjust to the hormone changes, naturally maintaining oestrogen from the adrenal glands and fat deposits.

Here are my basic hormone-balancing recommendations
Foods to include:
► Whole grains for fibre, B vitamin, magnesium and zinc content.
► Pulses for their phyto-oestrogenic effects, fibre and nutrients.
► Tempeh, miso, natural soya yoghurt and tamari for phyto-oestrogens, protein, calcium and magnesium.
► Linseeds (flax seeds) for their lignans, fibre, zinc and essential fats.
► Pumpkin seeds for zinc, magnesium and essential fats.
► Oily fish for their omega-3 fats and protein.
► Raw shelled hemp seeds for a balance of omega-3 and -6 and -9 fats that can help with female hormone balance.
► Sea vegetables for their high mineral content.
► Green vegetables for calcium and magnesium content.
► Wheatgerm, mung beans and their sprouts, spirulina, millet, black beans, kidney beans and black sesame seeds can all build energy which can be low at this time.
► Royal jelly can help to increase hormonal activity and release energy and a sense of wellbeing.
► Liberally eat oats, flax, barley, beets, cabbage, aduki beans, olive oils, split peas, yams, fennel and sesame seeds.

Foods and drinks to avoid

▶ Coffee and chocolate contain caffeine as well as methylxanthines that can affect female hormone balance. Avoid regular tea and coffee and alcohol, which overwork your adrenal glands, contributing to blood-sugar problems and oestrogen deficiency and increasing the risk of osteoporosis.

▶ Alcohol upsets blood sugar, female hormones and puts a strain on the adrenals.

▶ Added sugar and refined carbohydrates upset blood sugar and can lead to weight gain and cardio-vascular problems.

▶ Refined table salt can trigger hot flushes and water retention.

▶ Spicy hot foods can trigger hot flushes.

▶ Red meat and dairy products because of their potentially inflammatory saturated fats and acid-forming properties.
In order to neutralize the acid, minerals such as calcium may be taken from the bones, increasing the risk of osteoporosis.

Nutrients for menopausal women

▶ Your body needs **vitamin D** to utilize **calcium**, so it is important to get some sunlight.

▶ **Vitamin C** with bioflavanoids has been shown to help reduce hot flushes.

▶ **Vitamin E** can help reduce hot flushes and vaginal dryness.

▶ **B vitamins** reduce stress, anxiety, irritability, fatigue and poor concentration, giving the adrenals a rest.

▶ **Magnesium** is known as 'nature's tranquillizer', because it helps with symptoms such as anxiety and mood changes.

▶ **Dehydroepiandrosterone (DHEA)** can help to increase oestrogen levels. At present, DHEA supplements are available only on prescription. Check with your GP.

▶ **Gamma oryzenol** has made positive changes with my menopausal ladies.

Herbs for menopause

► **Agnus castus** is my top recommendation for my own clients. It acts as an adaptogen, balancing hormone production.

► **Black cohosh** may ease hot flushes and vaginal dryness.

► **Dong quai** can help to restore hormonal balance.

► **Sage** is helpful for hot sweats.

► **Milk thistle** helps to excrete old hormones and toxins.

► **Ginkgo biloba** has been shown to have a rejuvenating effect on the brain.

► **Angelica** for the female reproductive system, regulating hormones and improving the rhythm of the menstrual cycle.

► **Red clover** for balancing hormones because of its high B vitamin content.

► **Shatawari** is a popular Ayurvedic tonic used by some women to help to normalize the hormonal imbalances.

► **Valerian** can help with sleep. Drink a cup of camomile tea with a few drops of valerian an hour before bed.

Low thyroid function

Your thyroid may become sluggish around your menopausal years. This can cause a range of seemingly unconnected symptoms. Be aware of: thinning hair, constipation, dry skin, cold hands and feet, weight gain. (Of course each of these symptoms can occur from time to time even if your thyroid is healthy, so please get checked by your GP.) See page 301 in the A–Z for more information.

Specific menopausal symptoms and solutions

Hot flushes

▶ Avoid caffeine, alcohol, sugar and refined carbohydrates.

▶ Supplement with vitamin E daily. As much as 300iu three times daily may be needed but build up to this amount gradually. Do not take if you are on other medications.

▶ Citrus bio-flavanoids with vitamin C may also be helpful.

▶ Drink sage tea twice a day and if night sweats are a problem, have a cup before bed. Sage can reduce sweating.

▶ Red clover tea or tincture can also be helpful for its phyto-oestrogenic effects. You would need about 15 drops three times daily to see a difference.

Vaginal dryness or thinning

▶ Make sure you get plenty of essential fats in your diet daily: oily fish (mackerel, salmon, sardines, pilchards, herrings and trout), raw shelled hemp seeds, flax seeds, pumpkin seeds, sunflower seeds, walnuts and avocados are all good sources.

▶ Black cohosh tincture twice a day.

▶ Vitamin E daily. The foods listed above for their essential fat content are also good sources of vitamin E, as is olive oil.

▶ Dandelion leaf and oat straw teas can both be beneficial for their nutritive effects.

▶ Aloe vera gel can be applied topically to soothe and heal.

Osteoporosis

See page 337 in the A–Z.

Thinning hair

▶ Massage the scalp with olive oil containing a few drops of rosemary essential oil to stimulate the hair follicles.

▶ Avoid sugar, refined carbohydrates, alcohol and caffeine as these can all stimulate insulin. Excess insulin can result in hair loss.

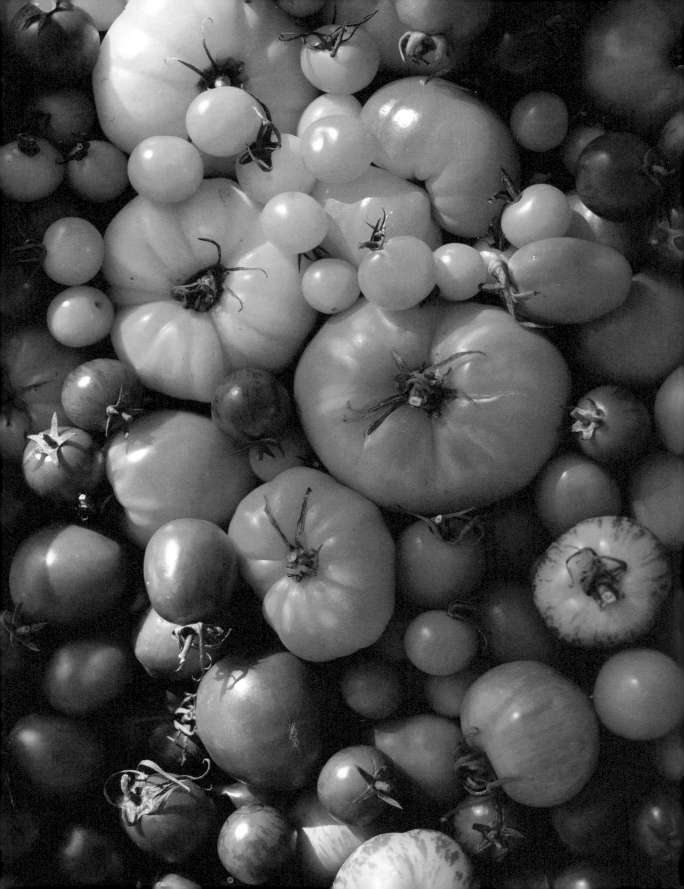

► Include sea vegetables such as nori or kelp in your diet to support the thyroid.

► Regular exercise helps to improve circulation to the scalp. The inverted postures in yoga may be particularly beneficial in increasing the circulation to the scalp. See page 181 in the A–Z for more information.

Mood swings

► Avoid low-fat diets. Good fats are needed for the production of hormones and neurotransmitters in the brain.

► Get outside every day as the action of daylight on the pineal gland helps to control our rhythms and moods.

► St John's wort has been shown to be as effective as anti-depressant medications without the side effects. Consult your medical practitioner before taking it especially if you are on any other medications.

► Black cohosh can aid mood.

► Motherwort is soothing.

► The spice saffron can be used in tiny amounts (just a few strands) to promote emotional stability; add it at the end of cooking to rice and vegetables.

► Acupuncture is balancing and can be extremely helpful, especially if you can find a practitioner who uses Japanese needles, which are small and gentle on the skin.

Ageing

You can be vital, useful, healthy and vibrant at all ages, right up to the end of your physical body. My friend Kitty used to teach me the Alexander Technique, giving lessons into her late nineties. She continued working until a couple of days before she passed away. This was a woman who emanated the most vibrant energy; who stood erect with sparkling eyes, and who told jokes with passion just a decade before her centennial. My mentor, Dr Sam Getlin, kept working with love and vigour until he was 102. And I recently saw my friend Norman at a health publishing exhibition. Norman, now in his mid eighties, assured me he still climbs the twenty-something floors of stairs every morning in his New Jersey apartment building.

My point here is that young, middle or elderly, if you take care of yourself, you are youthful at any chronological age. While people today may actually be living longer, they are living or rather existing in a much degenerative state. The hospitals are full. The UK's National Health Service is at breaking point. It is absolutely and utterly not necessary for us all to be subjected to the ills, the diseases and the overall bad health of modern society. You can live so much better, stronger and more nimble as you add years.

In fact, I will go so far as to say that the older you are, the better the chances you have to be fitter and healthier. The more years of chronology you add to your life, then the more years you have to build your muscles, to grow your stamina, expand your minds and free your soul. Even with my own physical body, I have had fitness instructors tell me that my abdominal core is like a rock. It wasn't like that when I was younger. My own emotional and spiritual quotients are far more developed today than when I was in my twenties because I have had the time to develop and evolve, to grow. This is the beauty and wisdom of ageing. So, you see, it is time and ageing that actually are not our foe, but a wonderful friend.

I am not oblivious to how the body may slow down as we get older; or how we may feel aches and pains, stiffness, lethargy, ails or even boredom as the years move on. I am no teenager myself; and I have consulted with hundreds if not thousands of clients of all ages to know how the body changes with time and gravity. But you must know whether we are talking about the abs, skin, hair, nails, mind or spiritual foundation, we have the power to excel forward to new advanced levels and heights of excellence if we take up the reins.

Long-lived populations

On the Japanese island of Okinawa the inhabitants are famous for their longevity. These people live to a phenomenally ripe old age and there are more centenarians in Okinawa than anywhere else in the world. The Okinawan Centenarian Study, which investigated these islanders for 25 years to discover their secret, describes how the islanders age much more slowly than the rest of us.

Death rates from stroke, cancer and heart disease are 59 per cent, 69 per cent and 59 per cent lower respectively of the average for the rest of Japan. They spend on average a breathtaking 97 per cent of their lives free from disease and disability. So what is their secret? The Okinawans eat healthy, natural food and they don't overeat. They do, however, manage to put away around seven servings of fruit and vegetables, seven servings of whole grains and two servings of soya and six glasses of water daily, plus oily fish three times a week on average, lots of green tea and no alcohol. They have a particular fondness for soya, sweet potatoes and watermelon and meat is eaten only occasionally.

And of course there's the lifestyle: unhurried, with plenty of exercise and a strong emphasis on spending time with family. They favour meditation, chi gung and t'ai chi.

It's not just Japan – other regions around the globe boast populations with long life expectancies and exceptional good health. The Hunza in the Hindu Kush Mountains, the

Georgians of the low Caucasus Mountains and the Greeks all have above-average life expectancy and exceptional wellness.

The common denominators between all these long-living populations are:

► Diet abundant and varied in fresh fruit, vegetables and natural foods.
► Low levels of animal protein or vegetarian.
► Absence of processed foods.
► Calm, peaceful living.
► Regular exercise.
► Usefulness right through old age.

Why do we age and what is the process?

The definition of ageing is hardly uplifting – 'the ever-increasing susceptibility to disease and death which accompanies advancing age'. But what, exactly, causes ageing and why do some people manage to look younger than their years? One of the most compelling, and scientifically accepted, theories is that it's down to oxidative stress. Stick with me and it will all make sense: although oxygen is essential to life, it is also a highly reactive chemical in the body, and it causes oxidation – a bit like rusting – in your cells. Compounds called 'free oxidizing radicals' (or just 'free radicals') attack the DNA of the cell, causing damage and affecting how your cells multiply. This cellular damage is a major contributor to the visible signs of premature ageing as well as the chronic disease that often comes with age, such as cancer, heart disease, Alzheimer's disease, cataracts, respiratory tract infections and many other conditions.

So, the fewer free radicals we have roaming about our bodies, the better. Unfortunately, you can no more avoid free radicals than you can revisit your youth. I wish I could promise you otherwise! What I can do is help you to arm yourself with the armour required to halt the action of these damaging chemicals.

You've probably already heard of them, but may not be quite sure what they are. They're called antioxidants and they literally deactivate free radicals. And your best source of antioxidants... surprise, surprise, is food.

Antioxidant vitamins, minerals and enzymes

▶ **Vitamin A (and its precursor, betacarotene)** is especially protective against diseases of the respiratory system, one of the major causes of death in the elderly.

▶ **Vitamin C** is one of the most important water-soluble antioxidants in cells and plays a protective role in just about every part of the body. It is essential for the formation of collagen, the intracellular 'glue' which holds cells together and keeps skin elastic and wrinkle-free. Highly concentrated in the eye, vitamin C protects against light damage and helps to prevent the development of cataracts. Not only is it a powerful antioxidant in itself, known to strengthen the immune system and prevent the growth of tumours, it also enhances the action of vitamin E, which in turn enhances the action of the antioxidant enzyme glutathione, an important liver protector.

▶ **Vitamin E** protects fats from oxidising (the brain is about 60 per cent fat so its protective role is vital) and is often found in healthy fatty foods, such as nuts. Like vitamin C, it plays an important role in guarding the eyes from age-related damage and is also involved in preventing free-radical damage to the cardio-vascular system.

▶ **Selenium** is linked to the prevention of cancer, especially breast and prostate, and decreased levels are also linked to cataract formation and age-related macular degeneration of the eye. This mineral is also vital for heart health, yet it is known that levels of selenium in the soil are widely deficient on a global scale. As well as being an antioxidant in itself, selenium is also necessary to make antioxidant enzymes in the body, such as glutathione.

What are the best sources of these wonderful nutrients which work to protect our health and delay the ravages of time? They tend to be found in the same foods, namely fruits, vegetables, nuts, seeds, legumes and just about any other plant food you can think of. The best sources of vitamin C are berry fruits (blueberries, strawberries, raspberries and so on), kiwi and citrus fruits. Potatoes are also a good source. Vitamin A is found only in animal foods, such as liver, oily fish and dairy foods, but its plant-based precursor, betacarotene, is widely found in fruits and vegetables with a yellow, red or orange pigment, such as carrots, peppers, apricots and oranges. Vitamin E – together with selenium – is found in nuts and seeds, particularly pumpkin seeds, walnuts, cashews and Brazil nuts. Nuts are also rich in the antioxidant enzyme glutathione. Another good source of selenium is garlic. Many raw foods contain food antioxidant enzymes which help you to break down and digest your food.

Antioxidant phytonutrients

The wide range of phytonutrients so far discovered is broadly categorized into two families: carotenoids and polyphenols. The most famous carotenoid is betacarotene, the plant-based precursor to vitamin A, and most people associate carrots with this carotenoid. There are plenty of other good sources, however, such as sweet potato, which also contains good levels of both vitamin C and vitamin E, red and yellow peppers and pumpkins. Other carotenoids, including lycopene, lutein and zeanxanthin, are just as important.

Tomatoes are particularly rich in the carotenoid lycopene, a high intake of which is associated with lowered risk of prostate cancer. Men are susceptible to developing benign prostatic hyperplasia – enlarged prostate – from the age of 50 onwards so would do well to make sure they eat plenty of lycopene-containing foods. Lycopene is thought to contain the greatest amount of antioxidant activity of all the carotenoids, and has been studied widely for its anti-cancer effects. Dark leafy greens are also rich in a variety of carotenoids – these include spinach, broccoli, Brussels sprouts, watercress and curly kale.

The retina of the eye contains particularly high levels of zeaxanthin and lutein. Eyesight is at particular risk of degeneration in later life because eyes are constantly exposed to light and free radicals. Carotenoids, together with vitamin C, have been shown to help to prevent the development of cataracts.

It's not only eyesight which light – especially sunlight – can cause to deteriorate prematurely. Nothing ages skin quite like prolonged exposure to the effects of the sun's rays. As well as looking like a wrinkled-up prune, sun overexposure is also firmly established as a major cause of skin cancer. Yet life would not exist without the sun, and all energy comes ultimately from it. The focus of preventative care has been heavily on either avoiding exposure – which means risking vitamin D deficiency – or slathering ourselves in sunscreen. Yet carotenoids have been shown to protect against the harmful effects of the sun's rays, both in terms of premature ageing and skin cancer, by blocking or inhibiting the effects of UV-induced free radicals. This makes sense when you consider that plants contain these compounds for their own protection: without carotenoids, all plant life on the planet would turn into a burnt mass shortly after sunrise.

Polyphenols

There are numerous types of polyphenols exerting powerful antioxidant effects, and more and more are being discovered. The best known are the flavanoids, which are powerfully antioxidant and can block the formation of cancer cells. One excellent flavanoid is quercetin, found in red onions and apples. Quercetin is anti-inflammatory and is used therapeutically to ease age-related inflammatory conditions such as arthritis.

Flavanoids are associated with a lower risk of developing coronary heart disease by helping to keep arteries clear of plaque.

You can spot a flavanoid-rich food by its colour – look for deep reds, purples and blues. Berries are particularly flavanoid-rich. What's more, they are especially rich in vitamin C. Bilberries are known to help to protect against sun damage to the eye as well as cataract formation. Blackberries help to prevent the build-up of plaque on artery walls and blueberries and strawberries are believed to have anti-cancer properties. Goji berries are also flavanoid packed and make an easy snack.

Another potent antioxidant polyphenol is ellagic acid, found in grapes, strawberries, blueberries and cherries. Other polyphenol-rich sources to look out for are green tea, herbs (especially rosemary and thyme), turmeric and mushrooms – in particular shitake, maitake and reishi. You should also aim to eat plenty of foods from the cruciferous family – kale, cabbage and broccoli are rich in glucosinolates, which can help prevent certain cancers, including those of the breast, stomach and colon.

There are a few other antioxidants which deserve special mention, namely alpha-lipoic acid (ALA), pycnogenol (extract of French maritime pine bark) and co-enzyme Q10. Alpha-lipoic acid is known as the 'universal antioxidant' because it has the extraordinary ability to regenerate other antioxidants, such as vitamins C and E, making them active again. The body makes ALA in small quantities but it is also available in supplement form. Pycnogenol is believed to help to prevent that most dreaded of age-related disorders, varicose veins, whilst co-enzyme Q10 is believed to help to strengthen the cardio-vascular system and prevent gum disease.

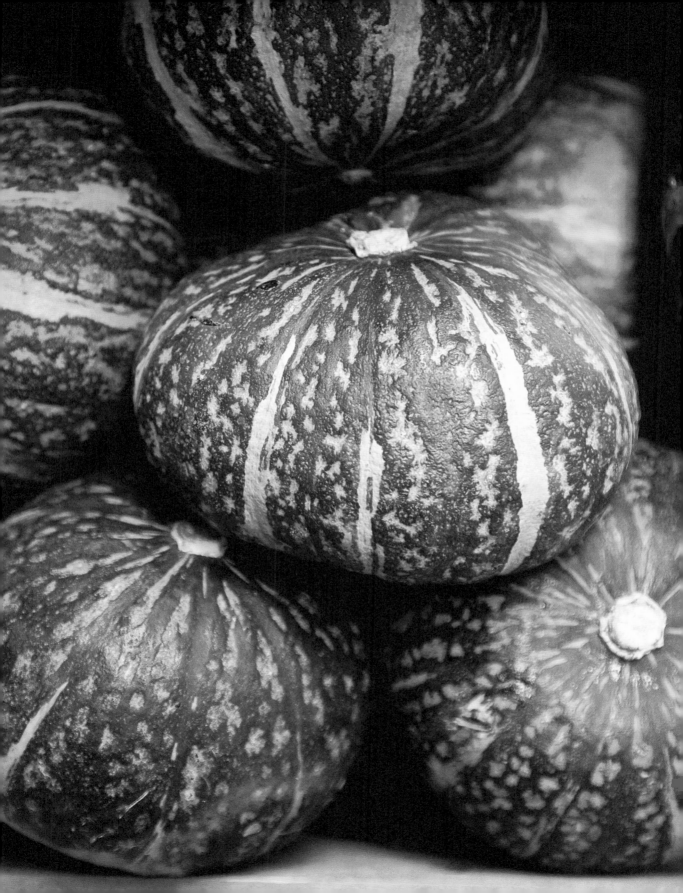

Essential fatty acids

It's not just antioxidants which help you to retain your youthful looks and organs. There are the essential fatty acids (EFAs): omega-6, and -3. These fats are converted in the body to anti-inflammatory prostaglandins. It is this effect which can help to prevent age-related disorders associated with inflammation, in particular arthritis and heart disease. Prostaglandins help to lower blood pressure and thin the blood, important for the prevention of blood clots. Omega-3 fats are known to be more deficient in the diet than omega-6 ones, and their protective effects are well documented. Numerous studies have found that the consumption of oily fish – the best source of omega-3 fats – protects against heart disease, and they are very good for the brain. It has also been found to be protective against other diseases associated with ageing, including rheumatoid arthritis and osteoporosis, cancer and diabetes.

Beauty comes from within, quite literally, and these fats keep the skin well oiled, helping to prevent dryness and wrinkling. As well as from oily fish, you can get your daily fats from seeds and their oils, including pumpkin, sunflower, sesame, raw shelled hemp and safflower.

Whole food

You need to consider whole foods as health-promoting and age-delaying. Beans, nuts and seeds are each a composite of nutrients, phytonutrients and fibre working synergistically to keep cells and organs functioning. Whole foods have been shown to have the potential to significantly reduce the risk of death from certain cancers and heart disease.

A review of studies on soya bean and heart disease found that this bean significantly lowers cholesterol and blood fats. You can even find frozen edamames (soya beans) in the freezer section of the supermarkets. Beans contain a wide range of potentially anti-carcinogenic compounds, namely fibre, vitamins and polyphenols. They release their sugars very slowly into the bloodstream. Regulating blood sugar has been shown in several studies to reduce the risk of stroke, heart disease, deterioration of eyesight, kidney infection and cognitive dysfunction.

Nuts are another longevity superfood. Associated with a reduced risk of heart disease, they have been found to almost halve the risk of heart attack in those who consume nuts more than four times a week, compared with those who rarely eat nuts. Walnuts, pistachios, macadamias, peanuts, almonds and pecans have all been found to reduce cholesterol and fats generally in the blood. I call almonds the Cholesterol Buster. Almonds are also high in the antioxidants, selenium and vitamin E. The antioxidants in almonds along with a substance called laetrile help to battle cell destruction in the body, which helps to protect the body from developing cancer. Finally, almonds have a cholesterol-lowering effect, since 70 per cent of the fat in almonds is the artery-clearing mono-unsaturated variety. Need any more convincing? Nuts are a good source of essential fatty acids, vitamin E, magnesium and folic acid – a B vitamin which helps to lower homocysteine, a risk factor in heart disease (see page 283).

The Fountain of Youth

One of the most important yet overlooked nutrients is water. The thirst mechanism diminishes as we get older, and the elderly are more prone to dehydration. Dehydration can lead to mental confusion as well as dry skin and fatigue, so it is vital to drink plenty of water throughout the day.

BRAIN FOOD

If you're forever losing your keys, your mobile, your handbag, forgetting people's names or losing the plot halfway through a simple episode of a soap opera, you need brain food (and, probably, a holiday!).

Foods that feed your brain

Your brain thrives on plenty of essential fatty acids, antioxidants, zinc, B vitamins and good protein. You also need the steady brain fuel provided by complex carbohydrates and the best nutrient of all, water.

- Salmon
- Tuna
- Sardines
- Chicken
- Lean white meats
- Tempeh
- Tofu
- Eggs
- Avocados
- Spinach
- Peas
- Pulses
- Beans
- Kelp
- Berries
- Brown rice
- Wheatgerm
- Whole-grains
- Quinoa
- Amaranth
- Millet
- Buckwheat
- Oats
- Rye
- Barley
- Nuts and seeds
- Turmeric

You could also take the following herbs and supplements:

▸ **Ginkgo Biloba** – This herbal supplement can help increase circulation to the brain and is known as the memory herb.

▸ **Liquid algae** – This is available from health-food stores as a nutritional supplement and is rich in protein and amino acids that may help to improve memory, mental clarity and concentration. The protein in algae nourishes the brain and nervous system because of its high level of amino acids and peptides (brain transmitters).

▸ **Choline** – Known as the 'memory vitamin', choline enhances brain function, mental acuity and neurological systems. Food sources of choline include soya beans, nuts, fish, especially sardines, and free-range organic eggs.

▸ **Lecithin** – 2 tablespoons of Lecithin granules sprinkled in your cereal or salad is the easiest way to restore creativity to your thoughts. Foods rich in lecithin (your brain is 20 per cent made up of lecithin) include eggs, plant foods, seeds, grains, legumes, soya beans and nuts.

Foods that are destructive to your brain

▸ Caffeine

▸ Sugar

▸ Chocolate

▸ Trans-fats – vegetable fats that have been hardened by hydrogenation; avoid all foods that list hydrogenated or partially hydrogenated fats or shortenings on their labels. They are often found in margarines, vegetable shortenings, low fat spreads and baked goods.

▸ Alcohol

Nutrition for older people

Foods to include

Vegetables of all types (except potatoes) can be eaten freely. Aim for a range of colours over the week and have something green every day.

Many older people cannot digest raw vegetables well. Raw foods can be hard to chew and may lead to gas and bloating if digestive function is not optimal. Steaming, baking and roasting are all good ways of preparing vegetables that make them easier to digest without the loss of too many nutrients. Soups are also a great way of getting lots of nutritious vegetables into one easily digested meal.

Steaming

To steam vegetables it's best to get a steamer; you can buy tiered saucepans or you can buy a steamer that will sit inside any pan. Otherwise, just putting a small amount of water in a pan and cooking the vegetables with the lid on is a simple way of largely steaming them. Most vegetables take only a few minutes to steam if chopped up into chunks beforehand. Try steaming carrots, broccoli, cauliflower, Brussels sprouts, swede, spinach, broad beans, peas or anything that you would normally boil. Do not oversteam or boil veggies to death.

Baking

There's more to life than just the plain old white potato. And potatoes are not the only vegetable that can be baked. Sweet potatoes and whole squash (such as butternut or red kuri) can be baked just as you would bake normal white potatoes. Other vegetables can be wrapped in tin foil and baked in the oven; beetroots and carrots work well cooked like this.

Roasting

Vegetables are delicious when roasted; the heat breaks down the carbohydrates in the vegetables into natural occurring sugars, meaning they taste sweeter and are easier to digest. Putting a small amount of olive oil on the vegetables actually helps to seal in the nutrients and enhances their flavour. Most vegetables can be roasted. The only preparation needed is washing, peeling (if necessary) and chopping into large chunks. Try parsnips, carrots, swede, celeriac, beetroots, squash, pumpkin, courgettes, marrows and mushrooms.

Fruit

Fruit is packed full of antioxidants that protect the body's cells from damage and disease. Soft fruits such as berries, apricots, nectarines and bananas may be easy enough to eat as they are. Others, such as apples or pears, may be better tolerated if cooked gently in a small amount of water with some cinnamon. Smoothies are easy to make if you have a blender; just put in any fruit (remove peel, stones and core where necessary) and blend. If you popped into my kitchen on any morning, you would find my blenders (yes. I have more than one) on overtime as I whip up smoothies for the whole family. In the McKeith household I'm the Smoothie Queen.

Juices

I recommend juicing vegetables. Veggie juices are nutrient power-houses, cleansing and easy to digest and absorb.

Whole grains

Fibre is vital for good digestion and elimination. Some of the best sources are whole grains. These include brown rice, millet, buckwheat, oats, quinoa, barley and rye. If you find grains difficult to eat, another easy way to benefit from the goodness of whole grains is by using the flakes. These can be soaked overnight with nuts, seeds and dried fruits to make a soft muesli or they can be made into a porridge. Buckwheat, millet and quinoa flakes are especially easy as they can be prepared without cooking.

Nut and seed butters

You will easily find them in most supermarkets and health-food shops. They are literally made from whole nuts and seeds puréed up. They provide a good way of getting the benefits of nuts and seeds if chewing the whole seeds is a problem. Rotate hazelnut, almond, pumpkin seed, sunflower seed and cashew nut butters. They can be stirred into porridge or whole grains after cooking to add flavour and essential fats. Use them as spreads on toast or sandwiches.

Beans and lentils

Tins of pulses can be added to soups as mentioned above and also to whole grains. Add them to grains towards the end of cooking and serve with salad or vegetables to make a nutritious meal. Sprouting pulses is a great way of rendering them more digestible. Sprouts can be added to soups at the end of cooking or stirred into cooked grains for easily digestible protein packed full of nutrients.

Eggs (if tolerated)

Eggs can be soft boiled, poached, scrambled or made into omelettes. They provide useful protein, B vitamins, essential fats (look for those high in omega-3 fats), zinc and lecithin (which aids fat digestion). They do not raise cholesterol but may be hard to digest for some people, so eat them in moderation.

Fish

Putting a piece of fish under the grill is so easy and can be the basis of a good meal. Serve with salad or vegetables for an easy lunch or dinner. Fish can also be steamed, poached or baked, so try these methods as well. The addition of herbs can help digestion and improve flavour. Fennel, dill and parsley all work well with fish. While fresh fish is ideal, canned fish such as mackerel, salmon, tuna, sardines and pilchards is a great, inexpensive and easy-to-use alternative.

Grilled chicken
All you need to do is pop a chicken breast under the grill to make a nutritious lunch or dinner. Serve it with lots of vegetables. Use miso broth as an easy delicious gravy to cook with the chicken.

Water and herbal teas
Hydration is vital for proper digestion, mental function and energy. Sip water and herbal teas throughout the day. Avoid drinking too much with meals as this can interfere with proper digestion. You could end up burping or bloated. Little sips are OK but best to do most of your liquid intake half an hour before you eat.

Foods to avoid
► Sugar, refined carbohydrates (white bread, white rice, white pasta, pastry, etc.) and processed foods can all upset blood-sugar balance leading to swings of mood and energy and cravings for more. They also contribute to tooth decay and are low in nutrients and fibre and they are usually high in calories.

► Caffeine and alcohol both affect blood-sugar levels, interfere with sleep and can be dehydrating due to their diuretic effect. Try herbal teas such as rooibosch, fennel, peppermint, nettle and camomile instead as these are good for the digestive and nervous systems.

► Added table salt. As you age, your sense of taste may decline. Taste loss can lead to the temptation to add salt to food to increase the flavour. Salt can lead to increased blood pressure and water retention. Use herbs to flavour foods instead. And if you really want a little salt, always use sea salt instead of table salt.

▶ Nightshade family: foods in this family include white potatoes, tomatoes, peppers, aubergines, chillies, paprika and tobacco. Those with arthritic or inflammatory disorders may do better without these in their diets as they can have an inflammatory effect. Try avoiding them for a few weeks and see how you feel.

▶ Citrus fruits can be irritating to the gut for some people, so if you suffer from digestive problems try replacing these with berries, cherries, apples, pears and apricots instead.

▶ Purines are found in shellfish, red meats and organ meats. If you suffer from gout you may be better off avoiding these foods as they can exacerbate the problem. Eat lentils and beans in moderation as these also contain small amounts of purines.

Reducing symptoms

Constipation

INCLUDE:
Soaked and ground flax seeds (linseeds), short-grain brown rice, oats, millet, quinoa, fruit (fresh and dried), vegetables, warm water with lemon, pure water, prunes, nettle tea.

AVOID:
Sugar, white flour, white pasta, white bread, white rice, processed foods.

High blood pressure (see page 291), high cholesterol (see page 294) and heart disease (see page 283)

INCLUDE:
Vegetables (especially green), fruit, beans and lentils, olive oil, garlic, onions, walnuts, almonds, flax seeds, fish, nettle tea, dandelion tea, water.

::: **AVOID**:

Salt, processed foods, tea, coffee, chocolate, alcohol.

Insomnia

::: **INCLUDE**:

Green vegetables, fish, chicken, brown rice, bananas, lettuce, celery, nuts, seeds.

::: **AVOID**:

Tea, coffee, alcohol, sugar, salt.

Osteoporosis

::: **INCLUDE**:

Green vegetables, tinned fish with bones, quinoa, chickpeas, haricot beans, almonds, figs, tahini, fruit and vegetables generally. Get regular weight-bearing exercise and get outside for at least 20 minutes a day with some skin exposed. Take care not to burn.

::: **AVOID**:

Excess animal protein, soft drinks, sugar, salt, tobacco.

Prostate problems

::: **INCLUDE**:

Tomatoes, watermelon, pink grapefruits, oily fish, pumpkin seeds, flax seeds, saw palmetto.

::: **AVOID**:

Sugar, refined carbohydrates, alcohol,

Arthritis

::: **INCLUDE**:

Oily fish, avocados, nuts, seeds and their butters and cold-pressed oils.

::: **AVOID**:

Potatoes (white), tomatoes, chillies, peppers, aubergines, tobacco, citrus fruits, rhubarb, dairy products, fatty meats.

Memory problems

⫶ INCLUDE:
Oily fish, pumpkin seeds, sunflower seeds, flax seeds, hemp seeds, fruit, vegetables, sage tea, ginkgo tea, algae.

⫶ AVOID:
Sugar, refined foods, burnt or fried foods, cigarettes, alcohol.

Poor circulation

⫶ INCLUDE:
Oily fish, flax seeds, pumpkin seeds, hemp seeds, berries, cherries, ginkgo biloba, horsetail tea.

⫶ AVOID:
Salt, sugar, caffeine and alcohol.

Eye Problems

⫶ INCLUDE:
Berries, cherries, carrots, apricots, nectarines, spinach, eggs.

⫶ AVOID:
Sugar, refined foods, alcohol, burnt or fried foods, heated fats.

Lifestyle tips

► Avoid over eating – this is a major cause of ageing.

► Do not eat late at night – have an early supper and if necessary a small snack such as a few soaked almonds or a natural soya yoghurt before bed to keep blood sugar stable and aid a full night's sleep.

► Make dietary changes gradually to give the body time to adjust.

► Get outside daily for 20 minutes in the sunlight. Vitamin D is vital for bone health and aids blood-sugar control.

► Get some exercise daily. If possible go for a walk or swim or do some gardening. Stretching increases blood circulation and oxygenation so have a good stretch twice a day.

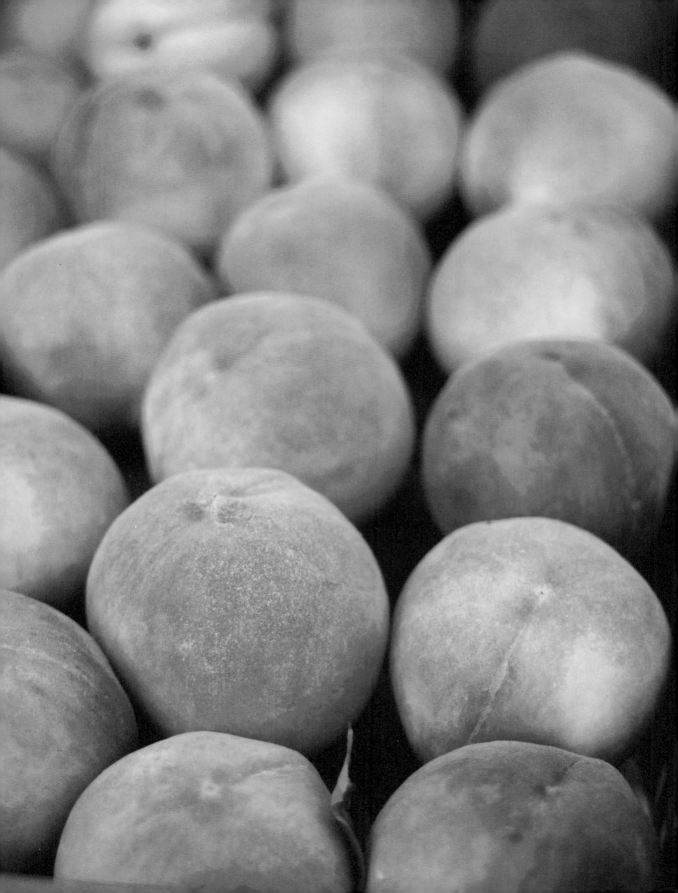

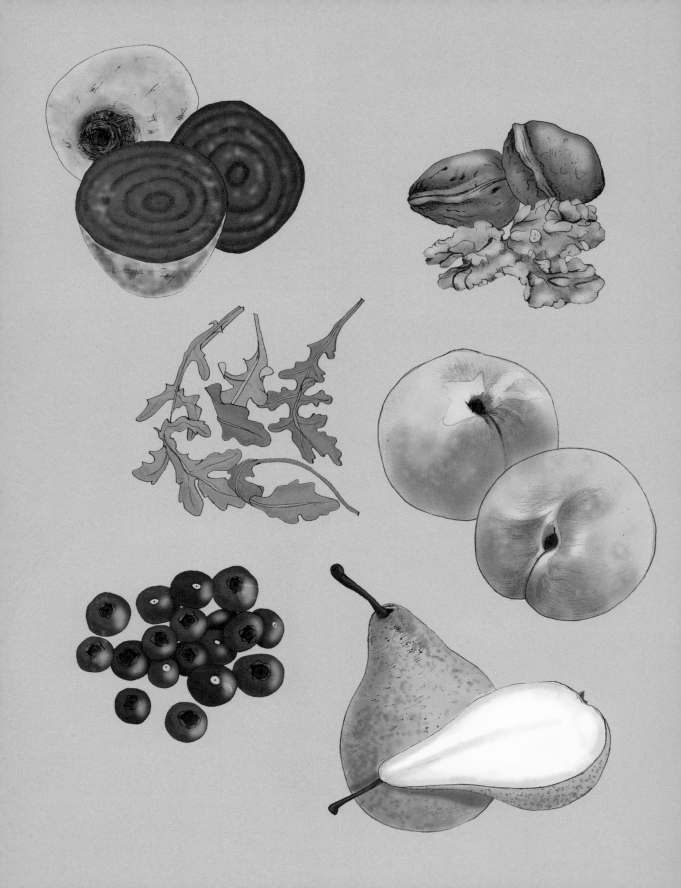

A–Z of conditions

ABSCESSES

Abscesses are usually an accumulation of pus caused by an infection consisting of dead white blood cells and micro-organisms. Abscesses can appear anywhere on the body, internally or externally, including ears, nose, throat, gums, abdominal wall, rectum or skin. If an abscess appears around a hair follicle, it is usually referred to as a boil. Boils notoriously appear on your bottom or in your armpit. It's another way for waste to make its way out.

Abscesses may appear in the form of red spots, raised red bumps, inflamed lesions, or yellow-white pustules. Fever, malaise and swollen glands may be experienced. The infected area around an abscess usually becomes swollen and tender. If you are diabetic, you need to keep your weight in check so that you are less at risk of leg abscesses.

It takes about two weeks for an abscess to open up and rid itself of its pus. When this happens, all pain and inflammation goes away.

Mouth abscesses can be particularly nasty and may require antibiotics (see page 188), so make sure you get to a dentist if you suspect you have one. You will also need to see a GP if you have a skin abscess that is streaked red, pus-filled or on the face.

Do not squeeze a boil or abscess. You will make it worse, may cause scarring, and the bacteria may spread through the bloodstream.

CAUSES MAY INCLUDE
► Depleted immune system.
► Injury to an area.
► Nutrient deficiencies, possibly zinc.
► Toxic overload and blood impurities due to unhealthy diet and lifestyle.
► Inefficient detoxification and elimination of toxins from the body.
► High-sugar diet and blood-sugar imbalances. Diabetics are at extra risk as are people who are overweight. It is not uncommon for diabetics to get leg abscesses.
► Viral infection.

Action plan
Abscesses require immediate attention. You may even need antibiotics so please see your GP. Your goal should be to strengthen immunity through your diet.

❖ EAT/DRINK
► Fresh, raw fruit and vegetables. These will help to build up the immune system and aid cleansing. Make sure that you eat some raw food with every cooked meal.
► Warm water – at least 8 glasses daily. The body cannot heal if it is dehydrated.
► Pressed, organic vegetable juice daily. Carrot, celery, cabbage, beetroot, radish and parsley all contain beneficial nutrients.
► Garlic (preferably raw) daily for its antibiotic, antibacterial properties. You can toss garlic into soups, dips, salads and stews.
► Soaked and ground flax seeds in water daily and dandelion-root tea or dandelion coffee three times a day to get your bowels moving regularly as good elimination is vital. The less your bowels move, the more compromised your immune system will be.

⠿ AVOID

▶ Sugar, refined carbohydrates, alcohol, caffeine, salt and processed foods. These all put a strain on the body and increase the toxic load.

▶ Pork products which are high in salt and fat that clog up the body. Abscesses indicate that the body's organs of detoxification and the immune system are struggling.

HERBS AND SUPPLEMENTS

▶ Liquid milk thistle, the liver-cleansing herb. Take daily to support detoxification and cleansing.

▶ Take echinacea tincture to support the immune system.

▶ Other useful herbs include burdock root, cayenne, dandelion root, red clover and yellow dock root.

▶ Take liquid chlorophyll drops as an internal cleanser.

▶ Astragalus – go on a six-month course.

▶ Take lactobacillus/probiotic in powder form.

▶ Supplements include zinc, vitamin C with bioflavanoids powder or capsules, vitamin A and vitamin E. You can also apply vitamin E directly to the abscess.

▶ Fish oil capsules.

⠿ EXTRA TIPS

▶ Apply manuka honey to external abscesses because it destroys viruses and bacteria and aids healing.

▶ For internal mouth/gum abscesses, swirl some aloe vera juice around in your mouth and then spit it out.

▶ Tea tree oil is a natural antibacterial that can be applied topically to external abscesses. Mix with water (1 part tea tree oil to 4 parts water) and dab onto external abscesses every few hours.

▶ Once the abscess has drained, apply calendula cream to help it to heal.

▶ Take showers instead of baths until the abscess has completely gone. This prevents the infection from spreading. Hygiene is critical. Wash your hands meticulously, too.

▶ Tissue cell salts of silica can help the healing process once the abscess has opened and the pus has gone. You can also get silica in gel form.

▶ Dry skin brushing daily followed by a hot and cold shower will help to get the lymph moving and will aid elimination through the skin. Lymph is the fluid that moves toxins out of the body. Avoid the actual area of the abscess.

ACID/ALKALINE BALANCE

To appreciate the importance of acid/alkaline balance (also known as pH, or potential hydrogen balance), understand that all of our billions of cells need to be alkaline in order to carry out nearly every bodily function.

As each cell performs its work, it secretes acid wastes that need to be neutralized for health to be maintained. In other words, we need to be alkaline to be healthy but are constantly creating acids in the body. The problem nowadays is that due to poor diet, a lot of people are more acidic than they should be. This is mainly caused by diet. As maintaining alkalinity is paramount for survival, the body will take minerals from other body parts if the diet does not supply adequate amounts; for example, magnesium and potassium may be taken from the heart causing cramping or strokes, and calcium may be taken from the heart causing cramping or strokes, and calcium may be taken from the bones leading to osteoporosis.

A body that has been overly acidic for a long time will be more susceptible to chronic or acute disease. For example, if excess acid is eventually dumped in the tissues and joints, arthritic symptoms could result.

CAUSES

All of the following tend to create an acidic state in the body:

► High-protein diet.
► Exercise/physical activity (this creates lactic acid).
► Sweating (this can lead to a loss of alkaline minerals).
► Stress.
► Drugs, both medical and recreational, tend to be acid-forming.

SYMPTOMS OF OVER-ACIDITY

An over-acidic person may present as grouchy, sensitive, exhausted and inclined to suffer aches, pains and headaches. Insomnia, skin problems, a sour stomach and acid sweat (which can discolour jewellery) are also indications of acidity. An acid environment in the tissues leads to an environment in which bugs can thrive, so an acidic person may be prone to cold sores and infections. Tell-tale acidic digestive signs are:

► burping after a meal
► indigestion (see page 308)
► heartburn
► flatulence

Action plan

Our body's first lines of defence against excess acidity are the minerals found in food. The aim is to eat a diet containing 80 per cent alkalizing foods and 20 per cent acid-forming foods. Most diets are the reverse of this.

EAT/DRINK

► Vegetables, especially asparagus, sea vegetables, endives, parsley, watercress, carrots, celery.
► Amaranth, millet, buckwheat and quinoa – other grains are acid-forming.
► Almonds, Brazil nuts, fresh coconut and chestnuts.
► Sprouted beans and seeds, fresh peas and green beans.
► Garlic.
► Freshly squeezed vegetable juices.

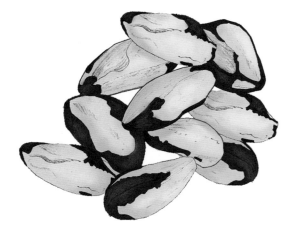

::: AVOID

▶ Red meat and processed meats, dairy products and eggs.

▶ Unsprouted beans and pulses.

▶ Refined sugars.

▶ Refined grains.

▶ Spirits, wine, beer, coffee, black tea, fizzy drinks, soft drinks and sweetened fruit juices.

▶ All drugs and tobacco.

HERBS AND SUPPLEMENTS

▶ Green superfoods such as wheat grass and herbal teas.

▶ Seaweed agar-agar (used to make desserts like jelly).

▶ Cayenne pepper.

::: **EXTRA TIPS**

▶ Deep breathing, meditation and relaxation techniques that reduce stress are helpful.

▶ Taking 2–3 teaspoons of apple cider vinegar before a meal can help people with overly acidic tummies.

▶ Bathing in Epsom salts (magnesium sulphate) can help to alkalize the skin and tissues.

▶ Chewing food thoroughly increases alkalinity as saliva is alkaline.

ACNE

Acne is the most common skin complaint. It can range from blackheads and red pimples to wide, reddened pores and noticeable, scarred tissue. If you scratch or squeeze pimples, you risk infection and spreading the acne.

Although acne most frequently occurs in the teenage years, many adults go through life with pimply faces as well as pimpled backs, chests and necks. New mums are susceptible, too, because of wildly fluctuating hormones and a tendency not to eat properly while taking care of the new baby. Acne is often due to a hormone imbalance which stimulates the sebaceous glands to increase oil output. Teens are supposedly victims of glands in overdrive. If traces of sebum become trapped inside skin pores, tissues can attract bacteria, resulting in inflammation and blemishes. But have you ever really looked at a spotty teenager's diet?

CAUSES MAY INCLUDE

▶ Zinc or vitamin A deficiency.

▶ Essential fatty acid deficiency.

▶ Congested colon and constipation.

▶ Yeast overgrowth and fungal infections.

▶ Overly stimulated sebaceous glands.

▶ Food allergies and food sensitivities, especially to milk.

▶ A high-fat diet and/or refined-food diet with too much white sugar.

▶ Hormonal imbalances, often caused by diet or hormonal changes such as puberty (see page 89), pregnancy (see page 104) or menopause (see page 138).

▶ Too much meat, hot spices, eggs, bread.

► Glucose intolerance.

► PMT (pre-menstrual tension, see page 347).

► Medications that contain bromides, iodides or steroids.

► The contraceptive pill can improve acne for some, but worsen for others, depending on the balance of oestrogen and progesterone in the brand of pill.

► Sluggish liver.

► Alcohol.

► Smoking.

Action plan

I want you to increase your fruit and vegetable intake to at least eight portions a day, and cut out any junk. I promise you'll notice the difference.

EAT/DRINK

► Fresh vegetable juices throughout the day – in particular carrot, lettuce, nettle, watercress, celery and dandelion.

► Vegetables, especially green leafy vegetables, carrots, onions and garlic.

► Seaweeds, liquid blue-green algae.

► Brown rice, mung beans, millet and wheat germ.

► Live sprouts.

► Herring.

► Sunflower seeds, raw shelled hemp seeds, sesame seeds.

AVOID

► Fatty or processed meats.

► Refined carbohydrates such as white rice, white bread and white pasta.

► Processed foods such as cakes, biscuits, processed ready meals and soft drinks.

► Dairy products.

HERBS

► Echinacea, dandelion, yellow dock, burdock root and red clover are all powerful internal cleansers.

► Kelp powder has a purifying effect on the blood and can be used in cooking.

SUPPLEMENTS

The nutrients I have used most successfully in helping to eradicate acne are outlined below. Do not feel compelled to take them all at once. You would be overwhelmed. You can rotate them and see what works for you.

► Zinc.

► Betacarotene.

► Vitamin A (do not take if pregnant). Try vitamin A drops, too. They won't solve the root cause but may improve appearance slightly.

► Vitamin B complex.

► Vitamin C which helps to counteract inflammation.

► Vitamin B6.

► Pantothenic acid.

► Propolis.

► Borage oil capsules.

► Acidophilus with bifidus, 'friendly' bacteria, which promotes colon health and elimination of toxins.

EXTRA TIPS

► Bathe the skin with a combination of tea tree and camomile (2 drops of each in a bowl of water) for a soothing, antibacterial wash.

► Try rubbing your face gently with pineapple chunks, or a natural face mask of rice milk, oats and a squeeze of lemon juice.

► Identify food sensitivities, if any.

One way to do this is to take your radial pulse (see page 180). Another way is to be tested for food sensitivities through an at-home blood test. Go to www.gillianmckeith.info for more details on food sensitivities and a home-test.

PIMPLE ANALYSIS

If you don't have full-blown acne, you may have a pimple problem. Here are some clues to help you get to the bottom of your little bumps.

► Pimples on the forehead relate to the intestines. They need a clean out. Take 1 tablespoon psyllium seed husks daily. I thoroughly recommend you go for a colonic – be brave!

► Pimples on the cheeks relate to lungs and breast. Drink mullein tea. Take the supplement co-enzyme Q10. Sprinkle lecithin granules on salads and cereals. Take astragalus twice daily. Eat brown rice. Take evening primrose oil. Take echinacea liquid twice daily. Avoid cow's milk, saturated fat and red meat.

► Pimples on the nose relate to the heart. Take hawthorn supplements or drink hawthorn tea, two cups daily. Eat barley grass (1 teaspoon daily).

► Pimples on the jaw relate to the kidneys. Eat quinoa. Drink dandelion tea. Take a magnesium supplement and B complex vitamin.

► Pimples on the shoulder relate to the digestion. Take digestive enzyme supplements. Drink 1 tablespoon of aloe vera juice daily. Eat avocados, fish and seeds.

► Pimples on the upper back relate to the lungs. Take astragalus twice daily.

Take germanium supplements. Eat basil, cayenne, fennel, fenugreek, garlic, ginger. Drink celery juice and mullein, nettle and peppermint teas. Eat simple, small meals avoiding dairy products and sugars. Cut out peanuts for a while.

► Pimples around the mouth relate to the reproductive organs. The herb agnus castus can help to correct hormonal imbalances that manifest as pimples around the mouth. Cut out full-fat dairy products for a while. Natural yoghurt is fine.

AIDS

AIDS stands for Acquired Immune Deficiency Syndrome. It can be caused when the Human Immune Deficiency virus (HIV) enters the immune cells and multiplies.

Generally there is a breakdown in the body's usual defences meaning infections are easily picked up and are hard to shake off. Sufferers of AIDS often die from infections and cancers that their immune systems can no longer deal with rather than from AIDS itself.

CAUSES

HIV is thought to be spread mainly through sexual contact or blood-on-blood contact such as from needles shared by intravenous drug users. Babies of mothers with HIV are also susceptible from contact in the womb and if breastfed.

It is important to get tested if you feel you are at risk. STD clinics offer free testing and counselling. It is also important to use protection in the form of condoms and spermicides.

SYMPTOMS

It is possible to be infected with HIV but not to develop any symptoms for several years. Symptoms are variable and may include digestive problems, diarrhoea, weight loss, skin lesions and swollen lymph nodes. Infections such as candidiasis, thrush, yeast problems, TB and various viruses are often part of the picture.

For full-blown AIDS to be diagnosed, the presence of specific infections or cancers associated with HIV need to be detected. It is thought that 50–60 per cent of people with HIV go on to develop AIDS. Individuals with compromised immune systems are far more likely to be the ones affected.

Action plan

There is a lot you can do to help, although your GP must always be your first port of call when making changes to your diet or lifestyle. The main aim is to support and nourish the immune system and to remove the challenges that compromise it. Changes to diet and lifestyle practices can make a huge difference to immune function. Make healthy living and what you put in your body your number-one priority.

⠿ EAT/DRINK

► Whole natural foods – fruit, vegetables, pulses, nuts, seeds, whole grains, sprouted seeds (especially sprouted broccoli seeds), broad beans and plenty of pure water.

These all help the immune system to prevent and fight off infections.

► Organic foods – conventional foods are higher in pesticides that challenge the immune system and are lower in nutrients that the body needs for health and healing.

► Freshly pressed vegetable juices which are a great way of getting vitamins, minerals and antioxidants into the body in a highly absorbable form.

► Colourful foods – the natural colour of food often indicates the presence of specific immune-building nutrients. Make sure you include plenty of greens every day.

► Unripe papaya and fresh pineapple which contain enzymes that aid proper digestion of proteins. Eat these between or before meals.

► Cabbage, kale and Brussels sprouts which contain the powerful antioxidant sulphoraphane that can really benefit the liver, which is important for the immune system. Instead of steaming the cabbage and sprouts, simmer them in water. When they are ready, strain the water off and drink it.

► Shitake and maitake mushrooms which have been found to contain substances that keep HIV from destroying the immune-strengthening cells.

⠿ AVOID

► Sugar, processed foods, refined foods, cigarettes, caffeine, alcohol, salt, additives and saturated fats – these all challenge the body and suppress the immune system.

► Anything to which you may be

intolerant – common culprits include wheat and other gluten grains (rye, oats, barley, kamut and spelt), dairy products, eggs, soya, chocolate and peanuts. It is probably worthwhile getting tested for food intolerances if you are not sure which foods affect you. See www. gillianmckeith.info for a home food-intolerance testing kit.

HERBS AND SUPPLEMENTS

► Cat's claw has been shown to be helpful.

► Pau d'arco, which can be drunk in tea form, has antibiotic and anti-fungal properties if infections are present.

► Astragalus helps to fight infections and enhance immunity. You can take it in either capsule or tincture form. I recommend 30 drops of the tincture four times daily.

► Use turmeric in your cooking for its immune properties.

► Drink aloe vera juice before each meal – this may inhibit the growth of HIV.

► To support the liver and cleanse the blood stream, useful herbs include dandelion root, milk thistle, black radish and burdock root.

► Eat ground and soaked flax seeds daily – they contain a mucilage that helps with the removal of toxins via the bowel.

► Take a strong multiple/mineral complex to make sure you are getting the basic foundational nutrients.

► Take vitamin C daily – it has been shown to inactivate the virus.

EXTRA TIPS

► Avoid stress, pollution and chemicals – these can all suppress the immune system.

► Engage in some form of relaxation such as meditation or breathing exercises to reduce the impact of stress on the body. Use only natural cleaning products in the home and on the body.

► Read the section on Candida (see page 219) as excess levels of intestinal yeast are common.

► Each morning, gently tap with your fist the thymus area above your chest, just under your neck. The stronger the thymus function, the better your immunity.

► For further information go to www.gillianmckeith.info/AIDS

ALCOHOLISM

Alcoholics are usually either physiologically or psychologically dependent on alcohol – often there is a combination of the two. Genetics and environmental factors can both play a part.

SYMPTOMS MAY INCLUDE

► Drinking early in the day.

► Binge drinking.

► Drinking to avoid withdrawal symptoms.

► You are way above the recommended weekly unit intake for your gender: males: 21; females: 14.

► You cannot get through the day without a drink, each and every day.

EFFECTS OF ALCOHOL ON THE BODY

Long-term heavy alcohol use can cause damage to the liver, kidneys, pancreas, brain and central nervous system. Alcohol suppresses the immune system, depletes the body of nutrients and removes water from the body.

Over time, alcohol can affect the body's ability to break down fats properly. This can lead to a fatty liver, hepatitis and cirrhosis of the liver which can cause death.

Alcoholics are at increased risk of high blood pressure, cardio-vascular disease, diabetes, osteoporosis, digestive problems, malnutrition and some cancers. The behaviour of alcoholics often has a negative effect on their relationships and on society generally.

Withdrawal from alcohol can cause symptoms such as hallucinations, convulsions, anxiety, perspiration, insomnia and more. Emotional and psychological support is needed during this time. Remember the symptoms will pass in a few weeks and you will feel better than you have in a long while. But you cannot ever go back to drinking alcohol. It is too great a risk.

Action plan

The first step is to choose not to drink and then to stop drinking alcohol completely. The following nutritional measures can help you through the process of recovery:

⁝ EAT/DRINK

► Fruits, vegetables, beans, grains, legumes, seeds, nuts, seaweeds.
► Alfalfa sprouts – these are high in many vitamins and minerals; alcoholics tend to have wide-ranging deficiencies, so high-nutrient foods are important.

► Oily fish three times a week and raw, unsalted seeds daily – alcoholics tend to be deficient in the essential fats needed for brain and central nervous system function.
► Water – 8 glasses a day. Alcoholics tend to be chronically dehydrated. Water and herbal teas can start to rehydrate your body and help to flush out toxins. So every time you feel like a drink of alcohol, go for herbal teas or water instead.
► Vegetable juices – they contain vitamins and minerals that are easily absorbed by the body and can help reduce withdrawal symptoms.

⁝ AVOID

► You absolutely must avoid sugar and refined carbohydrates at all costs if you are to beat the alcohol addiction. These will upset your blood-sugar control and create cravings, sometimes ravenous cravings. And of course, the alcohol you take in creates more swings of blood sugar. It's a vicious circle.
► Saturated, processed and fried fats – these all put a strain on the liver that your body may struggle to deal with.
► Coffee which causes blood-sugar swings that lead to cravings. Your cravings may then lead to alcohol.
► Cigarettes, which can upset blood-sugar levels.

HERBS AND SUPPLEMENTS

► Kudzu is a white root from the wild kudzu plant. Very few people have ever heard of it but it is invaluable because it can slow down the liver enzymes responsible for breaking down alcohol.

You may feel quite uncomfortable and experience nausea, swelling and redness if you attempt to drink any alcohol after eating kudzu. You can buy it in health-food stores.

► Green superfoods – spirulina, algae, wheat grass – mix them into smoothies for easier nutrient assimilation.

► Dandelion-root coffee – this can wean you from regular coffee and aid liver function.

► Camomile tea – camomile has a calming effect and can reduce feelings of anxiety that often arise during withdrawal.

► Fish oil and evening primrose oil supplements may be useful.

► Milk thistle extract which has been shown to aid the repair and regeneration of damaged livers. But make sure that it is an alcohol-free tincture otherwise you would be better off with capsules.

► Take an amino acid complex – amino acids have been shown to reduce withdrawal symptoms and to aid recovery from alcohol abuse.

► Take a good multivitamin with all the Bs and minerals – alcoholics are generally deficient in many nutrients. It has been found that the B vitamin niacin can help immensely in the early days.

► I also urge you to add extra zinc and magnesium.

⠿ EXTRA TIPS

► Find a support group near you – there are various organizations offering support such as Alcoholics Anonymous and Al-anon. Look in your local telephone directory or ask your GP about this. If you are drinking to bury emotional pain, you will need counselling and help.

► Avoid circumstances that trigger drinking – this may include people, places and activities. So, if you go to a bar to hang out with friends, it will be like self torture and you will probably end up drinking. Find other things to do with your time that you enjoy. Try sports, hobbies or learning new skills.

► Take time out to recover – the stresses of everyday life can make abstinence difficult, especially where alcohol has been used as a way of switching off from it all. Make giving up alcohol your main priority for as long as it takes.

► Hypnosis can help you to switch off the little voice in your head telling you that you need a drink.

► For further information go to www.gillianmckeith.info/alcohol.

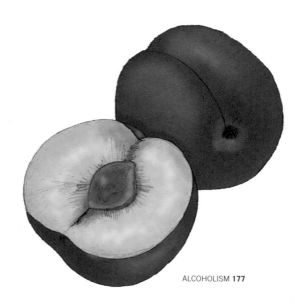

ALLERGIES

An allergic reaction is an abnormal reaction of the immune system to substances such as food, chemicals, dust, pollen or animal dander. The chemical at the heart of most allergic reactions is histamine. Excess histamine causes itching and inflammatory reactions. Histamine released in the nose will cause it to run; histamine released in the skin will cause itching and a rash; histamine released in the lungs will cause spasms and wheezing.

It is estimated that 60 per cent of the UK population suffer from unsuspected food reactions that can cause complicated health problems. A food allergy is when the immune system reacts immediately after ingestion or exposure to an allergen. Symptoms will occur very soon after exposure and include swellings, rashes and shortness of breath. Treatment with epinephrine (adrenalin) is needed as soon as possible to prevent anaphylactic shock and even death. If someone has an allergy they are unlikely to overcome it so will always need to avoid the food in any quantity. Even being near the food can provoke reactions in some people.
There are two types of reactions:
Type A – this is a classic allergy and reactions occur immediately after contact with an allergen.
Type B – this is a delayed allergy or intolerance and reactions can occur from 1 to 72 hours later.

Unlike food allergies, food intolerances generally produce very slow responses to foods. Food intolerances do not always involve the immune system in the first instance, though it may be implicated. Symptoms include tiredness, flatulence, bloating, constipation, diarrhoea, brain fog, water retention, mucus production, aching joints and muscles and headaches. These symptoms may appear several hours or even up to 48 hours after consumption. Usually the food or foods that cause problems are eaten so frequently that there is no obvious link between them and the symptoms, which makes it difficult to pinpoint when the food intolerances started.

For example, some adults do not produce lactase, the enzyme needed to digest the milk sugar lactose. They will often get digestive symptoms caused by the inability to break lactose down sufficiently. This would be considered an intolerance rather than an allergy as it is not caused by an immune response but by a digestive insufficiency. Other problem foods such as wheat contain large protein molecules that may create too much of a challenge for some people's digestive juices and these can lead to symptoms of intolerance or sensitivity such as digestive disturbances and mucus production. And food such as citrus fruits and tomatoes may irritate the gut lining causing digestive disturbances.

Testing for immuno-globulins can identify foods to which you are intolerant as it is these that build up when problem foods are eaten over a period of time (see Resources for how to find a nutritionist). Levels will often drop once the food has been eliminated for a few months. The sufferer may then be able to reintroduce the previously offending food in small quantities without adverse effects. This needs to be done with care.

CAUSES MAY INCLUDE
- Stress.
- Antibiotics.
- Antibacterial soaps.
- Pollution.
- Low-nutrient, high-sugar diets.
- Poor immune response.
- Calcium deficiency.
- Eating too much of the common allergens corn, wheat, dairy products, citrus fruits, shellfish.
- Lactose intolerance.
- Candidiasis (see page 219)
- Chemicals added to processed foods.
- Lack of stomach acid.

SYMPTOMS
Symptoms of allergies include eczema, asthma, hayfever, runny nose, itching, skin rashes, bloating, tiredness, migraines and arthritic-like complaints to name a few. Food intolerances can be extremely difficult to detect as they usually result from reactions to commonly eaten foods, but classic symptoms include diarrhoea, constipation, bloating, nausea/vomiting. Other symptoms can be irritable bowel syndrome (see page 314), frequent infections, mood swings, fatigue, aches, skin complaints, rhinitis and palpitations.

Action plan
You need to reduce histamine production and support your immune system to curb allergies.

EAT/DRINK
- Water – 2 litres a day. The body produces more histamine when it is dehydrated.
- Nettle tea. This can normalize the body's own production of histamine. It is particularly good to drink it in the spring to minimize hayfever.
- Different-coloured foods which have different immune-supportive properties (although don't consume if you know you are allergic or intolerant to any of these):
  * Red – tomatoes, strawberries, pink grapefruit, raspberries, cherries, watermelon, red peppers, goji berries, cranberries, pomegranates.
  * Orange – carrots, apricots, papaya, mangoes, orange peppers, pumpkin, squash.
  * Yellow – melons, yellow peppers, bananas, sweetcorn, yellow tomatoes.
  * Green – salad leaves, lettuce, broccoli, kale, cabbage, celery, avocados, Brussels sprouts, spinach, chard.
  * Blue/purple – blueberries, blackberries, red cabbage, beetroot, red grapes, red kale, purple-sprouting broccoli.
- Vitamin C-rich foods. Vitamin C has an anti-histamine effect and there's lots of it in berries, cherries, kiwi fruit, peppers, broccoli and goji berries.
- Foods high in quercetin which has an anti-histamine effect such as apples, onions, parsley, kale and buckwheat.
- Hemp seeds. Raw shelled hemp seeds contain the omega-3 and -6 essential fats that have an anti-inflammatory effect. Many people with allergic reactions do not break down fats particularly well. Hemp seeds contain GLA, the broken-

down form of the omega-6 fats as found in evening primrose oil. You can also use hemp seed oil in salad dressings.

► Oily fish which contain the broken-down form of the omega-3 fats EPA and DHA. These are great for reducing symptoms of eczema and asthma.

▓ AVOID

► Mucus-forming or allergenic foods.

► Tea, coffee and alcohol which all dehydrate the body.

► Sugar, refined carbohydrates and processed foods. These foods are devoid of nutrients and suppress the immune system.

HERBS AND SUPPLEMENTS

► Get some horsetail tincture (do not worry, it is not actually horse's tail). It is a good source of calcium and calcium is often low in allergy-prone individuals.

► Green superfoods: blue-green algae, spirulina and sprouted barley grass all contain immune-strengthening nutrients.

► Take L-glutamine powder before meals which may help to lessen reactivity to foods.

► Supplement with probiotics. These are the beneficial bacteria that reside in your gut. Go for capsules or powders (often kept in the fridge section of a health food store) rather than the probiotic drinks, as the drinks may contain sugar which can worsen allergies.

▓ EXTRA TIPS

► Keep a food diary to see if you can track any reactivity to a particular food or beverage.

► Take the do-it-yourself pulse test to see where you may be food sensitive:

(a) First thing in the morning, when you wake up, take your radial pulse. Place your pointer finger on the radial pulse (on your wrist). Count the number of beats in a 60-second period. Your reading should be somewhere between 50 and 70 beats per 60 seconds.

(b) After eating a meal, take your radial pulse again. If the pulse reading score has increased by more than 10 beats, then you may have a sensitivity to a particular

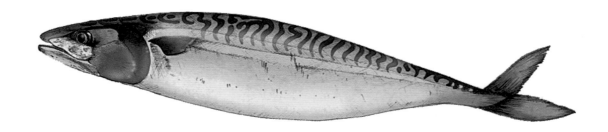

food you have just eaten. You will then need to separate out the foods to find the one to which you are reacting, using the same method.

► Chew food really well until it becomes liquid to aid digestion.

► If you eat a variety of foods you are less likely to develop food sensitivities.

► Learn to manage stress. Consider relaxation techniques such as meditation, tai chi, yoga or breathing exercises.

► Get to bed early. You will be more reactive when tired and you need proper sleep to allow the gallbladder and liver to detoxify properly.

► Get tested for parasites as that can often be a root cause of food allergy. Home-testing kits are available on www. gillianmckeith.info. It's worth going on a course of black walnut tincture to clear out parasites.

ALOPECIA

Alopecia basically means hair loss. There are different degrees of hair loss, including alopecia areata, which refers to patches of hair loss; alopecia totalis, which refers to the loss of all hair on the head (baldness); and alopecia universalis, which refers to the loss of all body hair.

Alopecia can often lead to bouts of depression and anxiety due to changed physical appearance. And that's why I applaud TV presenter Gail Porter, who has managed to take the stigma out of alopecia by appearing in public without a wig. This brave step has made it easier for sufferers everywhere to ask for help and to get to grips with dealing with the condition.

CAUSES

There are many possible underlying causes behind alopecia, with some sort of stress nearly always being implicated. Other contributory factors include:

► Female hormone deficiency.

► Androgens (male hormones).

► Low stomach acid or digestive enzyme insufficiency.

► Imbalance in gut bacteria.

► Rapid weight loss; yo-yo diets and years of constant dieting.

► Diabetes or high insulin levels.

► Nutrient deficiencies, particularly iron, protein, biotin and other B vitamins.

► Underactive thyroid.

► Emotional issues.

► The menopause, pregnancy or discontinuing the contraceptive pill.

► Skin diseases such as ring worm and eczema.

► Chemicals in cosmetics.

► Anti-cancer drugs.

► Poor circulation to the scalp.

► Ageing.

► Excess vitamin A intake.

► Genetic predisposition.

► Auto-immune reaction whereby immune system attacks hair follicles.

Action plan

It is important to find out the underlying causes behind the hair loss. Testing for thyroid function, iron and B vitamin status and hormone levels may be useful so that these can be addressed if necessary.

A

⠿ EAT/DRINK

► Brown rice, lentils, sunflower seeds, oats and quinoa. These all contain B vitamins and biotin needed for healthy hair growth.

► Seaweed hijiki. Its properties are helpful for maintaining healthy hair.

► Dark green leafy vegetables and green herby leaves.

► Oily fish, nuts and seeds. These contain essential fats needed for healthy hair and follicles. Aim to eat fish 2–3 times a week and eat 2–3 tbsp of seeds daily. Be sure to include some pumpkin and flax seeds as these contain zinc, also needed for hair growth.

► Sprinkle kelp flakes onto soups and salads. Kelp is rich in iodine needed for thyroid function. An underactive thyroid is sometimes implicated in cases of hair loss.

⠿ AVOID

► Sugar, refined carbohydrates and alcohol. These can all raise blood-sugar and insulin levels which can have a negative effect on the hair follicles.

► Wheat bran, tea and coffee. These can interfere with the absorption of minerals, such as iron, needed for hair growth.

HERBS AND SUPPLEMENTS

► Take warming herbs and spices to improve circulation, such as cayenne pepper (in small amounts), ginger, cinnamon and cumin. Add them to soups, stews and casseroles.

► Take the herb astragalus which is a very good source of Vitamin B.

► Add the contents of a multivitamin to a smoothie, daily.

► Take vitamin B complex daily. Make sure it contains biotin as this is particularly important for hair growth.

► Iron supplements should be taken only if you are diagnosed with iron deficiency.

► If digestive symptoms are present, take digestive enzymes with meals to aid absorption of nutrients. You may also benefit from taking probiotics as the beneficial bacteria in the gut produce some B vitamins that are needed for hair health.

► If there is a female hormone imbalance, supplementing with agnus castus can help. Magnesium is also needed for hormonal balance.

⠿ EXTRA TIPS

► Do everything possible to strengthen your immune system because a poor immune response may cause an auto-immune reaction resulting in widespread hair loss (see page 181).

► Lie on a slant board (head down) for 15 minutes each day, although check with your doctor before trying this. You can create a slant board by using any board that will take your body size and weight and propping it up against the sofa or a chair. Make sure it is really secure. Lie down and relax. You can also massage the scalp while in this position. The inverted postures in yoga are also helpful.

► Massage the scalp with a mixture of 1 tbsp of olive oil and 15 drops of rosemary essential oil. This helps to improve circulation to the scalp and nutrient flow to the hair follicles.

► Treat your hair gently. Try not to use chemical hair dyes, use only natural products and a soft brush and do not towel dry or heat dry your hair. Rinse your hair two or three times a week with a combination of sage and rosemary tea.

ALZHEIMER'S DISEASE

Alzheimer's disease is a condition which attacks the brain function, affects memory, especially short term, and alters intellectual capacity to the point that simple daily tasks become impossible. It is heartbreaking to watch the deterioration of a person with Alzheimer's, but there are steps you can take.

CAUSES

To date, no factor has been proven to be a specific cause of Alzheimer's disease. A combination of factors, including age, genetic inheritance, environment, diet and general health, is likely to be responsible.

Action plan

The key is to get a good supply of nutrients to the brain cells to produce the all-important neurotransmitters.

⠿ EAT/DRINK

► Whole foods with plenty of fresh fruit and vegetables to keep blood-sugar levels stable and the brain nourished.
► Foods plentiful in antioxidants, including berries.
► Foods that contain cysteine, methionine and sulphur which naturally help to rid the body of heavy metals. So, fish, eggs, chives, horseradish, garlic and onions, asparagus, nuts and seeds should be on the menu.
► Good fats found in salmon, herring, mackerel, linseeds, raw shelled hemp seeds, pumpkin seeds, gold of pleasure seed oil, sunflower oil.
► See page 156 for more information on foods that feed the brain.

⠿ AVOID

► White stuff. That means white bread, white pasta, white rice and sugar. For brain function, you need a good supply of nutrients, especially the B vitamins, and you won't get enough living on the white stuff.
► Coffee and alcohol as they affect the brain negatively.

HERBS

► Astragalus, red clover and nettle are good sources of B vitamins and other helpful nutrients.
► Add liquid algae to smoothies to help in the removal of heavy metals from the body.
► Ginkgo biloba has been found in studies to help increase circulation to the brain. It increases brain function due to its effect on acetylcholine, the brain chemical that allows the communication between nerve cells for reasoning and memory.
► Hawthorn improves blood flow to the brain.
► Club moss has been found to improve memory in Alzheimer's sufferers.
► Biota seed is known in Chinese medicine for helping with age-related memory loss. You would have to see a specialized practitioner for this.
► Coptis has been found to help prevent negative effects of aluminium.

SUPPLEMENTS

► You absolutely must take a good all-round multivitamin/mineral complex. There are usually numerous nutrient deficiencies with this condition.

► Take B vitamins: B1, B3, B12. Neurotransmitters in the brain depend on B vitamins.

► In Alzheimer's patients, there is usually insufficient stomach absorption. Take betaine with HCL before meals to help the assimilation and absorption of nutrients.

► If zinc is low, the brain nerve cells may be affected. And zinc is a critical nutrient which in normal situations would be at high levels in the hippocampus, the memory centre.

► Soya lecithin in high dosages can make a huge difference to brain function. It helps to prevent the destruction of brain tissues.

► Take DHA omega-3 oil to provide the brain with the essential fatty acids.

► Supplements of DHEA may improve brain power. DHEA is a hormone which is usually found in high levels in the brain but as we age it seems to decline markedly. Low levels have been linked to memory problems.

EXTRA TIPS

► I believe it is worth looking into Chelation Therapy, a method of removing toxic metals from the blood. I recommend getting your mercury fillings analysed for leakage and possible replacement. See a holistic dentist who understands the issues surrounding mercury poisoning and the negative effects on the brain.

To learn more, go to www.gillianmckeith.info/holisticdentist.

► I believe there is a connection between the absorption of aluminium and Alzheimer's. Use only stainless-steel pots and glass cookware. Aluminium can be found in processed cheeses, pickles, cake mixes, baking soda and some processed foods. Read the labels and avoid deodorants, douches, shampoos and medicines such as antacids that contain aluminium.

► Keep your brain active. Learn a new language. Do crossword puzzles.

► Keep stress at bay. If you don't, you may have too much circulating cortisol hormone which will affect brain function.

► For further information, go to www.gillianmckeith.info/alzheimers.

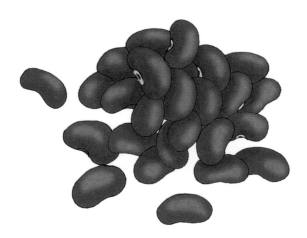

ANAEMIA

Anaemia is diagnosed when there are insufficient red blood cells or there is a lack of haemoglobin in the blood, resulting in reduced oxygen getting to the cells. Cell function and energy levels decrease as the cells become deficient in oxygen.

Sickle-cell anaemia: this is an hereditary disorder that has no cure. Sufferers can be helped by improving their nutritional status through diet and supplements.

Pernicious anaemia: this refers to a deficiency in B12. Some older people present themselves as senile when, in actuality, they may be seriously B12 deficient.

Signs and symptoms include a yellow tinge to the skin, oedema, indigestion, a red, beefy and sore tongue, bleeding under the skin, depression, weak heartbeat and numb feet. Pernicious anaemia can be caused by poor absorption, low stomach acid and a vegan diet as B12 is mainly found in animal foods such as fish, meat and eggs. Nutritional yeast flakes and the green superfood spirulina and sea veggies are vegetarian sources of B12.

Iron-deficiency anaemia: iron is needed to make haemoglobin that carries oxygen to the cells. About 15 per cent of women are thought to suffer from this type of anaemia. Heavy menstrual bleeding, pregnancy, malabsorption and poor diet are all common causes.

SYMPTOMS MAY INCLUDE

► Lack of energy.
► Breathlessness on exertion.
► Dizziness.
► Loss of appetite.
► Constipation.
► Brain fog.
► Reduced muscular strength.
► Poor bodily repair.
► Increased susceptibility to infections.

COMMON SIGNS TO LOOK OUT FOR

► Enlarged flabby tongue with teeth marks.
► Very pale tongue.
► Poor hair condition.
► Brittle and ridged finger nails.
► Cold hands and feet.
► Pale lips, eyelids and skin.

Action plan for iron-deficiency anaemia

Have a blood test – it is important to ascertain whether your symptoms are caused by a lack of iron. Supplementing with iron is not recommended if you are not deficient in iron. It is also important to find out what has caused the deficiency in the first place.

⁙ EAT/DRINK

Iron-rich foods, such as:

► Eggs.
► Amaranth.
► Oily fish.
► Beans and pulses such as lentils, chickpeas, haricot beans, kidney beans, pinto beans, baked beans, butter beans, peas.
► Nuts, such as almonds, cashew nuts, Brazil nuts, walnuts.

▶ Sesame seeds.

▶ Dried fruit, such as apricots, figs, dates.

▶ Green vegetables, such as watercress, spinach, kale.

▶ Kelp flakes – sprinkle them onto soups and salads with beetroot.

▶ Ginger – add to soups or steep with lemon for a delicious hot drink.

⠿ AVOID

▶ Tea and coffee – these can both interfere with the absorption of iron.

▶ Wheat bran – bran contains phytates that reduce mineral absorption.

▶ Spinach, chocolate, rhubarb and sorrel – these are rich in oxalic acid which interferes with iron absorption.

▶ Processed foods, beer, confectionery, ice cream and soft drinks. The additives in these interfere with iron absorption.

HERBS

▶ Anise, caraway, cumin, mint, parsley, watercress, thyme, cinnamon, and the seaweed dulse all improve iron absorption.

▶ Gentiana, a little-known herb, has been shown to increase digestive juices and digestive enzymes and thus stimulate digestion.

▶ Nettles are rich in iron and other minerals so drink nettle tea. Dandelion-root coffee or dandelion tea are also a good source of iron.

▶ Yellow dock is packed with iron and can be found in tincture or tea form. Take along with the herbal tincture red clover.

▶ Ginseng in the form of tea can be helpful if you are feeling really tired and exhausted.

SUPPLEMENTS

▶ Iron – as prescribed by your doctor; use in ferrous gluconate form or yeast-free floradix as some iron supplements can cause constipation. Iron is best absorbed on an empty stomach.

▶ Vitamin C.

▶ Folic acid which is also needed for red blood cell formation.

▶ Vitamin B complex, including biotin. B vitamins aid red blood cell production and iron absorption.

▶ Sublingual vitamin B12.

▶ Digestive enzymes or hydrochloric acid to aid absorption. If poor absorption is one of the causes, you might be bloated or gassy.

▶ The tissue cell salt ferr phos (iron phosphate) for low haemoglobin.

⠿ EXTRA TIPS

▶ Avoid antacids and antibiotics unless absolutely necessary – these can interfere with iron absorption.

▶ Eat iron-rich foods (see above) with vitamin-C rich foods at the same meal (vitamin C helps with absorption of iron). For example, eat fish, lentils and eggs with vegetables and salads.

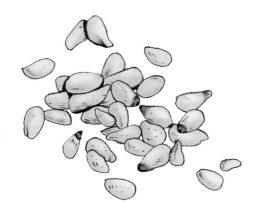

ANOREXIA NERVOSA

The term anorexia originally meant loss of appetite. Now it is generally used to describe someone who denies themselves food, even when they are hungry. Anorexics have an irrational fear of body fat and weight gain and a constant desire to get thinner. They have misperceptions of body image, often feeling fat even when underweight.

SIGNS AND SYMPTOMS

► Dramatic weight loss; 15–25 per cent below normal weight is the definition for being anorexic.

► Eating only a few foods that are low in fat and calories.

► A preoccupation with body shape and image.

► Wearing baggy clothes to hide thinness.

► Avoidance of social gatherings where food is involved.

► Making excuses for not eating and secretiveness around food.

► Missing three consecutive periods.

► Loss of sexual desire.

► Malnutrition and failing health.

► Obsessive exercise.

► White spots on nails which indicate a marked zinc deficiency.

CAUSES MAY INCLUDE

► A culture where thinness is associated with attractiveness.

► Emotional and psychological imbalances; common character traits of anorexics include obsessiveness, low self-esteem, perfectionism, approval seeking.

► Trauma or abuse in early life.

► Relationship problems.

► The need to gain control. Feeling powerless can trigger the need to have control of some aspect of life; the food that enters the body is one thing that can be controlled.

► Nutrient deficiencies (particularly zinc) and neurotransmitter imbalances.

Action plan

The aim is to restore a healthy attitude towards food with three regular meals a day and to restore the body to a state of health. Nutritional therapists can help to devise eating plans to aid weight gain and restore health. Don't try to do it alone.

⋮⋮ EAT/DRINK

► Liquid algae and liquid zinc. You will have more of an appetite for food once you normalize zinc levels. Zinc supplementation can go a long way towards helping you to get well. So eat raw shelled hemp seeds, pumpkin seeds, sesame seeds, sunflower seeds, wheat germ and herring.

► Nutrient-packed foods, including avocados, miso soup, watercress, bananas, brown rice, quinoa, nut butters, oat cakes and hummous.

► Smoothies with superfood powders or flax-seeds thrown in.

HERBS AND SUPPLEMENTS

► Gentiana, from health-food stores, will help digestion and stimulate appetite and digestive juices.

► A combination of ginseng and astragalus can aid recovery.

► Burdock helps to stimulate appetite.

► Zinc, magnesium, fish oils, B vitamins, probiotics and digestive enzymes may all be useful.

► Look for a liquid multivitamin/mineral supplement, too.

EXTRA TIPS

► Psychotherapy: this is important for addressing the underlying emotional issues such as low self-esteem and irrational fears. There are many different types of psychotherapy including cognitive behavioural therapy, family therapy and group therapy. But unless you address the nutritional deficiencies, it will be a fight to get better. Please do not ignore the nutritional side of anorexia.

► For further information, go to www.gillianmckeith.info/anorexia

ANTIBIOTICS

Antibiotics can kill off the beneficial organisms in the gut, putting extra stress on the liver. If you are taking, or have recently completed, a course of antibiotics then the following action plan is useful.

Action plan

The aim is to keep a balanced level of good bacteria in your gut so that you don't end up with another common condition called candidiasis (see page 219).

EAT/DRINK

► Fruit and vegetables; at least 8 portions a day to support the immune system.

► Fermented foods. Yoghurt, kefir, sauerkraut, miso and natto are all fermented foods that contain beneficial bacteria.

► Organic animal products. Unlike organically reared animals, conventionally farmed animals are often routinely given antibiotics. This means that antibiotic residues may be in the meat or animal products that you eat which can give you an extra dose of antibiotics that will challenge your system further.

► Fibre which is needed by the bowel to clear out unwanted toxins and also to provide fuel for the good bacteria. Fibre is found in whole grains, pulses, nuts, seeds, fruit and vegetables, specifically artichokes, bananas, onions and celery.

► Garlic and onions. These have antibacterial properties so can enhance the effectiveness of the antibiotics and speed recovery.

► Water: at least 8 glasses a day. This will help the immune system to deal with the infection and help to clear out unhelpful toxins and organisms.

AVOID

► Sugar, refined carbohydrates and dairy products. These can all encourage yeasts that tend to take hold after antibiotics have reduced the good bacteria in the gut.

► Alcohol.

HERBS AND SUPPLEMENTS

► Echinacea, astragalus, Siberian ginseng, barberry root, burdock root, oregano leaves, pau d'arco and elderberries are all useful for your immune system. They can be taken as teas or tinctures.

► Take milk thistle daily to aid the liver in its work.

► Probiotics contain beneficial bacteria that tend to get killed off when antibiotics are taken. Look for high-potency, good-quality products.

⠿ EXTRA TIPS

► Avoid pesticides and environmental chemicals. These can all challenge the immune system. Eat organic foods when possible and use only natural household products.

ANXIETY DISORDER

Anxiety disorder can be either chronic or acute. Acute anxiety can manifest itself in the form of intermittent panic attacks. These may last from a few minutes to half an hour or so. Symptoms include increased heart rate, difficulty in breathing, dry mouth, feelings of impending disaster, chest pain, dizziness, shaking, nausea and difficulty in thinking clearly. Those who suffer from panic attacks often become fearful about going out and avoid certain situations. I am seeing an increasing number of anxiety-ridden individuals and one thing they all have in common is a magnesium deficiency. Chronic anxiety involves more general feelings of unease and tension with an inability to relax. Sufferers tend to overreact to small stresses.

CAUSES MAY INCLUDE

► Chronic or acute stress and adrenal imbalance.
► Food allergies.
► Poor blood-sugar control.
► Use of stimulants: caffeine, alcohol, nicotine and drugs.
► Nutrient deficiencies.
► Hyperthyroidism.
► Depression.

Action plan

Pack your diet with lots of anti-stress nutrients and eat regularly throughout the day; ideally six small meals.

⠿ EAT/DRINK

► Whole grains such as brown rice, oats and quinoa. These supply B vitamins and magnesium, both of which get used up during stress. Magnesium, in particular, is necessary for muscle and nerve relaxation.
► Lots of green vegetables such as kale, chicory, broccoli, savoy cabbage and pak choi.
► Foods high in calcium and magnesium which also calm the body: wheat germ, soya products, lentils, nuts, leafy greens, celery, lettuce, sesame seeds and steamed almonds.
► Foods that comfort the nerves: B-vitamin-packed brown rice, mashed sweet potatoes, natural yoghurts, oatmeal and

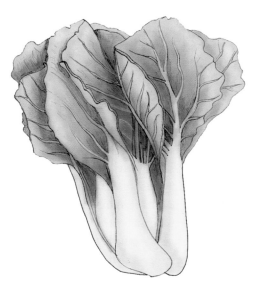

steamed veggies help. Rice pudding is a soother, too.

► Goji berries, one of the richest sources of vitamin C. Goji berries also contain vitamins B1, B2, B6 which can help the body to deal with stressors more effectively.

AVOID

► Caffeine, sugar, alcohol, nicotine and drugs, all of which stimulate the adrenal glands to produce stress hormones and upset the blood-sugar balance.

► Wheat, intolerance to which is commonly implicated in mood disorders.

HERBS AND SUPPLEMENTS

► Good sleep is necessary for normal stress reactions. Hops, passionflower, skullcap and lime flowers may all be taken as tinctures or capsules before bed.

► Ginkgo biloba tea which also lowers anxiety and increases nutrients to the brain.

► Camomile, lime flowers and lemon balm teas are all good for promoting feelings of relaxation.

► Siberian ginseng can help to reduce feelings of anxiety and stress.

► The superfood spirulina can supply you with a full array of nutrients. Anxiety sufferers usually test deficient in nerve-nourishing minerals and vitamins so tend to respond well to superfoods and supplements.

► Supplement with magnesium citrate. Magnesium is a natural muscle and nerve relaxant that gets used up during stress.

► Supplement with chromium picolinate to keep blood-sugar levels stable.

► Take vitamin B complex each morning. The B vitamins also tend to get used up by the adrenal glands when under stress and are important for blood-sugar control. Do not take B vitamins in the evening as they can be over-energizing.

► Take vitamin C for optimum adrenal function. Eat lots of berries and fruits for naturally occurring Vitamin C.

► Take niacinamide with meals to nourish the nerves and make you feel less jumpy.

► Gaba (gamma amino butyric acid) can also ease panic attacks.

EXTRA TIPS

► Get regular, moderate exercise. Brisk walking, swimming and dancing are all good activities. Aim for at least 20 minutes a day.

► Learn relaxation techniques. There are many ways of learning to relax including yoga, meditation, tai chi, breathing exercises and listening to relaxing music.

► Use lavender essential oil. Lavender is an excellent relaxant. You can add a few drops to the bath or put some in an oil burner.

► Eat small, regular meals and snacks to stabilize blood-sugar levels. It is also important to avoid sugar and refined carbohydrates as these raise blood-sugar level rapidly followed by a slump when the adrenal glands kick in with stress hormones to bring levels up again. This can trigger a panic attack or feelings of anxiety.

ARTHRITIS

See OSTEOARTHRITIS, RHEUMATOID ARTHRITIS.

ASTHMA

Asthma is characterized by spasms in the airways in the lungs. This impedes the exhalation of air causing coughing, wheezing, tightness in the chest and difficulty in breathing. The spasms are caused by chronic or excessive inflammation or by sensitivity of the airways to outside stimuli such as cold air, pollution, pollen, chemicals, cigarette smoke, animal dander, etc. Other triggers include stress, exercise, laughing and respiratory infections.

UNDERLYING CAUSES MAY INCLUDE

► Hereditary factors.

► Fatty acid imbalance – essential fats can have an anti-inflammatory effect whilst saturated and processed fats can have a pro-inflammatory effect.

► Nutritional deficiencies – magnesium, vitamins B6, B12, vitamin C and selenium are often found to be low in asthmatics.

► Food intolerances or allergies – mucus-forming foods are a particular problem. Dairy products, eggs, soya, chocolate, corn and wheat may all be culprits. (See page 178.)

► Sensitivity to chemicals in food additives, preservatives and colourings or in household cleaning products, carpets, etc.

► Inhalant allergies – pollen, animal hair, smoke and dust mites.

► Insufficient stomach acid – asthmatics often have low stomach acid and this in turn can lead to food intolerances and nutrient deficiencies.

Action plan

Many asthmatics are put on various medications by their GP. However, there is much the asthmatic can do to reduce or relieve symptoms through diet.

▦ EAT/DRINK

► Fruit and vegetables – these are high in potassium which counteracts the effects of sodium. They are also the best sources of vitamin C needed to reduce inflammation.

► Oily fish such as salmon, sardines, trout, herring and mackerel. They have an anti-inflammatory effect which is good for the inflamed asthmatic.

► Garlic, red onions and apples – these contain quercetin, which inhibits inflammation.

► Brazil nuts which are rich in selenium. This trace mineral has an anti-inflammatory effect and several studies have linked its consumption with relative protection from asthma.

► Green leafy vegetables, nuts and seeds, which are all good sources of magnesium: constriction of the airways in the lungs is a feature of asthma. The mineral magnesium can help to prevent this by promoting relaxation in the muscles that line the airways.

► Organic foods as they do not contain chemicals and preservatives that can trigger attacks and challenge the immune system.

▦ AVOID

► Dairy products, as these are famously mucus-forming for many people.

► Wheat, soya, chocolate and eggs can also be mucus-forming.

► Salt – high salt intake is linked to respiratory-tract disorders. Salt is in all processed and packaged foods, so avoid these.

► Cold food and drinks – these can cause the airways to go into spasm.

HERBS AND SUPPLEMENTS

Note: For children under the age of 12, consult a herbalist for a herbal programme.

► The herb astragalus has been found to strengthen the lungs.

► Other good herbs include peppermint, lobelia, skullcap, ephedra and liquorice.

► Drink mullein tea. It can help to expel excess mucus and make breathing much easier. Pau d'arco tea is also helps.

► Take a few drops of lobelia during an attack to reduce the spasm and open the airways.

► Magnesium to relax muscles and nerves.

► Fish oils for their anti-inflammatory effect.

► Vitamins B6 and B12 may help to reduce symptoms.

► Vitamin C for anti-allergenic and anti-inflammatory effect.

► N AcetylCysteine helps to thin out bronchial secretions and sinus mucus.

► Hydrochloric acid – particularly if you have digestive symptoms as well. This can aid absorption of nutrients and reduce food intolerances over time. Take meadowsweet daily before meals to increase production of hydrochloric acid.

⁝⁝ EXTRA TIPS

► Identify environmental allergens and avoid them – most asthmatics will have some idea what triggers their attacks. Pollen, dust, animal hair, chemicals,

cigarette smoke and other triggers should be avoided as much as possible.

► To avoid dust mites, vacuum regularly and use anti-allergenic bedding. If you can afford it, get rid of carpets and put in ceramic, stone or hardwood floors.

► Take up singing – singing is great for improving lung capacity and oxygen flow without conscious effort.

► Massage the chest with 6 drops of rosemary or eucalyptus oils mixed with 2 tsp of almond oil to open up the airways. These oils can also be used in the bath.

► Practise yoga which is great for improving breathing. Find a class where breathing exercises are incorporated into the session.

► Swimming in the sea or lakes is good for the lungs, but less so in chlorinated pools.

► Avoid nuts with young children. Use nut butters instead.

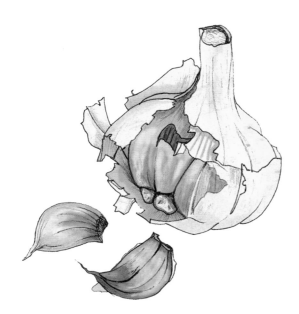

ATHEROSCLEROSIS

Atherosclerosis occurs when the arteries become filled with fatty cholesterol deposits called plaque. These fatty deposits line the artery walls causing mild circulation impairment initially but the plaque can get worse and clog the arteries over time, making them stiff and narrow. Gradually these deposits can cause a total obstruction of the arteries leading to heart attack or stroke. Smoking is one of the easiest ways to clog your arteries or harden them.

Warning signs may include leg cramping, exhaustion after only a little exertion, dizzy spells, memory problems, headaches, chest pain, tightness known as angina, breathing difficulties, fainting fits, inability to speak and shortness of breath. Unfortunately, there aren't always any warning signs.

CAUSES MAY INCLUDE
- ► Smoking.
- ► Diet high in saturated fat.
- ► High blood pressure.
- ► High cholesterol.
- ► High triglycerides.
- ► High levels of blood lipoprotein.
- ► Lack of fibre.
- ► Sedentary lifestyle.
- ► Stress.
- ► Excess iron.

Note: Diabetics are at high risk of atherosclerosis as they often have higher levels of cholesterol and triglycerides.

Action plan

If you smoke, you must stop. And anyone with this diagnosis should include plenty of anti-inflammatory foods in their diet.

⋮⋮ EAT/DRINK
- ► Tofu, tempeh, chestnuts or almonds instead of meat.
- ► Oily fish such as salmon, mackerel, trout and herring. They are a good source of omega-3, an artery protector and anti-inflammatory.
- ► Virgin olive oil or gold of pleasure seed oil.
- ► Onions and garlic for their cholesterol-reducing and blood-thinning properties.
- ► Almonds and pecans since the fat they contain is the artery-clearing mono-unsaturated variety.

⋮⋮ AVOID
- ► Rubbish and you know what that is: cakes, pies, pastries and foods containing trans-fatty acids. These foods do not keep blood-sugar levels stable.
- ► Red meat, milk and cheese.
- ► Butter and margarine.
- ► Refined oils in plastic bottles. Use olive oil for cooking and cold-pressed oils like flax and hemp in dressings.

HERBS
- ► Add ginger to your meals.
- ► The herb astragalus can keep macrophages from creating plaque once the artery walls have been damaged.
- ► Turmeric may have a salutary effect on heart health.
- ► Cayenne pepper is known as an artery saver as it can help to dilate arteries.
- ► Ginkgo biloba herbal fluid extract.
- ► Hawthorn leaf tea is a must. Hawthorn contains flavanoids which have antioxidant and anti-inflammatory effects. It also helps the liver to convert bad LDL cholesterol to good HDL.
- ► Siberian ginseng tea.

► Take 2 tablespoons of flax oil daily for its beneficial omega-3 content. Squirt a wee bit of lemon into the flax to make it more palatable.

► Sprinkle lecithin granules over salads and into soups. Lecithin, a source of cholesterol-busting phosphatidylcholine, helps to break down fat and remove cholesterol deposits.

► Alfalfa powder, a source of saponins, is an easy way to bring down cholesterol.

► Vitamin C is very important as it helps to break down plaque.

► Take the following supplements in rotation:

* Co-enzyme Q10
* Vitamin E
* Magnesium
* Vitamin B complex
* Niacin
* Borage oil or evening primrose oil
* Tocotrienol antioxidants

EXTRA TIP

► I believe it is worth looking into Chelation Therapy as a way of removing plaque.

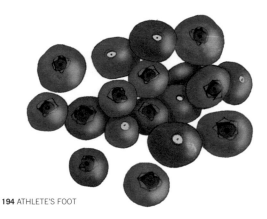

ATHLETE'S FOOT

Athlete's foot is a fungal infection of the skin. It's tough to get rid of so you have to keep at it. Symptoms include scaling, redness, itching and cracking of the skin. It can easily be picked up in swimming pools, spas and public showers.

CAUSES MAY INCLUDE

► Localized infection caused by the warm, moist environment inside shoes where fungus can thrive.

► Systemic fungal overgrowth. See *Candida albicans*, page 219.

► Antiobiotic use, see page 188.

► Diet high in sugar, refined carbohydrates and alcohol.

► Suppressed immune system.

Action plan

People often ignore this condition, but left to its own devices it will tend to get deeper. Follow my plan and you will address the root causes.

EAT/DRINK

► Garlic. It contains antimicrobial compounds that can protect your skin from fungal infections. If you're prone to athlete's foot or other skin conditions, add one or two cloves of chopped raw garlic to your food daily. And even chuck a clove into your shoes. When you are walking, the garlic will be crushed and enter your bloodstream.

► Whole natural foods with plenty of fresh vegetables – these will help to support your immune system in its fight against the fungus.

AVOID

▸ Sugar.

▸ Refined carbohydrates.

▸ Soft drinks.

▸ Alcohol.

▸ Dairy products.

HERBS AND SUPPLEMENTS

▸ Drink 3 cups of pau d'arco tea daily – this has anti-fungal effects. You can also soak your feet in the tea for further effects.

▸ Try grapefruit seed extract. If you can't stand the taste, get the capsules.

▸ Supplement with zinc, as zinc levels are often low in those with athlete's foot.

▸ Probiotics replenish the beneficial bacteria and help to crowd out the yeast.

EXTRA TIPS

▸ Keep your feet dry and well aired – wear cotton socks and take your shoes off as much as possible.

▸ After a shower, dry your feet thoroughly and then cover them in cornstarch, baking soda or arrowroot powder. These powders will help to absorb the extra moisture on your feet so there will be no damp between your toes.

▸ Apply tea tree oil or thuja oil – try using it diluted first to check for reactions; it is quite powerful and can cause soreness on sensitive skins.

ATTENTION DEFICIT HYPERACTIVITY DISORDER

ADHD or ADD primarily affects children. It is characterized by an inability to concentrate or pay attention. Often there are associated learning and behavioural problems. There can be a tendency to medicate without first checking whether there might be simpler, often diet-related answers.

CAUSES MAY INCLUDE

▸ Food allergies and chemical sensitivities. Food additives, processed foods, soft drinks, sugar and refined carbohydrates are common culprits. Wheat and dairy products and other allergenic foods may also play a part.

▸ Nutritional deficiencies or imbalances are also implicated. In particular, there may be deficiencies in essential fats, B6, magnesium and zinc.

▸ Unstable blood-sugar levels which can affect concentration, mood and behaviour.

▸ Hereditary factors.

▸ Trauma during pregnancy.

▸ Oxygen deprivation at birth.

▸ Exposure to fluorescent lighting.

▸ Dental fillings.

▸ Stress.

▸ Pollution.

Action plan

The action plan is a guide for parents with hyperactive children. Monitor what your children are eating and drinking; it could make life a great deal easier for you if you are able to spot potential dietary triggers.

GET YOUR CHILD TO EAT/DRINK

► Small, regular meals and snacks – large meals upset blood-sugar levels more than smaller meals. Good snacks include fruit, oat cakes with nut butter (if not allergic to oats or nuts), carrot sticks with hummous, unsulphured dried fruit and avocados.

► Fruit and vegetables – these are good sources of vitamins and minerals and are needed to stabilize behaviour and mood.

► Lettuce which contains natural plant chemicals that aid relaxation.

► Linseed oil on salads or stirred into cooked grains and vegetables.

► Magnesium-rich foods such as green vegetables, nuts, seeds and whole grains.

► Zinc-rich foods such as pumpkin seeds, linseeds, fish, meat, whole grains and pulses.

GET YOUR CHILD TO AVOID

► Sugar, soft drinks, processed foods, preservatives, colourings and additives, refined carbohydrates, caffeine (in tea, coffee, colas and chocolate) and salt. It's far better to try this first before subjecting your child or yourself to years of medication.

► Almonds, apples, grapes, peppermint, apricots, cherries, currants, berries, peaches, plums, prunes, tomatoes, cucumbers and oranges which contain salicylates which have been found to aggravate ADHD in some children.

► Sulphites – these are often used as preservatives in dried fruit so buy organic when possible.

SUPPLEMENTS

► Magnesium which is a natural muscle and nerve relaxant.

► Zinc – low zinc levels are often a factor in ADHD and zinc can combat the effects of high lead and copper.

► Fish oils – these are needed for brain function and mood stability.

► Evening primrose oil.

► Vitamin B complex.

► Vitamin C.

EXTRA TIPS

► Check for food intolerances which are strongly implicated in children with behavioural disorders. This is because eating foods to which we are intolerant is thought to stimulate the release of endorphins. These are feel-good chemicals in the brain that become addictive leading to cravings for the problem foods. Identification of food intolerances can be done by a test or by eliminating the foods that are craved or eaten most often. Wheat, dairy, chocolate, yeast, soya and eggs are all common culprits. For home-testing kits, go to www.gillianmckeith.info or visit a nutritionist.

► Have a hair mineral analysis – this will highlight the presence of toxic metals and nutrient deficiencies. Lead and copper are both implicated in ADHD. High levels of phosphorus and low levels of magnesium and calcium may also be a problem.

► Provide lots of opportunities for physical activity.

► Give your child a lavender oil massage or bath – just put a few drops of lavender essential oil in the bath and encourage your child to sit or play in the bath for 20 minutes.

► For further information, go to www.gillianmckeith.info/attentiondeficit.

AUTISM

There is no single definition of autism as it is not a single disorder but rather a spectrum. Characteristics of autism include limited speech, lack of facial expression, difficulty with social interactions, impaired understanding of others' feelings and points of view, solitary play, hypersensitivity to sound, smell or colour, hyperactivity, need for routine, obsessive-compulsive disorders, rocking, head banging, loud pitched screams and poor eye contact.

Often sufferers will only eat a narrow range of foods and may have obsessions with certain foods. Digestive problems are also common.

UNDERLYING CAUSES

There are likely to be a number of underlying causes behind autism. Each autistic is likely to have a unique set of circumstances that have triggered the onset of the symptoms. Autistics often have a family history of:

► Auto-immune diseases.
► Allergies.
► Behavioural problems.
► Coeliac disease.
► Exposure to organo-phosphates (used in agriculture).
► Irritable bowel syndrome.
► Migraines.
► Obsessive-compulsive disorders.
► Attention deficit hyperactivity disorder (ADHD) (see page 195).

Action plan

Although autism is not really a disease and may not be 'curable', quality of life can be vastly improved if some of the underlying causes are identified and when possible removed. It is a complex disorder but the following suggestions may be worth trying. A diet plentiful in natural, wholefoods whenever possible is key.

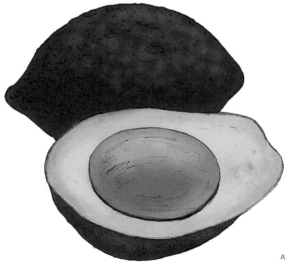

A

⣿ EAT/DRINK
► Oily fish (three times a week or supplement with fish oils daily). Oily fish contain omega-3 fatty acids that are important for a healthy brain and nervous system. In a pilot study, supplementing the diet of autistic children with fish oils led to better sleep patterns, more eye contact, improved cognitive and motor skills and sociability. Children were also found to be less aggressive, irritable and hyperactive. Good sources of the omega-3 fats used in the trial are salmon, trout, herrings, sardines and mackerel.
► Brown rice, quinoa, avocados, nuts, seeds, legumes, bananas. These are good sources of B vitamins.

⣿ AVOID
► Gluten and dairy foods. These can trigger the release of opioids (endorphin-like substances) in susceptible individuals. Autistic sufferers tend to have excess levels of opioids which have a profound effect on behaviour.
► Limit tomatoes, aubergines, peppers and white potatoes. These foods contain solanine, to which autistic children may be sensitive.
► Citrus fruits, soya, corn, chocolate and foods containing yeast can worsen symptoms.
► Eliminate all possible trigger foods for one month. Reintroduce gradually and monitor symptoms using a food diary.
► Food additives, preservatives, artificial sweeteners and processed foods – these can all challenge the body and affect mood and behaviour.

► Sugar, refined carbohydrates and caffeine – these upset blood-sugar levels leading to emotional upset, cravings and behavioural problems.

HERBS AND SUPPLEMENTS
► Vitamin B6 seems to be sorely deficient in those with autism as does magnesium. They should be supplemented but taken with an additional B complex for best results.
► Take digestive enzymes with meals – these aid digestion and absorption of nutrients and reduce the likelihood of food intolerances. Better breakdown of food is very important to avoid the build-up of the behaviour-altering opioids in the urine and spinal fluid.
► Take probiotics – these aid digestion and gut immunity. Problems with digestion and immunity are both implicated in autism.

⣿ EXTRA TIPS
► Have Epsom salts baths twice a week – some autistics have difficulty metabolizing sulphur and this can contribute to symptoms. Epsom salts contain magnesium sulphate so bathing in the salts can increase levels of sulphur as well as magnesium in the tissues. Both of these are beneficial. Use 2 cups of salts in a warm bath and soak for 20 minutes. Do not rinse off; pat dry and go to bed. Sulphur tissue salts can also be taken to improve sulphur levels.
► For further information, go to www.gillianmckeith.info/autism.

BACKACHE

Backache can be a very tiring experience as pain is such a drain on the body's energy system. You may feel aches, sharp pains, gnawing pain. Back pain can radiate anywhere from the neck, right down the spine to your tailbone. The pain can even move into the buttocks and hips too. Lower-back pain is the most common back complaint and a huge problem for many.

CAUSES MAY INCLUDE

- Spinal malformation.
- Scoliosis.
- Sedentary lifestyle.
- Obesity.
- Poor posture.
- Heavy lifting.
- Pregnancy.
- Kidney weakness.
- Back injuries.
- Congesting foods.

Action plan

EAT/DRINK

- Quinoa barley, aduki beans, black beans, kidney beans, salmon, trout, fennels, onions, parsley, beetroot, spring onions, chives, blackberries, mulberries, blueberries. They are nourishing to the kidneys if that is the source of your back pain, and also high in magnesium, which can help relieve pain and tension.
- Oily fish, raw shelled hemp seeds, flax seeds, walnuts and avocados contain anti-inflammatory essential fats.
- Water: 6–8 glasses daily are required to flush out toxins and hydrate the body.

AVOID

- Peppers, aubergines, tomatoes and white potatoes. They may promote congestion in the kidneys due to the release of the compound solanine. In weak individuals, solanine can interfere with the enzymes in the back muscles, causing pain.
- Saturated fats and trans-fats found in margerine and baked goods because these can increase inflammation.

HERBS AND SUPPLEMENTS

- Teas of mint, camomile, sage, thyme, yarrow and elderflower can induce a free flow of perspiration. This should help to release a build-up of lactic acid that can cause pain.
- Take the herb St John's wort or hypericum for pain caused by nerve injury.
- Teas of ginger, cinnamon bark, fenugreek, raspberry, blackberry, rose hips, dandelion and uva ursi (15 drops in hot water) all help to nourish the kidneys.
- Take 3 drops of pine tincture 4 times daily to relieve nerve pain.
- Tincture of willow bark can be a natural pain reliever as can the herb horsetail.
- Magnesium supplements are important for bone and muscle strength, and magnesium is a natural muscle and nerve relaxant. Magnesium is the mineral that mobilizes calcium into the bones, so make sure that you get enough of it as well as adequate calcium and vitamin D.
- Vitamin B12 injections have been shown to reduce lower-back pain.
- Silica can also help bone structure. You can get silica in liquid form or as capsules and tablets.

⠿ EXTRA TIPS

► A poultice of linseed meal may help to soothe the area.

► Apply capsicum cream for pain relief.

► Lie down with a hot-water bottle placed under your lower back. The heat is soothing to the kidney area and gives warm relief to your sore back.

► Do gentle stretches to release stiffness and prevent muscle spasms.

► Do not sit for long periods of time. If you have a desk job, make sure that you get up every hour, on the hour and move around. Dance on the spot, go for a walk, just move your body. If you sit all day, you can really stiffen up and pain can feel more intense.

► Lose weight if you need to. When you are overweight, the intestinal area weakens and you end up with your belly sticking out. This extra frontal weight will pull your posture out of line and cause undue back strain.

► Strengthen your centre core. You can do this with an exercise regime called Pilates. When the muscles from stomach through to back are strong, there is less likelihood of injury or spinal shift. And you get a washboard stomach as a bonus so that can't be bad! Once you learn the movements, you can do the mat work at home.

► Correct posture and bending are worth learning. The Alexander Technique teaches a series of movements and proper usage of the body.

► Get regular massages. This can help to soften muscle tissue and release pain. It is critical that the buttocks be massaged,

too, as back pain can be exacerbated by tension and holding in the buttock muscles.

► Acupuncture has been shown to relieve pain in many sufferers.

► Rolfing can be helpful for spinal misalignment, scoliosis and other back issues. It helped me a great deal. It is a deep, muscle-tissue and fascia massage which can help pain and posture.

► For further information go to www.gillianmckeith.info/backpain.

I suffered a slipped disc following a mountain biking accident and had to take painkillers to be able to do anything. Anyway, I knew that there was something seriously wrong with my digestion at the time (due to the drugs), and through using Gillian's book, I helped myself get back into step. I still constantly refer to it now, when I am aware something is not right (low energy, mood swings, etc.) and it works really well for me. To note, I'm young, fit and healthy, and have never been overweight . . . I use the book to keep me away from the doctors and away from additives and junk food!

BLOATING

It is normal to have wind occasionally. But continual bloating, farting and/or burping is not the norm. For the sake of yourself and those around you, do something about it now. Junk diets, too much sugar, wheat and dairy make the problem worse. Those who suffer from this affliction will testify to its untimely, unwelcome arrival at critical moments. The good news is that it's completely avoidable.

CAUSES

► Eating the wrong foods at the wrong time or in the wrong combination.

► Eating too much salt and not drinking enough water.

► Food intolerances. These can cause water retention. Wheat and dairy are common culprits.

► Stress. This leads to poor digestive function meaning food will sit in the gut for longer than it should. Fermentation, putrefaction and gas are the result.

► Not chewing your food really well. This results in an increase of bacteria and yeast, which produce gas.

► Strenuous exercise straight after a meal.

Action plan

The following plan should help aid digestion.

⁛ EAT/DRINK

► Warm water. Drink a glass of room-temperature water before meals and only take little sips or no sips at all during meals to avoid bloating. Ice-cold water will give you gas. Drink 1½–2 litres daily. You need to drink more not less if you have water retention and bloating to help your body dilute the salt in your tissues and allow you to excrete more salt and fluid.

► Celery which contains sodium and potassium needed for water balance.

► Chicory which contains prebiotics that feed the good bacteria in the gut.

► Miso which contains enzymes to aid proper digestion.

► Raw sauerkraut which contains enzymes and beneficial bacteria to aid digestion.

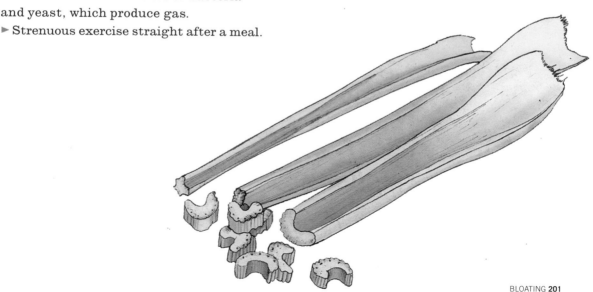

► Brown rice and millet which contains fibre to encourage good bacteria and improves bowel function generally.

► Ground flax seeds which contain a mucilaginous fibre that soothes and lubricates the intestines. Pop in a smoothie.

AVOID

► Refined carbohydrates – white rice, white bread, white pastry, white pasta, white flour products.

► Alcohol and sugar.

► Wheat and dairy products.

► Salt and spices.

► Caffeine from coffee, tea, colas and chocolate.

► Carbonated drinks.

► Processed or packaged foods.

► Fruit combined with other foods.

► Animal proteins combined with grains and starches.

HERBS AND SUPPLEMENTS

► Fennel, dill, coriander, basil, mint, chervil, parsley, sage, rosemary and thyme in your cooking to aid digestion.

► Ginger, fennel, peppermint or slippery elm tea mid morning and/or before meals to relax the stomach.

► Nettle or dandelion tea have a slight diuretic effect without depleting nutrients.

► Drink ¼ glass aloe vera juice and a teaspoon of liquid chlorophyll before your largest meal to stimulate digestion.

► Take a digestive enzyme supplement with meals.

EXTRA TIPS

► Combine food à la Gillian. That means eat fruit on an empty stomach but never for dessert. Wait 30 minutes after eating fruit before you eat any other foods.

► Do not mix dense proteins and dense carbohydrates at the same meal. That means no meat and potatoes at the same meal, no fish and chips, no pasta and tuna together. Mixing too many different types of foods together at the same meal makes it tough on digestion. Bloating, abdominal pain and stomach distension may result, not to mention plenty of gas from both ends.

► Eat at more or less the same times each day if possible otherwise you can end up bloated. Breakfast, snack, lunch, snack, dinner, snack. Missing breakfast and then catching up with a croissant makes you bloated.

► Eat dinner early. Eating late at night depletes the stomach of fluids at a time when its energy is at its weakest. You could end up with indigestion and will not absorb nutrients properly.

► Eat when relaxed. Total relaxation while eating renders maximum digestion.

► Food needs to be chewed thoroughly until it becomes liquid in your mouth for proper digestion to occur.

► Close your mouth when you eat. If you take in too much air with your food, the gases from the air travel to your stomach along with your food.

► If your stomach is in agony from the bloated feeling, lie down on your back and draw your knees in close until the stomach pressure eases.

BOWEL CANCER

see also CANCER, page 215.

Also known as colon or colorectal cancer, bowel cancer is a malignant disease of the large bowel (colon) or rectum. It is the second largest cause of cancer death in the UK and the third most common cancer after breast and lung cancers. Every year over 35,000 people in this country are diagnosed with the disease, which affects men and women equally. Although around one in 20 people will get bowel cancer at some point in their life, if caught early enough it is highly treatable.

CAUSES AND RISK FACTORS

► Age: About 83 per cent of cases occur in people over the age of 60. However, bowel cancer incidence in younger people is on the increase.

► A strong family history of bowel cancer.

► People with a history of inflammatory bowel disorders such as Crohn's disease or ulcerative colitis.

► People who have had previous polyps removed.

► Eating a diet high in meat.

► Eating a diet low in fibre, and high in saturated fat.

► Regular consumption of alcohol, especially beer.

► Cigarette smoking.

► An inactive lifestyle.

► Overweight or obesity.

► Chronic constipation.

SYMPTOMS

Although symptoms may vary, the most common to look out for include:

► Changes in bowel habits such as loose stools or constipation for several weeks.

► Bleeding from the bottom for no apparent reason.

► Blood in the stools.

► Severe abdominal pain.

► A lump in the abdomen.

► Extreme tiredness with no known cause.

► Unexplained weight loss.

Action plan

Diet and lifestyle changes can help reduce your risk for the disease or improve your chances of recovery. You will need to take time out for you. If you are being treated for bowel cancer, make sure you check with your GP before taking any of the suggested supplements.

EAT/DRINK

► A high-fibre diet, as this aids regular bowel movements and provides protection against bowel cancer. Opt for whole grain cereals such as whole grain brown rice, millet, quinoa and amaranth. Avoid refined grains that have had their fibre removed. Other excellent sources of fibre include beans and pulses, vegetables, fruit and sprouted beans and seeds.

► Fresh fruit and vegetables, if possible seven to nine portions a day. Besides being a good source of fibre, these food groups are abundant in phytonutrients – powerful plant antioxidants that have anti-cancer activity.

► Vegetables from the cruciferous family such as broccoli, cauliflower, Brussels sprouts, cabbage, collard greens and kale. Cruciferous vegetables contain several cancer-protective substances including indole-3-carbinol, glucaric acid and sulphoraphane. Research suggests people who eat cruciferous vegetables regularly have a reduced risk for bowel cancer.

► Tomato-based foods. Tomatoes contain a phytonutrient called lycopene, consumption of which has been associated with a reduced risk of bowel cancer. It is thought that lycopene is better absorbed from cooked tomatoes as opposed to raw. So tomato sauces or tinned tomatoes are a good source of lycopene but watch for the sugar content, so best to get them from a health-food store or the wellbeing or wholefoods sections of supermarkets. And of course, you could make your own if you're trying to increase your intake of this powerful antioxidant.

► Selenium-rich foods, including Brazil nuts, broccoli, oily fish, asparagus, brown rice, dulse, garlic, kelp and wheat germ.

► Chickpeas for their anti-carcinogenic compounds.

► Garlic has been found to lower the risk of bowel cancer, which may be due to its ability to reduce the development of cancer-forming compounds in the body. So try to include garlic, preferably raw, in your diet regularly.

► Freshly pressed fruit and vegetable juices. These are packed with cancer-fighting antioxidants and help to detoxify and supercharge the body.

► Water, to help keep the motions soft and moving through the colon. Drink at least eight glasses of bottled or filtered water daily.

► Nettle and dandelion teas help to keep stool soft and moving regularly.

⠿ AVOID

► Meat, especially red meat, processed meat products such as sausages, and well-done/charred meat as it contains more cancer-forming compounds than lightly cooked meat. People with bowel cancer are best to avoid meat altogether and eat mainly plant-derived sources of protein instead. Good sources of these include tofu, beans, whole grains, quinoa, nuts, seeds, eggs (no more than five a week) and natural live yoghurt.

► Foods high in saturated fat such as full-fat dairy products (butter, cream and cheese).

► Foods that contain toxic trans-fats such as hard margarine, biscuits and anything that has been deep-fried.

► Refined grains such as white bread and white rice as they are devoid of fibre.

► Refined sugar and all foods that contain it as some studies have reported associations between sugar intake and bowel cancer risk. Opt for fresh and dried fruit (unsulphured) instead.

► Processed foods as these will add toxicity to your body and contribute little nutritional value.

► Alcohol. Several studies have found a link between alcohol intake and an increased risk of rectal cancer. Beer appears to be the worst for increasing precancerous changes in the colon, probably due to cancer-promoting chemicals in it known as nitrosamines.

► Caffeinated drinks including coffee and black tea. Instead, drink grain coffee substitutes, green tea which contains an antioxidant compound called epigallocatechin gallate (EGCG), and herbal teas like nettle, fennel, camomile, peppermint, ginger and rooibosch.

HERBS AND SUPPLEMENTS

► Garlic. Studies have found people who eat more garlic have a lower incidence of bowel cancer, so taking it in supplement form may be worthwhile.

► Reishi mushroom (can be taken in capsule form) for its anti-cancer and immune-boosting effects.

► Vitamin C has been demonstrated to reduce the risk of bowel cancer in women, but not men. However, being a common antioxidant nutrient its supplementation is recommended in both sexes.

► Vitamin E. Some studies have shown that people who take vitamin E supplements may have a decreased risk of precancerous colon polyps and bowel cancer, compared to those who do not supplement with it. This is likely to be due to its antioxidant effect.

► Selenium. As blood levels of this antioxidant mineral have been found to be low in people with bowel cancer and other cancers, supplementation is advisable. It also appears to boost immune function in bowel cancer patients.

► Salvestrols. These natural plant compounds indirectly target cancer cells and may help to destroy them.

► IP-6, a compound present in oat and wheat bran that you can also take in supplement form, has been shown to have anti-cancer properties, especially in relation to bowel cancer.

► Vitamin D supplements may help protect against colon cancer.

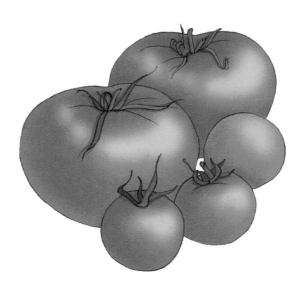

::: EXTRA TIPS

► Deal with any emotional issues that may be a problem. Talk to someone. Get help or counselling.

► Regular exercise cuts the risk of bowel cancer compared to a sedentary lifestyle, so try to get out and about for a while every day.

► Take up relaxation exercises or meditation.

► Do not smoke as the effects of smoking increase the risk of bowel cancer.

► For further information go to www.gillianmckeith.info/cancer.

BREAST CANCER

See also CANCER, page 215

One in nine women will develop breast cancer at some point in their life, and it is now the most common cancer in the UK, excluding non-melanoma skin cancer. Most cases occur in post-menopausal women. Breast cancer can also occur in men, although it is comparatively rare. Although breast cancer in British women is on the rise, cure rates are also rising slowly and steadily, probably due to increased breast awareness, earlier detection and improved treatment.

Interestingly, the incidence of breast cancer varies dramatically in different parts of the world. For instance, it is six times more common in Britain and the US than in Japan. However, when women move from low- to high-risk countries, over time they acquire the same risk as women in the country they have moved to. This strongly suggests links to dietary, lifestyle and environmental factors.

CAUSES AND RISK FACTORS

▶ Age: about 80 per cent of cases occur in women aged over 50 years.

▶ Starting your period at a young age (under 12).

▶ A late menopause (after 55).

▶ Having no children or having them late in life.

▶ Taking the contraceptive pill or hormone replacement therapy (HRT).

▶ Being overweight (especially after the menopause).

▶ A strong family history of breast cancer.

▶ Carrying a breast cancer gene (this accounts for fewer than 10 per cent of breast cancer cases).

▶ Eating a high saturated-fat diet.

▶ Regularly drinking more than one unit of alcohol per day.

▶ Cigarette smoking.

▶ Having dense breast tissue.

▶ Having certain benign breast conditions such as atypical hyperplasia.

▶ Radiation exposure.

SYMPTOMS

▶ A lump in the breast or armpit.

▶ Change in size or shape of the breast.

▶ Nipple inversion or puckering.

▶ A rash around the nipple.

▶ Nipple bleeding or discharge.

▶ Puckering of the breast skin.

▶ Swelling of the arm.

▶ Persistent breast pain (although pain is not always present).

▶ Breast inflammation.

▶ Prominent veins on the breast.

▶ If the breast cancer has spread to other parts of the body symptoms will include weight loss and fatigue.

Action plan

This Action Plan can help you to boost your immune system, cleanse your body and balance your hormones – important factors in both preventing and fighting this condition. If you are being treated for breast cancer, make sure you check with your GP before taking any of the suggested supplements.

⠿ EAT/DRINK

▶ Fresh fruit and vegetables (preferably raw) every day – seven to nine portions are ideal. Eat produce from all colour spectrums as this will help to ensure you get a variety of phytonutrients – powerful plant antioxidants that help to protect the body against cancer.

► Vegetables from the cruciferous family – broccoli, cauliflower, Brussels sprouts, cabbage, kale, turnips and swede. Cruciferous vegetables contain a substance called indole-3-carbinol, which stimulates the conversion of oestrone, the bad form of oestrogen that promotes breast cancer, into an inactive form.

► Sprouted seeds and legumes. Sprouted broccoli seeds are particularly beneficial as they contain sulphoraphane glucosinolate, a precursor to sulphoraphane, in amounts up to 50 times higher than those found in regular broccoli. It has been shown that sulphoraphane blocks the formation of mammary tumours.

► Kohlrabi contains many important anti-carcinogenic properties.

► Purple sprouting broccoli. This is a good source of the phytochemical sulphoraphane that has cancer-preventing properties. It is great steamed or stir fried. The stem, head and leaves can all be used and are all beneficial to health.

► Freshly pressed fruit and vegetable juices. These are concentrated in cancer-fighting antioxidants and help the body to cleanse and revitalize. Try a vegetable cocktail made from carrot, celery, beetroot, fennel and parsley.

► Fibre-rich foods. Researchers have found that a high-fibre diet reduces the risk of breast cancer. Good sources include brown rice and other whole grains, muesli, oats, beans and pulses.

► Foods that contain phyto-oestrogens. Phyto-oestrogens are plant-based compounds that have mild oestrogenic effects and have the ability to block the action of some of the body's naturally occurring and more potent oestrogen by competing with it. Many studies have found this mechanism to be cancer-protective. Phyto-oestrogens are present in soya products (such as soya milk, tofu, tempeh and miso), linseeds, celery, fennel, wheat, oats, chickpeas and lentils.

► Foods containing good fats. Sources of these include seeds, nuts, dark leafy green vegetables, tofu, avocados, and unrefined vegetable oils such as flax seed oil and extra virgin olive oil. Oily fish is a good source of omega-3 fats.

► Water, to keep your body cleansed and hydrated. Drink at least eight glasses of bottled or filtered water daily.

⠿ AVOID

► Processed foods as these will make your body more toxic.

► Refined sugar, and all foods that contain it. Eat fresh and dried fruit (unsulphured) instead, to satisfy sweet cravings.

► Salt.

► Alcohol. The liver helps to break down oestrogen, preventing excessive levels from accumulating in the body.

► Coffee and black tea. Instead, drink grain-based coffee substitutes and herbal teas such as nettle, fennel, camomile, peppermint, ginger and rooibosch.

► Meat. Eating a meat-free diet is believed to be beneficial. Female vegetarians have lower oestrogen levels than meat-eaters, so this could be one of the reasons for lower incidence of breast cancer. In addition, charred meat contains cancer-promoting compounds, as does non-organic meat which would have been treated with artificial hormones and growth factors. Good vegetarian sources of protein include tofu, beans, whole grains, quinoa, nuts, seeds, eggs (no more than five a week) and natural live yoghurt (with no added sugar).

► Foods high in saturated fats such as fried foods and red meat.

► Dairy products.

► Foods that contain trans-fats such as hard margarine, biscuits, cakes and crisps.

HERBS

► Milk thistle supports liver function and may reduce the growth of breast cancer cells.

► Siberian ginseng may help the body to recover from chemotherapy and radiation therapy more quickly.

► Echinacea, red clover and astragalus all help to support the immune system.

► Polyphenols (antioxidants) in green tea have been associated with a reduced risk of several types of cancers, including breast cancer.

SUPPLEMENTS

► Betacarotene, buffered vitamin C (look for vitamin C combined with a mineral like magnesium ascorbate or calcium ascorbate, as ascorbic acid is harsh on the digestive tract), vitamin E and selenium are all antioxidant

nutrients which help protect the body against cancer-forming agents.

► Vitamin B complex. B vitamins help to boost energy levels.

► Vitamin D. This may help to curb the development of breast cancer.

► Co-enzyme Q10. This is produced naturally in the body, helps cells to produce energy and acts as an antioxidant. It also stimulates the immune system.

► Calcium D-glucarate. Animal studies suggest that this compound lowers oestrogen levels in the body, an effect that may reduce the risk of breast cancer.

► Inositol hexaphosphate (IP6). This has been reported to have anti-cancer properties.

EXTRA TIPS

► Being overweight increases your risk of breast cancer, especially if you are post-menopausal. Oestrone and oestradiol, both cancer-promoting oestrogens, can be produced to excess by fat cells.

► Reduce your exposure to xeno-oestrogens – chemicals that mimic oestrogen. Buy organic food, chemical-free toiletries and cleaning products, and avoid wrapping food in clingfilm.

► Don't smoke.

► Being active cuts your cancer risk, probably by reducing hormone levels. On average, women who regularly walk, swim, jog and cycle for 35–45 minutes five times a week are less likely to develop breast cancer than sedentary women.

BRONCHITIS

Bronchitis is an inflammatory disorder which may start as a dry cough followed by catarrh, phlegm and a rattling cough. Inflammation in the bronchials is a sign that the immune system is struggling to keep things in balance. Bronchitis is more likely to occur after a cold and when you are run down.

Chronic bronchitis can cause enormous discomfort to the lungs as you are always coughing. You may experience difficulty in breathing. If you are or have been a smoker it may not be bronchitis, but a condition called emphysema (see page 258). Acute bronchitis should not last more than two weeks.

CAUSES MAY INCLUDE
► Smoking.
► Weakened immune system.
► Viruses.
► Allergies.
► Asthma.
► Bad colds.
► Hospital stays.

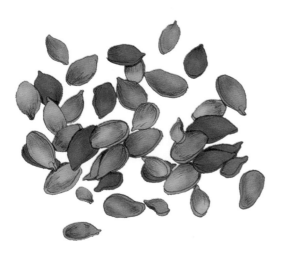

Action plan

Breathing will be easier if you can break up and dissolve the mucus.

⁛ EAT/DRINK
► Immune-supportive foods that are rich in antioxidants. These are the tools the immune system uses to deal with invaders and to help repair damage in the body. Fresh fruit and vegetables are powerhouses of antioxidants. Eat different coloured fruits and vegetables as each colour represents the presence of a different antioxidant.
► Essential fats as they have an anti-inflammatory effect. They are found in oily fish such as mackerel, sardines, salmon, trout and herrings as well as nuts and seeds.
► Hemp seeds, flax seeds, sunflower and pumpkin seeds. They contain vitamin E needed to protect the immune system. Olive oil and avocados are another rich source.
► Home-made soups such as chicken or miso broth to help thin out mucus.
► Carrots, sweet potatoes, spinach, spring onions and cantaloupe melon because they contain betacarotene (pro-vitamin A), vitamins C, E and the mineral zinc, all of which are needed for the proper functioning of the immune system.
► Garlic for its natural antiviral and antibacterial qualities.
► Shitake mushrooms to increase the infection and bacteria-fighting cells. A strong immune system is essential to prevent secondary infection.
► Vegetable proteins such as beans and lentils.

► Water – vital for immune function and healthy lungs. Drink a large glass of warm water 20–30 minutes before each meal and drink herbal teas between meals (Rooibosch tea is a good substitute for black tea as it does not contain caffeine but has a tea-like taste).

► Sulphur-rich foods such as leeks, Brussels sprouts and cabbage. Sulphur is partially eliminated through the lungs so this eases the mucus build-up in the bronchial tubes.

AVOID

► Immune-suppressive and challenging foods. These include sugar, refined grains (white bread, white rice, white pasta, pastry, etc.), salt, processed and packaged foods, additives, caffeine and alcohol.

► Red meats and dairy products because they contain saturated fats which can be pro-inflammatory.

HERBS AND SUPPLEMENTS

► Many herbs and gentle spices have beneficial properties for bronchitis; they are often anti-inflammatory, antibacterial and antiviral. They also support digestive function which often becomes weaker as we age. Good ones to try would be turmeric, cayenne pepper, cumin, coriander, oregano, parsley, mint, fennel, nettle, cinnamon, chives and ginger.

► The herb astragalus should be taken for a period of six months to strengthen your immune system and to fortify the lungs.

► Echinacea tincture can help to prevent secondary infection and dry up excess mucus.

► Expectorant herbs such as chickweed, coltsfoot, comfrey, elecampane, eucalyptus, horehound, hyssop, liquorice, mullein and pleurisy root can all help to discharge phlegm and mucus.

► The herbal tincture mullein can work wonders. It can help to bring up the phlegm so you don't cough as much.

► If fever is present, add foods that make you sweat such as catnip, cayenne, camomile, elder flowers, garlic, ginger, horseradish, lemon balm, sage, spearmint and yarrow.

► Anti-inflammatory bioflavanoids can be taken as a supplement with vitamin C.

► Bromelain supplements in between meals can act as anti-inflammatories, too.

► Supplements of n'acetyl cysteine can help to lessen mucus and break it up.

EXTRA TIPS

► Poultices of hot linseed and bran placed across the chest can help. Pulped onion between layers of muslin will help to break up congestion.

► Inhaling eucalyptus oil, friars balsam or thyme oil mixed with water can bring relief.

BRUISING

Bruising is purplish marks on the skin caused by the bleeding of capillaries under the skin. Pain and swelling may also result.

CAUSES

Any injury or blow to the body can cause a bruise. Bruises can also be triggered by steroid therapy, haemophilia, anaemia, smoking, anti-clotting drugs and deficiencies in vitamin K or bioflavanoids.

Action plan

If the bruises do not go away, see your GP.

EAT/DRINK

▶ Citrus fruit pith, kiwi fruits, berries, blackcurrants, elderberries, goji berries, apricots, onions, alfalfa, peppers, buckwheat and green vegetables for their bioflavanoids and vitamin C content to protect the capillaries. Vitamin C helps to build collagen tissues (that is, skin tissue) around the blood vessels in the skin.

▶ Liquid algae. If bruising occurs without any fall or knock to the body, then it may be a sign of other nutrient deficiencies as well as possible bioflavanoid lows.

▶ Buckwheat. Buckwheat contains rutin that can protect the capillary walls.

▶ Asparagus, broccoli, Brussels sprouts, cabbage, cauliflower, egg yolks, natto, oatmeal, alfalfa, kelp and nettles all contain vitamin K which is needed for proper blood clotting.

▶ Sweet potatoes and cauliflower which are high in vitamin C.

SUPPLEMENTS

▶ Vitamin C with bioflavanoids to strengthen capillary walls.

▶ Probiotics to improve vitamin K absorption.

EXTRA TIPS

▶ Apply arnica cream to the bruise to aid healing. Do not use arnica on open wounds.

▶ Apply a cold-water compress to reduce swelling and speed healing.

▶ Avoid non-steroidal anti-inflammatory medications when possible because they can cause bleeding. These include aspirin and ibuprofen.

BULIMIA NERVOSA

Those suffering from bulimia generally have episodes of binge eating followed by purging that often involves vomiting or laxative abuse. Usually this is done in secret and bulimia can go on for years without anyone knowing. Often bulimics are obsessed with exercise and will engage in vigorous exercise to atone for the binge episodes. They may also try and starve themselves after a binge to make up for the excessive intake of calories. This is counterproductive as it tends to lead to further bingeing and so the cycle goes on.

A bulimic's weight often remains the same but there may be other signs and symptoms of the condition. These may include swollen salivary glands, erosion of tooth enamel, frequent or constant sore throats, ulcers, blood-sugar problems, erratic heart beat, cessation of or disrupted menstrual cycle, hair loss, premature ageing, weakness, and low blood pressure. Mineral imbalances, rectal bleeding and dehydration may also result from bulimia.

CAUSES

Usually there are psychological issues at the root of the bulimia. Bulimics often use food to divert attention from difficult emotional issues. Low self-esteem lies at the root of the problem for many. Many bulimics suffered abuse or neglect as children. For others it may be a result of being or feeling rejected by a member of the opposite sex. Some bulimics are perfectionists and high achievers.

There may also be biochemical imbalances such as blood-sugar fluctuations and hormonal or neurotransmitter imbalances that affect mood and behaviour.

Action plan

Seek psychological help – you can ask your GP about what is available. Cognitive Behavioural Therapy works well for many.

⠿ EAT/DRINK

► Protein. Good-quality protein is needed to keep blood-sugar levels stable. Include lentils, beans, nuts, seeds, fish, lean white meats and eggs.

► Vegetable juices – vomiting and laxative abuse both lead to electrolyte imbalances. Vegetable juices are rich in minerals that can correct this imbalance.

⠿ AVOID

► Sugar, refined carbohydrates, junk foods, caffeine and alcohol which can upset blood-sugar balance, are unsatisfying and lead to cravings for more. You may experience withdrawal symptoms when you first cut these out but it is worth persevering.

► Wheat – especially in bread, cereals and cakes that you crave or binge on. Bulimics often become intolerant to wheat because of eating it excessively. Endorphins are released when you eat something to which you are intolerant, leading to cravings for more.

SUPPLEMENTS

► Supplement with acidophilus capsules. Purging and eating sugar and refined carbohydrates both disrupt the gut bacteria and encourage yeasts and unhelpful bacteria to grow.

Supplementing with some good bacteria can help to replenish the good guys and restore gut function.

► Take a good-quality multivitamin/ mineral complex. You are likely to be low in many nutrients. The vitamin supplement will help to restore levels and aid physical and biochemical recovery.

► Take extra zinc.

⠿ EXTRA TIPS

► Aim to eat small, regular meals and snacks throughout the day – this will keep blood-sugar levels balanced and will reduce cravings and the likelihood of bingeing.

► See a homeopath. Homeopathy can go a long way to helping this condition.

Food has made a positive change in my life, after battling with eating disorders for over a decade. I have been recovered for about two years now. I have educated myself about food and nutrition and I am still learning loads. Eating healthily has brought a positive change to my life as I have more energy, generally feel better, my mind is more balanced, and I have energy to help others, which I love doing. Destroying my body all those years has left me with osteoporosis, digestive problems, intolerances and I now have faith in good, nutritious food that will help me on the road to proper healing and recovery!

BURNS AND SCALDS

Burns are caused by dry heat and scalds are caused by moist heat. Burns are classified according to degrees of severity. First-degree burns are identified by the skin not being broken. Second-degree burns are when the skin is broken and blistered. Burns more severe than this need hospital treatment.

Action plan

This action plan is designed to help the healing process through boosting your nutrition.

⠿ EAT/DRINK

► Water: rehydration is important.
► Carrot juice, a fantastic source of beta-carotene which can aid the healing of the skin.
► Cucumber juice is also useful as a topical treatment for burns.
► Brightly coloured fruit and vegetables – these contain antioxidants needed for healing. Vegetable juices would also be recommended for their high nutrient and healing properties.
► Foods rich in vitamin C, such as berries, broccoli and bell peppers, to help your skin to heal.

⠿ AVOID

► Alcohol suppresses the immune system, depletes nutrients and is dehydrating, which may slow the healing process.

HERBS AND SUPPLEMENTS

► Astragalus to help the body adapt to the stress of dealing with the burns.
► Take 1 tbsp of flaxseed oil daily – for anti-inflammatory and healing effects.
► Take 50mg zinc once or twice daily.
► Vitamins A, C, E and B complex.
► L-glutamine.

⠿ EXTRA TIPS

► Do not remove clothing that is adhering to the wound; cut round it if necessary.
► First- and second-degree burns should be immediately cooled under cold running water for at least 10 minutes.
► Raw white potato slices can be cooling to burns.
► Never put butter or greasy creams on burns. The heat of the burn will get worse and the pain will increase.
► Apply aloe vera gel or the pulp from aloe vera leaves after cooling to ease pain.
► Apply manuka honey with lint – manuka honey has traditionally been used in the treatment of burns to prevent infection and speed healing.
► Apply nettle tea to reduce pain. This can also be taken as a drink.
► Make a paste of slippery elm powder mixed with milk and apply to aid healing.
► Keep the burnt area elevated to prevent swelling and lightly covered to reduce the danger of infection.

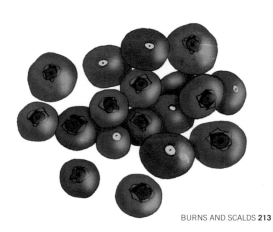

B

BURSITIS

Bursitis is inflammation of the fluid-filled sacs called bursae that provide a cushion between the tendons and bones. Common areas to be affected include the elbows, knees, hips and shoulders. Other names for bursitis include tennis elbow, frozen shoulder, bunions and weaver's bottom!

Symptoms include inflammation, swelling, dull, persistent pain and reduced range of motion.

CAUSES
► Injury.
► Wear and tear.
► Rheumatism or arthritis.
► Food intolerances.
► Calcium deposits.

Action plan

The following nutrition advice is to aid any conventional treatment you may need for your condition. It focuses on anti-inflammatory foods and plenty of antioxidants to help repair damaged tissue.

⠿ EAT/DRINK
► Essential fats for their anti-inflammatory and healing effects. Good sources include oily fish, nuts, seeds and cold-pressed oils.
► Raw fruit and vegetables and juices for their antioxidant content. Antioxidants are needed by the immune system for repairing damaged tissue.
► Fresh pineapple between meals. The core of pineapple contains the enzyme bromelain which can help to reduce inflammation.

HERBS AND SUPPLEMENTS
► Horsetail tea which contains silica needed for tissue repair.
► Other good teas to drink include nettle and celery seed as they remove excess fluids, and pau d'arco for its anti-inflammatory effect.
► Take devil's claw extract for its anti-inflammatory, analgesic and anti-rheumatic properties.
► Take magnesium citrate if there are calcium deposits. Magnesium is needed for the proper utilization of calcium in the body. Without sufficient magnesium relative to calcium, calcium can be deposited inappropriately.
► Take sublingual (placed under the tongue for quick, maximum absorption) supplements of vitamin B12. Magnesium, calcium and vitamin D are important, too. You need more magnesium than calcium.
► Use turmeric liberally in your cooking. It contains curcumin which has powerful anti-inflammatory effects.

⠿ EXTRA TIPS
► Apply cold packs to affected areas.
► Get outside in daylight with some skin exposed for at least 20 minutes a day. Daylight is the best source of vitamin D which is needed for proper calcium utilization and healthy bones.
► Stop any activity that aggravates the pain and take it easy physically.

CANCER

Among the most feared of diseases, cancer begins with just one abnormal cell that multiplies out of control. Clusters of these cells form tumours, which can interfere with healthy tissues and spread to other parts of the body.

Cancer cells are caused by substances called carcinogens – cancer-forming compounds that are present in foods, in the air, and are even produced inside our bodies. Most of these compounds are neutralized before they can do harm, but continual exposure may eventually lead them to damage the genetic material inside healthy cells, which over time can manifest as cancer.

It is estimated that more than one in three people will develop cancer during their lifetime. Although there are at least 200 different types of cancer, breast (page 206), lung (page 321), bowel (page 203) and prostate (page 349) cancers account for over half of all new cases in the UK, with breast cancer being the most common.

The good news is that because as much as 80 per cent of all cancers are due to known factors, the disease is highly preventable. Smoking is responsible for 30 per cent of cancer cases, while as much as 35 to 50 per cent are linked to unhealthy eating habits.

CAUSES AND RISK FACTORS
► Age: the chances of developing cancer increase with age.
► High saturated-fat diet.
► High intake of red or processed meat.
► Being overweight or obese.
► Alcohol.
► Smoking and passive smoking.
► Inactivity.
► High levels of hormones such as oestrogen and testosterone.
► Air pollution.
► Ionizing radiation.
► Ultraviolet radiation from the sun.
► Industrial chemicals.
► Medications.
► Viruses.
► Family history.

SYMPTOMS MAY INCLUDE
► Lumps or swelling
► Bleeding
► Pain (although pain is not always present in the early stages).
► Enlarged lymph nodes.
► Poor appetite.
► Fatigue.
► Weight loss.
► Night sweats.
► Anaemia.

Action Plan

The following plan is based on scientifically proven ways to reduce your cancer risk. It can also be used as a holistic food and lifestyle guide alongside conventional cancer treatments or other chosen forms of cancer therapy. If you are being treated for cancer, make sure you check with your GP before making any of the suggested dietary changes and/ or supplements.

❖ EAT/DRINK
► Vegetables and fruit in abundance. These food groups are rich in vitamin C

and phytonutrients and reduce the risk of many cancers. Eat eight to nine portions. Five a day is not enough. Variety is the key, so include fruit and veg from all the colour spectrums to ensure you get a wide range of nutrients and antioxidants. Besides eating plenty of salads and fresh fruit, you can increase the amount you eat by adding extra vegetables to soups, stir fries and casseroles, and piling them into sandwiches. When cooking vegetables, choose methods that limit nutrient loss such as steaming, water stir frying and baking.

► More raw food. That means eating more fruit and vegetables in an uncooked state.

► Betacarotene-rich foods including carrots, sweet potatoes, kale, spinach and winter squash. Betacarotene is an antioxidant and immune booster. In addition, the body is able to convert it into vitamin A, which helps cells reproduce normally.

► Tomatoes. This fruit contains a carotenoid antioxidant called lycopene (also found in sweet red peppers) that has been found to inhibit the proliferation of cancer cells and may help protect against cancers of the prostate, lung, stomach, pancreas, bowel, oesophagus, mouth, breast and cervix. However, some people are sensitive to a compound called solanine in tomatoes. If you have arthritic-like symptoms and/or joint pain, it is not a food that I would feature in high amounts in an anti-cancer regime. It is possible to get supplements of lycopene from a health-food store.

► Cruciferous vegetables including broccoli, cabbage, Brussels sprouts, cauliflower, cabbage, kale, swede, turnips, pak choi and watercress. You can obtain several anti-cancer compounds from this family of foods such as indole-3-carbinol, glucaric acid and sulphoraphane.

► Sprouted seeds and legumes as they are an excellent source of vitamins, minerals and enzymes. Sprouted broccoli seeds are especially good as they contain sulphoraphane glucosinolate, a precursor to the anti-cancer compound sulphoraphane, in amounts of up to 50 times higher than those found in broccoli.

► High-fibre foods, particularly those rich in insoluble fibre such as whole grains (brown rice, millet, wholemeal bread) and cereals. Other good sources of fibre include beans, lentils, peas, fruit and vegetables. People who eat a high-fibre diet have been reported to have a low risk of many cancers.

► Phyto-oestrogen-rich foods such as soya (tofu) and flaxseed, and to a lesser extent sesame seeds, oats, barley, chickpeas, lentils, alfalfa, apples, wheat germ and fennel. These foods have a mild oestrogenic effect which appears to be protective against some cancers (breast, prostate and colon).

► Foods high in essential fatty acids including seeds like raw shelled hemp seeds, nuts, dark leafy green vegetables, tofu and unrefined vegetable oils such as flaxseed oil.

► A small handful of raw almonds daily as they contain anti-cancer properties.

► Garlic has been found to lower the risk of oesophageal, stomach and bowel cancers, which may be due to its ability to reduce the development of carcinogenic compounds in the body. So try to include garlic in your diet regularly.

► Oily fish as it is a good source of cancer-protective omega-3 fats.

► Freshly pressed fruit and vegetable juices as they are concentrated in anti-cancer phytochemicals and help to boost the immune system. They also cleanse, nourish and hydrate the body.

► Include sea vegetables in the diet: kombu, wakame, dulse, nori once or twice a week.

► Water, to help keep the cells cleansed and hydrated.

► Compounds in green tea called polyphenols (antioxidants) have been associated with a reduced risk of several cancers.

⁘ AVOID

► Red and processed meats as they are high in saturated fats, devoid of fibre and contain toxins.

► Foods high in saturated fat including meat, eggs, cheese, milk, butter and cream. High intakes of this type of fat increase cancer risk.

► Fried foods, margarine and foods containing margarine such as pies, cakes and biscuits. These generally contain lots of saturated fat, hydrogenated fat and trans-fats.

► Refined grains and white flour products such as white rice, white bread and white pasta, as they lack fibre and have been robbed of many nutrients.

► Processed foods as they will increase the body's toxic load.

► Sugar and foods that contain sugar, as they lack nutrients and deplete the body of essential vitamins and minerals. Opt for naturally sweet foods such as fresh and dried fruit instead. Make sure dried fruit is free of sulphur dioxide.

► Salt.

► Alcohol as it lacks nutritional value and has a negative impact on the liver, which is the main organ of detoxification. Too much alcohol has been linked to an increased risk of cancer of the mouth, larynx, oesophagus, liver, breast and possibly bowel.

► Black tea and coffee. Instead, drink grain-based coffee substitutes and herbal teas such as nettle, fennel, camomile, peppermint and ginger.

HERBS

► Echinacea, red clover and astragalus all help to support the immune system.

► Cat's claw enhances immune function and has antioxidant activity.

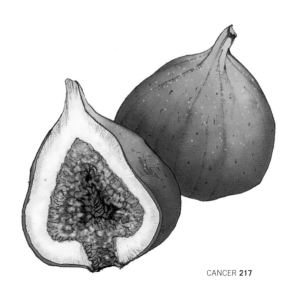

C

▶ Reishi mushroom has anti-cancer and immune-boosting effects.

▶ Siberian ginseng may help the body to recover from chemotherapy and radiation therapy more quickly.

SUPPLEMENTS

▶ Betacarotene, buffered vitamin C, vitamin E and selenium are all antioxidant nutrients which help protect the body against cancer-forming agents.

▶ Vitamin B complex to boost energy levels and aid normal cell function.

▶ Co-enzyme Q10. This is produced naturally in the body and improves cellular oxygenation. It also has antioxidant properties and stimulates the immune system.

▶ IP-6, also known as inositol hexa-phosphate, has been reported to have anti-cancer activity.

▶ Vitamin D supplementation may help protect against cancer of the breast, colon, prostrate, ovary, lungs and pancreas.

▶ Salvestrols. These natural plant compounds indirectly target cancer cells and help to destroy them. Cells affected by cancer contain an enzyme called CYP1B1. Salvestrols get converted by this enzyme into chemicals which can kill the diseased cells. Because the CYP1B1 enzyme is not present in healthy cells, salvestrols exert no effects there.

⠿ EXTRA TIPS

▶ Opt for organic food whenever possible.

▶ Going vegetarian or vegan is an option to seriously consider as studies have found that vegetarians are less likely to develop cancer.

▶ Buy natural organic cleaning products, toiletries and cosmetics instead of chemically based ones.

▶ Reduce your exposure to xeno-oestrogens – toxic man-made compounds present in pesticides, weedkiller, paints, adhesives and plastics.

▶ Don't smoke and avoid passive smoking.

▶ Maintain a healthy body weight as overweight and obesity are associated with an increased cancer risk.

▶ Get regular exercise as this will help to keep your weight in check and has a cancer-preventive effect.

▶ Try to avoid stress and practise relaxation techniques such as meditation.

▶ Reduce exposure to air pollution, industrial chemicals and ionizing radiation.

▶ Protect yourself from the sun with regular use of sunscreen and sun-protective clothing.

My wife, Josie, is recovering from breast cancer, having completed all her hospital treatment. Following the chemotherapy and radiation she felt less and less well, with backaches, a loss of energy and her taste not fully returned. We purchased Gillian's *You Are What You Eat* and upon checking Josie's tongue it appeared she had a vitamin B deficiency. So off I went to purchase vitamin B supplements together with an aloe vera drink. The change in Josie within two hours was remarkable; she felt more energetic, her backache was reduced (not 100% gone but certainly loads better) and she has now returned to her part-time work after 11 months off!

CANDIDIASIS

Everyone has a certain amount of yeast growing within the body. But an overgrowth or excess of yeast can lead to conditions including thrush, vaginal infection and candidiasis. Candidiasis occurs when the unhealthy bacteria or yeast take over the healthy bacteria in the gut, and the proper balance of intestinal flora is upset.

Certain events in a life might trigger these overgrowth yeast problems: for example, stress, divorce, job loss, illness or death of a loved one. Pregnancy and giving birth can trigger candidiasis in women. And even a poor diet of junk food can bring it on, especially if the liver is not working optimally.

Candidiasis is frequently misdiagnosed or ignored. Symptoms might include chronic fatigue, headaches, digestive disorders, bloating, oedema, mental dullness, confusion, severe and multiple allergies and chemical or food sensitivities.

Primary diagnosis is through a test that shows abnormal production of the alcohol ethanol in the gut. It is best to have blood, stool and other biochemical tests to evaluate the presence and extent of candidiasis.

Study the following Candida Self Check so that you may evaluate your own symptoms. If you think that you may have candidiasis, I urge you to consult your GP and a nutritionist or herbalist.

SYMPTOMS
- Athlete's foot.
- Bloating.
- Clogged sinuses.
- Confusion (brain fog).
- Constipation.
- Diarrhoea.
- Digestive disturbances.
- Easy bruising.
- Excessive mucus.
- Exhaustion.
- Flaky skin.
- Flatulence.
- Food allergies.
- Headaches/migraines.
- Hypoglycaemia (low blood-sugar levels).
- Sensitivity to odours, fumes.
- Joint/facial/ear pain.
- Loss of libido.
- Mucus in stools.
- Night sweats.
- Persistent cough.
- Premenstrual tension.
- Recurrent sinusitis.
- Insomnia.
- Sick feeling all over.
- Sore, burning tongue.
- Vaginal/anal itching.

Action plan

Improving the strength of the liver is critical in preventing and combating candidiasis.

STAGE ONE: MODIFY DIET (MONTH 1)
EAT/DRINK IN ABUNDANCE
- Wheat grass and barley grass.
- Kale and collards.
- Radishes, parsley and watercress.
- Dandelion greens.
- Chard and celery.
- Broccoli and cabbage.
- Brussels sprouts.
- Runner beans and aduki beans.

- Horseradish and ginger.
- Squashes and pumpkins.
- Scallions, onions and garlic.
- Sea vegetables: nori, kombu and dulse.
- Grains: millet, buckwheat, rye, amaranth, quinoa.
- Sprouts: sprouted barley, rice, millet, quinoa.

⠿ AVOID
- Alcohol.
- Sugar and sweets.
- Breads or baked goods with added yeast.
- Mushrooms.
- Dairy products.
- Coffee and conventional teas.
- Sodas or carbonated drinks.
- Wheat.
- Citrus fruits.

⠿ EAT/DRINK IN MODERATION
- Potatoes, sweet potatoes and yams.
- Fruit.
- Red meat.
- Eggs.
- Fermented foods (vinegar, soy sauce, mustard).
- Tomatoes.
- Nuts.

STAGE TWO: BUILD NUTRITIONAL FOUNDATION (MONTH 2)
SUPPLEMENTS
- Take wild blue-green algae – the algae essentially dries the excess mucus and helps to drain dampness from the body. It also helps to raise the levels of micronutrients including zinc, selenium, iron, magnesium and calcium.
- Take biotin which prevents the yeast from budding full circle.
- Drink aloe vera juice which is anti-fungal and anti-parasitic.
- Take superfood powders, such as Gillian McKeith's Organic Energy Powder, which strengthen digestive organs, rebalance healthy flora, and contain active enzymes, antioxidants, vitamins, minerals and essential fatty acids.

STAGE THREE: STRENGTHEN LIVER (MONTH 3)
SUPPLEMENTS
- Silymarin stimulates the manufacture of new liver cells and increases the production of glutathione and bile.
- Lipotrophic formula contains the nutrients choline, betaine and methionine, which enhance liver function and increase the levels of two important liver compounds: S-adenosylmethionine (SAM) and glutathione.

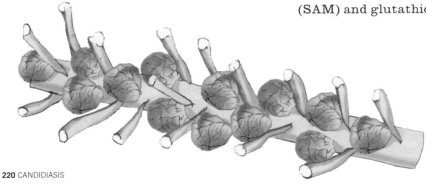

STAGE FOUR: ROTATION OF ANTI-FUNGAL HERBS (MONTH 4) HERBS

Use one herb only per week. At the end of the week, move on to the next herb. My top four (for a course of a month) recommendations are caprylic acid, gentiana, pau d'arco and barberry.

► Barberry (berberis vulgaris).
► Oregon grape.
► Black walnut.
► Burdock root.
► Caprylic acid.
► Chaparral.
► Echinacea/golden seal combination.
► Grapefruit seed extract (liquid drops).
► Garlic (liquid).
► Suma (pfaffia paniculata).
► Gentiana.
► Tanalbit.
► Pau d'arco.
► Wormwood.
► Red clover.
► Plus propolis.*

For example, use pau d'arco every day for one week. Then stop the pau d'arco and start red clover the next, and so on. If you use these herbs in tea form, then drink 2 to 3 cups a day. If you are using herbal capsules, tablets or tinctures, then please follow directions on the label.

*Propolis should be taken during the entire herbal rotation in addition to one other herb.

STAGE FIVE: STRENGTHEN DIGESTIVE SYSTEM (MONTH 5)

► Guar gum helps to promote good bowel movements.
► Triphala helps to promote good bowel movements.

► Digestive enzymes complex contain proteases which help to keep intestines free of parasites and yeasts.
► Betaine w/HCL before meals.

FINAL STAGE: INTRODUCE FRIENDLY BACTERIA (MONTH 6)

► Lactobacillus acidophilus and bifidobacteria bifidus.

CANKER SORES

Also called apthous ulcers, they are small, painful ulcers on the lips, gums, tongue and inside the cheeks. They are usually red but can be filled with yellowish fluids containing white blood cells and bacteria. The development of the ulcer is usually preceded by burning and tingling in the area.

CAUSES

► Being run-down and stressed.
► Fungal infections.
► Dental problems.
► Food intolerances.
► Viral infections.
► Nutrient deficiencies.

Action plan

Building immunity is the main goal here, plus ensuring that you eat a varied diet as eating the same foods, day in, day out, can contribute to intolerances.

::: EAT/DRINK

► Brightly coloured fruit and vegetables.
► Whole grains: rye, oats, millet, quinoa and brown rice.
► Turkey, chicken and fish.

▶ Legumes.

▶ Watermelon, celery and cucumber which have cooling properties for reducing the pain of canker sores.

▶ Burdock-root coffee to cleanse the blood stream.

⠿ AVOID

▶ Acidic fruits such as citrus fruits, tomatoes, apples and plums as these may irritate the area.

▶ Spicy foods, alcohol and caffeine as these can act as local irritants.

▶ Sugar and refined foods as these are low in nutrients and suppress the immune system.

▶ Any foods to which you may be intolerant. Wheat is a common culprit.

HERBS AND SUPPLEMENTS

▶ Pau d'arco tea for its anti-fungal and anti-inflammatory effects.

▶ Take probiotics, especially if there is a fungal overgrowth. These help to balance the gut bacteria and support the immune system.

▶ Take vitamin C. Canker sores can indicate a vitamin C deficiency.

▶ Take L-lysine before meals. This is an amino acid that is often deficient in those with canker sores and ulcers.

⠿ EXTRA TIPS

▶ Consult your dentist if dental problems or oral hygiene may be contributing.

▶ Use tea tree oil mouth wash – add 3 drops of tea tree oil to a small glass of water.

▶ Apply tea tree oil directly to the sores.

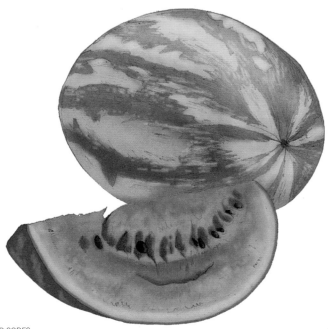

CARPAL TUNNEL SYNDROME

Carpal tunnel syndrome is characterized by numbness, weakness and pain along with burning or tingling in the fingers and wrists that may be worse at night. Flexion of the wrist may worsen symptoms. The pain may radiate up to the arm and shoulder.

CAUSES

Carpal tunnel syndrome is caused by compression of the nerves between the ligaments and carpal bone in the wrist. Repetitive and strenuous activities may trigger the syndrome. Injury or trauma to the wrist can sometimes be the cause. Nutrient deficiencies are also part of the picture, in particular vitamin B6 and omega-3 fats. People taking anti-depressants or oral contraceptives are at increased risk as these medications increase the requirements for vitamin B6.

Other linked conditions include arthritis, tendonitis, menopause, Raynaud's, hypothyroidism, diabetes and water retention, so these may need to be addressed as well.

Action plan

The aim is reduce potential fluid retention in the body, which when high contributes to pain.

EAT/DRINK

▶ Fresh pineapple between meals. The core of pineapple contains the enzyme bromelain, which has anti-inflammatory effects.
▶ Foods rich in vitamin B6. Nutritional yeast flakes, eggs, fish, peas, sunflower seeds, brown rice and alfalfa are all good sources.
▶ Essential fatty acids daily. These have an anti-inflammatory and lubricating effect. Salmon, mackerel, sardines, trout, herrings, hemp seeds, pumpkin seeds, flax seeds and avocados are all good sources.
▶ Add turmeric to beans, grains and vegetables during cooking. Turmeric has well-researched anti-inflammatory properties.

AVOID

▶ Oxalic acid found in spinach, chard, rhubarb, asparagus, beet greens and eggs.
▶ Salt, coffee, tea, alcohol, sugar and processed foods. These can all aggravate the condition through increased water retention or depletion of vitamins.
▶ Food containing additives. These can interfere with the utilization of vitamin B6 in the body. Especially avoid yellow dyes.
▶ Excessive consumption of meat protein.

HERBS AND SUPPLEMENTS

▶ Herbs such as cramp bark, butcher's broom, capsicum, marshmallow root, black cohosh, St John's wort and skullcap can be taken as tinctures or capsules.
▶ Supplement with vitamin B complex and B6. Carpal Tunnel Syndrome (CTS) can be a sign of B6 deficiency so supplementation can make a big difference.

EXTRA TIPS

▶ Identify whether the cause is due to specific activities and change your way of working, if necessary. Nowadays, CTS is often linked to computer use so get your posture and chair looked at. Changes in the way we sit can often make a huge difference. Your back should be relatively straight with your forearms parallel to the floor and feet flat on the ground.

C

▶ To prevent CTS, make sure you take regular breaks from tasks that affect the hands and wrists. Shake the hands out every hour and make circular movements in either direction with the wrists. Massage the wrists and hands to improve circulation to the area.
▶ Apply St John's wort oil or aloe vera gel to aid healing.
▶ Be careful of your position when sleeping. Sleep on your back with your hands by your side.

CELLULITE

A dimpled, chicken-skin appearance on the thighs and buttocks, cellulite is caused by clumps of unmetabolized fat, water and trapped wastes beneath the skin that push up against surrounding fibrous connective tissue. When these waste materials harden, dimples appear and you get what seem to be clumps of fat under your skin, creating a puckering effect. Once you have it, it is a fight to get rid of it. But what you don't want to do is add to it.

CAUSES MAY INCLUDE
▶ Lack of sleep.
▶ Poor diet.
▶ Lack of fibre.
▶ Too many saturated fats.
▶ An overworked liver.
▶ Hereditary factors.
▶ Poor blood circulation.
▶ Poor lymphatic flow, possibly due to lack of adequate water intake.
▶ Hormonal imbalance.

Action plan

Reducing the amount of fat in the body, increasing circulation of the lymph, taking care of your liver, eating a nutritious diet and treating unbalanced oestrogen levels can all contribute to helping you finally be free from the bonds of cellulite!

⠿ EAT/DRINK
▶ Cruciferous veggies: these are rich in lecithin, a nutrient that can help to repair tissue damage in skin cells. Research has shown that cabbage-leaf protein can help to break down toxins in the liver. A build up of toxins in the blood is thought to trigger or cause cellulite.
▶ Kale.
▶ Collards.
▶ Broccoli.
▶ Cabbage.
▶ Brussels sprouts.
▶ Kohlrabi.
▶ Cauliflower.
▶ Pak choi.
▶ Chinese cabbage.
▶ Turnip root.
▶ Rutabaga.
▶ Mustard greens.
▶ Radishes.
▶ Daikon.
▶ Horseradish.
▶ Wasabi.
▶ Arugula.
▶ Watercress.
▶ Berries: a potent source of antioxidants and protective nutrients that can combat the free radicals and tissue damage that cause cellulite. Goji berries are particularly beneficial as they are packed with nutrients and flavanoids that

support liver health and aid cellulite-beating detoxification.

► Sprouted broccoli seeds: sulphoraphane, an active compound found in broccoli and highly concentrated in broccoli sprouts, has been shown to boost liver and skin cells' detoxifying abilities.

► Grapefruit which significantly increases the production and activity of liver detoxification enzymes.

► Foods containing good fats such as flaxseed, flaxseed oil, walnuts, Brazil nuts, raw shelled hemp seeds, oily fish and omega-3 enriched eggs.

► Balance your oestrogen levels through diet. Make sure your diet is rich in fruits, vegetables, fibre and essential fatty acids.

► Remember to drink up to two litres of still, NOT fizzy, water daily.

⠿ AVOID

► Caffeine and carbonated drinks.

► Any foods that contain trans-fatty acids (cakes, biscuits) or are overcooked (this destroys vital nutrients).

► Red meat and dairy products as they are known to trigger oestrogen excess.

► Sugar, saturated fats and processed refined foods can also upset blood-sugar balance and trigger hormonal imbalance.

► Salt.

HERBS AND SUPPLEMENTS

► Liquid algae contains phytochemicals and plant pigments that are nourishing to the liver. A strong liver, nutritionally speaking, is a weapon in the war against cellulite.

► The herbal supplement gotu kola.

► Milk thistle also helps the liver to deal with its toxic load.

► Agnus castus in capsule or tincture form to help balance hormone levels.

⠿ EXTRA TIPS

► Stop smoking (it reduces blood flow to the skin, destroys vitamin C and is loaded with pollutants).

► Avoid exposure to excess sun, pollution or too much stress.

► Avoid liposuction as it may take away the cushion of fat under the skin. This may allow cellulite to settle.

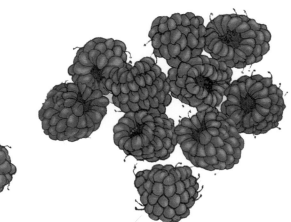

► Get a good night's sleep – around eight hours suits most of us. If you sleep for less than four hours a night, you are more likely to be overweight and have a flabby backside and wobbly thighs. Being tired slows your metabolism and can affect your food choices, making you go for high-calorie, fatty foods for a fast energy spurt.

► Brush the skin dry with a dry skin brush before you have a bath or shower. This action gets the lymph fluid moving which carries toxins out of the body, so reducing the chance of cellulite building up.

► Move your body. Exercise is one of the best ways to shift cellulite as it boosts blood and lymph circulation, encourages sweating and removal of waste materials and restores a slim subcutaneous fat layer. Aerobic exercises that raise your heart rate combined with gentle toning is the best type of anti-cellulite exercise prescription. BUT avoid excessive exercise (which stresses the body to form free radicals).

► Tone areas of the body such as the buttocks and thighs, which are prime areas for cellulite, with leg curls and squats. You don't need to lift heavy weights to get rid of cellulite. Consistent, frequent exercise is the key.

CHLAMYDIA

Chlamydia is one of the most common sexually transmitted diseases (STDs). It is caused by the chlamydial trachomatis micro-organism and can affect both men and women. Symptoms include irregular bleeding, vaginal or urethral discharge, problems with urination, genital inflammation, itching and some pain. However, you can have the disease with no apparent symptoms. If left untreated, women may develop pelvic inflammatory disease (PID), damage to the fallopian tubes and infertility. Men may suffer prostatitis and problems with their reproductive organs.

CAUSES

Being sexually active without taking precautions puts you at risk of contracting the infection. Babies can also acquire it at birth, when it can cause eye disorders.

Action plan

It is important to see your GP or visit a health clinic. Nutritionally, it will help to include foods that give extra support to your immune system.

EAT/DRINK

► Three portions of fresh fruit and five portions of fresh vegetables daily.

► Raw garlic which has potent antibacterial properties.

► Foods high in zinc such as pumpkin seeds, raw shelled hemp seeds, sesame seeds.

► Raw vegetable juices to help the immune system.

HERBS AND SUPPLEMENTS

► The immune-supportive herbs, echinacea, astragalus, goldenseal and barberry can all be taken as tinctures.
► Drink pau d'arco tea daily to support the immune system.
► Drink dandelion-root tea to support liver and bowel function.
► Supplement with acidophilus; beneficial bacteria can crowd out unhelpful bacteria and support immune function.

⠿ EXTRA TIPS

► Get tested if you suspect you may have chlamydia. Both partners must be tested and treated if necessary to avoid re-infection.
► Douche with 10 drops of golden seal extract in 30ml of witch hazel daily.

CHRONIC FATIGUE SYNDROME

Chronic fatigue syndrome (CFS) – also called Myalgic Encephalomyelitis (ME) – is characterized by chronic, unexplained tiredness. The criteria that would lead to a diagnosis include debilitating fatigue, not relieved by rest, lasting more than six months. Medical test results for hormonal imbalances, nutrient deficiencies and psychiatric problems are generally normal. The fatigue may be preceded by an illness such as glandular fever or flu but often the cause is unknown. Some people suffer with it for years and then get better. Others may have bouts that recur after an illness or period of stress.

SYMPTOMS

► Tiredness.
► Aches and pains.
► Loss of appetite.
► Anxiety.
► Depression.
► Headaches.
► Fever.
► Digestive problems.
► Poor concentration.
► Swollen glands.
► Brain fog.
► Sensitivity to light and noise.
► Poor sleep patterns.

CAUSES

Each individual diagnosed with CFS will have a different set of underlying causes. Contributory factors may include:
► Compromised immune system.
► Poor blood-sugar control.
► Viral or bacterial infections such as glandular fever.
► Use of antibiotics or other medication.
► Food intolerances.
► Compromised digestive function; parasites, bacteria, yeasts, digestive enzyme and stomach acid insufficiency and intestinal permeability may all be part of the picture.
► Chronic stress and adrenal fatigue.
► Malfunctioning general endocrine (hormonal) system.
► Diet low in nutrients and high in toxins.
► Chemical and environmental sensitivities.
► Pollution and heavy-metal poisoning, e.g., from mercury amalgam fillings.
Conditions that may be mistaken for chronic fatigue include anaemia (see page 185), fibromyalgia (see page 270),

Lyme disease, hepatitis, cancer (see page 215) and depression (see page 243).

Action plan

It is advisable to consult a medical practitioner in order to ascertain and address all the possible underlying imbalances. It is often too difficult to try and manage this condition on your own. You need weekly guidance and help.

⁛ EAT/DRINK

► Organic foods which are higher in nutrients and lower in toxic chemicals that can stress the immune system.
► At least two litres of water or herbal teas a day.
► Vegetable juices. They provide easily available nutrition without creating any challenge for the digestive system. Good vegetables to include are carrots, beetroots, radishes, celery, cabbage, chard, fennel, parsley, ginger and alfalfa sprouts. Apples can be added for sweetness.
► Fruit and vegetables which provide antioxidants needed for a well-functioning immune system. Aim for 2–3 pieces of fruit a day plus 6 servings of vegetables.
► Oily fish three times a week. These contain the anti-inflammatory essential fats.
► Seeds such as hemp, pumpkin, sunflower and flax. Aim for 2–3 tbsp daily.
► Sea veggies. Seaweeds contain much needed minerals. Brown-rice sushi, for example, is packed with minerals and much needed vitamin B.
► Foods that are not mucus-producing such as adzuki beans, celery, turnips, kohlrabi, amaranth, lettuce, squash and pumpkin.

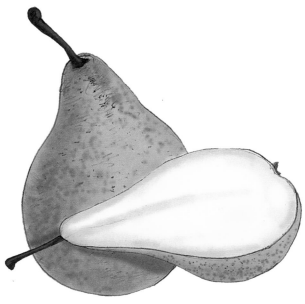

C

⠿ AVOID

▶ Sugar, refined carbohydrates, alcohol, caffeine and processed foods. These can all lead to highs and lows of blood-sugar levels.

▶ Food to which you are intolerant because they stress the immune system leading to fatigue. Take the pulse test (see page 180) to determine what you may be reacting to. Common culprits include gluten grains (wheat, rye, oats, barley, kamut and spelt), dairy products, soya, nightshade family vegetables (potatoes, tomatoes, peppers, aubergines, chillies and tobacco), eggs, chocolate and peanuts. For an in-depth food intolerance analysis, go to www.gillianmckeith.info.

HERBS AND SUPPLEMENTS

▶ Herbs that can help to improve energy, immune function and mood include Siberian ginseng and astragalus. Seek advice before taking these.

▶ Green superfoods such as chlorella, wheat and sprouted barley grass, algae and spirulina can help with nourishment and cleansing.

▶ Supplement with evening primrose oil and fish oils. These can help to improve energy and overall functioning.

▶ Supplement with magnesium malate. Magnesium is needed for energy as well as relaxation.

▶ Take co-enzyme Q10. This can help to oxygenate the tissues and improve energy.

⠿ EXTRA TIPS

▶ Support your digestive system. Digestive enzymes taken with meals can improve absorption of nutrients needed for energy. It is also important to chew thoroughly and to relax when eating.

▶ Take probiotics to normalize gut bacteria. Healthy gut bacteria play a big role in immunity and digestion.

▶ Support your liver. An overloaded liver can lead to feelings of toxicity and tiredness. The liver plays an important role in digestion and absorption as well as detoxification. Milk thistle is a great liver regenerator. Take this daily and drink dandelion-root coffee.

▶ Drink pau d'arco and camomile teas which help to combat yeast overgrowth and reduce intestinal damp.

▶ Make sure your bowels are moving 2–3 times a day. A clogged-up colon will only contribute to toxicity and fatigue. Soaked figs and prunes can be eaten before breakfast to promote bowel function.

▶ Get plenty of rest. It is important not to overexert yourself. You may have days when you feel you have more energy but overdoing it on these days can wipe you out for the next few days. Pace yourself. Take herbs to aid sleep if necessary. Camomile, lime flowers, hops, passionflower and skullcap are all good for promoting restful sleep.

▶ Use only natural products around the home and bathroom. Those with chronic fatigue are often more sensitive to the chemicals found in most household products. Visit your health-food store for natural and organic cleaning products, shampoos and soaps.

▶ Useful therapies may include cranial osteopathy, manual lymphatic drainage and aromatherapy massage.

▶ For further information, go to www. gillianmckeith.info/chronicfatigue.

CIRRHOSIS OF THE LIVER

Liver cirrhosis refers to a condition in which, over time, liver cells have become hardened and fibrotic. Scar tissue builds up and blood cannot flow freely into or out of the liver, reducing liver function. The liver has many important functions in the body including detoxification; blood-sugar and cholesterol control; digestion and absorption of protein, fats and carbohydrates to name a few. The liver is an organ that can usually regenerate well but in cases of cirrhosis, the liver cells may not be replaced in the way they would be in a healthy liver.

SYMPTOMS

► Nausea.
► Constipation.
► Diarrhoea.
► Loss of appetite.
► Indigestion.
► Low-grade fever.
► Fatigue.
► Muscle weakness.
► Eye problems.
► Jaundice.

CAUSES

The most common cause is chronic and excessive alcohol use. Other factors include damage from gallstones, drugs, previous bacterial or viral infections, such as hepatitis, obesity and poor diet generally.

Action plan

Your liver needs support, and there is much you can do to help through changing your diet and lifestyle.

EAT/DRINK

► Dandelion-root coffee to help to get the bile flowing from the liver to the gallbladder and into the bowel. This is needed for proper digestion of fats and bowel function and is often reduced in those with cirrhosis of the liver.
► Regular cups of warm water and lemon are helpful.
► Low-fat, sugar-free food. Fat digestion is dependent on good liver function. Small amounts of healthy fats such as olive oil, flaxseed and hemp seed oils can be used in salad dressings.
► Fish and vegetable proteins such as pulses, nuts, seeds and soya.
► Raw fruits and vegetables. These foods will take the strain off the liver and provide abundant antioxidants needed for healing. Try consuming only freshly pressed juices and raw fruits and vegetables for three days.
► Globe artichokes containing cynarine which has been shown to increase the flow of bile, aiding the digestion of fats and improving bowel function.
► Beetroot is rich in antioxidants and is cleansing and detoxifying.
► Foods from the onion family, such as garlic, spring onions and chives. These contain sulphur, an important nutrient for the liver.
► Green foods. These contain chlorophyll and vitamin K as well as sulphur. Chlorophyll is excellent for cleansing and rejuvenating the cells. Vitamin K is needed to reduce bleeding and bruising. Cabbage, broccoli, Brussels sprouts, kale, cavolo nero, pak choi, chicory, watercress and salad leaves are all beneficial.

► Plain foods rather than heavily spiced or flavoured food. Brown rice or quinoa with steamed vegetables or fish with green salads are good examples.

⠿ **AVOID**

► Sugar, margarine, heated fats, fried foods, processed meats, pastries, dairy products, crisps, caffeine, refined carbohydrates and foods containing additives.

► Alcohol. If you carry on drinking, your liver function will just deteriorate further. If necessary, seek help. It is easier to give up alcohol if the rest of the diet is nutritious so work on this as well.

HERBS AND SUPPLEMENTS

► Sprinkle turmeric on food to help to regenerate liver tissue and aid liver function. It can also get the bile flowing.

► Other useful herbs and spices include ginger, rosemary and cayenne pepper in small amounts.

► Take milk thistle which has excellent liver rejuvenating properties.

► Supplement your diet with green superfoods. Blue-green algae, spirulina and wheat and barley grasses all contain an abundance of nutrients needed for detoxification and cell renewal.

► Supplement meals with digestive enzymes. Look for those containing lipase as this will aid fat digestion.

COELIAC DISEASE

Coeliac disease is caused by an intolerance to gluten found in wheat, rye, oats and barley. In coeliacs the gliadin protein in gluten damages the lining of the intestine. This impairs the absorption of nutrients and can cause serious malnutrition. About 1 per cent of the population are thought to be coeliacs. It may be diagnosed in babies when they are first given cereal grains. However, many people do not get diagnosed until they are in their forties. If untreated, more serious health problems can develop, such as infertility and osteoporosis.

SYMPTOMS

► Diarrhoea.

► Abdominal swelling.

► Weight loss.

► Pale, foul-smelling stools that float and don't flush easily.

► Muscle and joint pain.

► Inability to gain weight.

► Fatigue.

► Nutrient deficiencies.

CAUSES MAY INCLUDE

► Genetic components.

► Food allergies.

► Gluten intolerance.

► Abnormal auto-immune reaction.

Action plan

If you suspect you may have coeliac disease, get your GP to run a test. And you must make changes to your diet, otherwise you will be miserable.

⊞ EAT/DRINK

▸ Gluten-free grains such as brown rice, red rice, wild rice, buckwheat, quinoa, millet, amaranth, polenta and corn.

▸ Bananas: mashed with slippery elm powder and arrowroot, they provide good nourishment for babies and children with coeliac disease.

▸ Beans, nuts and seeds.

▸ Fruit, vegetables, fish, lean white meats, eggs and sea vegetables.

⊞ AVOID

▸ Alcohol containing glutens such as beer, wine, whisky and vodka.

▸ Icecream and packaged foods, especially soups, which contain glutens.

▸ Wheat, rye, barley, kamut, spelt and oats which contain glutens.

▸ Seasonings and sauces when eating out. Foods you would not expect to contain gluten often do.

HERBS AND SUPPLEMENTS

▸ Take aloe vera juice before each meal to aid digestion and bowel function.

▸ Drink alfalfa tea. This is extremely nourishing and is particularly useful when digestion has been compromised.

▸ Drink blood-nourishing yellow dock tea.

▸ Slippery elm powder can help to soothe the gut.

▸ Take protein-digesting enzymes with meals. Papein, from papayas, has been found to help in the digesting of wheat gluten once you have had gluten out of your system for at least six months.

▸ Liquid superfoods such as liquid algae, spirulina and other green foods can give you much needed minerals and vitamins.

▸ Liquid B vitamins, especially vitamin B6.

▸ Zinc.

▸ Pyridoxal 5 phosphate.

⊞ EXTRA TIPS

▸ Don't avoid restaurants but do have the confidence to always ask about food on the menu and whether a dish is gluten free.

▸ Check whether you are sensitive to the wheat husk and not just to the gluten part of the wheat. Some gluten-free foods are not wheat free and you may suffer the same reaction. It is also worth checking if you are lactose intolerant as this often goes hand in hand with wheat/gluten intolerance.

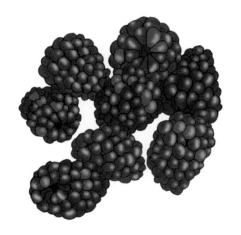

COLD SORES

Cold sores are caused by the herpes simplex virus which is related to the herpes virus that causes chickenpox and shingles. It can remain dormant in the body for years. Many people carry the virus but do not suffer from cold sores. They usually appear on the lips, around the mouth or nose and sometimes the eyes.

Early symptoms include burning or tingling, then a blister usually forms from which pus may emerge. Cold sores can be extremely painful and may last 2–3 weeks.

CAUSES MAY INCLUDE
► Bright sunlight.
► Stress.
► Compromised immune function.
► Poor diet.
► Hypothyroidism.
► Low iron levels.
► Menstrual period.
► Hormonal imbalances.
► Amino acid imbalances.

Action plan

Cold sores are often a sign that you are run down, so you need to look after yourself and your diet.

EAT/DRINK
► Fresh fruit and vegetables and vegetable juice. Fruit and vegetables contain antioxidants needed by the immune system to help to fight infections.
► Water – up to two litres daily.
► Mung beans, mung bean sprouts, lima beans and fish. These contain lysine which inhibits the growth of the cold-sore virus.

► Zinc-rich foods, including fish, pumpkin seeds, raw shelled hemp seeds, brown rice, chicken and sesame seeds.

AVOID
► Sugar, coffee, alcohol, refined foods, spices, saturated fats and fried foods. These can irritate and suppress the immune system.
► Chocolate and peanuts. These contain arginine which can perpetuate the virus.
► Wheat, carob, soya, oats, meat, dairy products, coconut, gelatine, pineapples, tomatoes, walnuts and shellfish.

HERBS AND SUPPLEMENTS
► Pau d'arco or lemon balm tea. Both have immune-boosting and anti-viral properties.
► Drink aloe vera juice and swoosh it around in your mouth so that the cold sore comes in contact with the aloe juice.
► Astragalus for general immunity. This will speed recovery.
► Supplement with L-lysine (take on an empty stomach 20–30 minutes before meals) and vitamin C with bioflavanoids.
► Zinc citrate.

EXTRA TIPS
► Apply a cut garlic clove to the sore twice a day. Garlic has antiviral properties. It is also beneficial to include raw garlic in the diet.
► Do not share towels or face cloths. The virus is contagious.

COMMON COLD

Keeping colds to a minimum is about strengthening immunity, especially through the winter. Runny noses, stuffy noses, sneezing, dull headache and sore throat are some of the symptoms of a common cold. Feeling under the weather and lethargic goes with these stuffed-up symptoms.

CAUSES MAY INCLUDE

▶ Poor immune system.

▶ Lack of zinc.

▶ Poor diet.

▶ Too much added sugar and sweeteners.

▶ Too many late nights.

▶ Being run down.

▶ Chronic stress.

▶ Air travel.

▶ Lack of ventilation indoors.

Action plan

If you really want to stop catching colds, you have to mean business and if you want the cold to not linger, you have to attack it, not just tickle it.

⦂⦂ EAT/DRINK

▶ Garlic. The compounds allicin and allium in garlic help to get rid of germs. Use garlic in soups, spreads, stews and, if you are brave, add it to veggie juice.

▶ Chicken which contains selenium and zinc, both needed for immune function. Research shows that chicken soup has an anti-inflammatory effect. Get organic chicken for the soup and add lots of vegetables to provide antioxidants and vitamins. Sipping the hot soup and inhaling the steam may clear congestion. Soup also provides hydration which is important for thinning mucus. Cook your soup with added garlic and onions for stronger effect.

▶ Eat hearty vegetable soups, too, and blend them for easy digestion. You can pack them with onions, ginger, scallions and garlic as well as other herbs and vegetables which are full of nutrients. Onions contain virus-fighting compounds. Eat them raw, too.

▶ Peppers can clear out your stuffy nose. You can use the fresh jalapeno type pepper or try a ¼ teaspoon of ground pepper (the red one) in some water.

▶ Use shitake mushrooms in your cooking. They have been shown to improve immune response.

▶ Add radishes to soups and salads.

▶ Lots of liquids. Teas are great to sweat it out of you. Ginger, camomile, peppermint, lemon and honey, elderflower and linden teas are all good. Peppermint tea can help to bring relief to a stuffy nose. Add some cinnamon powder to ginger tea for extra effect.

⦂⦂ AVOID

▶ Dairy products and sugary foods. They are mucus-producing and clog your organs. You will just feel worse.

▶ Sugar. When you overeat on sugar, you decrease the white blood cells and that weakens your immune fighting ability. You need to have a strong immunity to keep colds at bay.

HERBS AND SUPPLEMENTS

▶ Use pickled daikon in your stews or salads. You can get it from health-food stores. It has properties that help to reduce mucus.

- Drink nettle tea.
- At the first sign of a cold, place one or two drops of frankincense on your tongue (not if pregnant). Sometimes this is just enough to nip a cold in the bud.
- Yerba mate tea is also good for stopping a cold early in its tracks.
- Echinacea extract liquid is a must. (Contraindication: Echinacea may not be recommended for those with auto-immune disorders such as rheumatoid arthritis and lupus as it can increase immune activity and it is thought people with these conditions already have overactive immune systems.)
- My favourite herb of all time is astragalus. I like it in extract liquid form but you can get it in capsules, too.
- If you are under chronic stress, then it is a good idea to use Siberian ginseng herbal extracts alongside the astragalus through the winter. Constant stress exposure weakens immunity.
- Mullein tincture can help to bring out mucus.
- Suck on a zinc gluconate lozenge. Do not go over 125mg of zinc in a 24-hour period, though. You can take lozenges for up to 7 days but after that stop as you can end up suppressing the immune system if you overdo the zinc.
- Sage tincture may help to relieve a sore throat that can sometimes accompany a cold.
- Drink sage tea, marshmallow tea and red raspberry, too, for throat relief.
- Take vitamin C powder, half a teaspoon in some warm water every hour until you get relief or possibly diarrhoea! Do not keep taking the C if the bowels get loose. Vitamin C has been shown to reduce the severity and the duration of a cold.
- Take vitamin A for three days at the first sign of a cold. But then stop. Or betacarotene. Do not take vitamin A if you are pregnant.
- Gargle with sea-salted water to help to relieve a cold. Gargling with aloe vera juice is beneficial, too, as is gargling with echinacea and sage extracts.
- Willow bark extract can help to break a fever that often goes with a cold, or that hot, sticky feeling.
- If you have a ton of mucus, try the age-old remedy of thyme infusion. That means 1 teaspoon of the loose herb in a cup of hot water or put it into a tea ball.

EXTRA TIPS

- Any sinus congestion can be helped by inhaling. Boil some water, put it into a big bowl with a few drops of eucalyptus and add some peppermint, too, place a towel over your head, and breathe in the oil and steam with your mouth closed if possible.
- Dry skin brush once or twice a week to keep lymph moving. This will help to improve the circulation.
- Have a bath with a few drops of the essential oil frankincense (not if pregnant). Or have a lavender bath. This is another good way to help strengthen the body's natural defences. Just 4 drops is enough.
- Get to bed early. That means before 10pm. Sleep is a fantastic healer. Don't worry if you don't fall asleep right away; just resting early is fantastic. You will feel so much better in the morning.

► Wear a hat on cold days. A lot of body heat can escape from the head, leaving you more vulnerable.

► Bathe your feet in mustard water. This is thought to draw congestion away from the nose and down through the body.

► Treat yourself to a reflexology session. Ask your reflexologist to work on the toes in particular as twiddling the toes and rubbing the sides may help to relieve some congestion. You may find them quite sensitive if you have a cold.

► Flushing out the nasal passages with saline water using a neti pot can reduce colds and infections. The warm salty water loosens and dissolves any build up of virus-laden mucus from the nose and sinuses.

► If you can't breathe at night, put a humidifier in your room for a few nights to help you breathe better. Keep your window open a little to get some fresh circulating air.

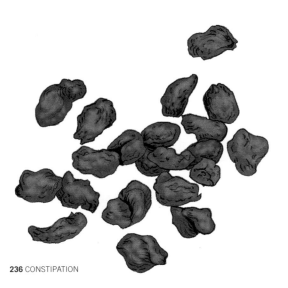

CONSTIPATION

Constipation is difficulty in moving the bowels. A proper functioning bowel should empty out regularly, approximately twice daily, without effort. Difficult bowel movements such as sitting on the toilet for ages, trying to force something out, or dropping little 'rabbit pellets' are signs that you may be constipated, and that your liver is most certainly congested. Blocked bowels can be the start of a litany of serious, sometimes irreparable, health problems but most bowel problems can be eliminated if treated in time.

CAUSES MAY INCLUDE

► Poor diet.

► Lack of fibre.

► Lack of exercise.

► Not enough water.

► Internal toxaemia.

► Imbalance of good and bad bacteria.

Action plan

The following plan should help to get things moving.

⁙ EAT/DRINK

► Foods to get things moving include soaked figs and prunes, soaked flax seeds, ground flax, flaxseed oil, olive oil, brown rice, oats, apples, grated raw carrot or pumkin and pine nuts.

► Start the day with a mango smoothie.

► Cauliflower, cabbage, sauerkraut, Brussels sprouts, broccoli, sprouted seeds, raw shelled hemp seeds which are liver strengtheners.

► Dark green mineral-rich leafy vegetables.

► At least one litre of still water or other fluids daily. Your fluid intake should consist of mostly still spring water, some herbal teas, vegetable juices, and perhaps pure fruit juices now and again.

⠿ AVOID
- Red meat.
- Saturated fats.
- Dairy products.
- Spicy, hot foods.
- Sugar and sweets.
- Tea and coffee.

HERBS AND SUPPLEMENTS
- Drink herbal teas such as nettle, dandelion and fengugreek, and dandelion coffee.
- Supplement with magnesium. The mineral magnesium is essential for both bowel regularity and liver function.
- Slippery elm powder.
- If there is no movement at all, try the herbs cascara sagrada, senne or turkey rhubarb.

⠿ EXTRA TIPS
- Drink a cup of warm water with some lemon squeezed in it when you wake in the morning; do it again about two hours before bedtime. It's very cleansing.
- Take moderate exercise. Not getting any form of exercise contributes to constipation. Gentle exercise stimulates the peristalsis of the large intestine, the wave-like motion which helps to move the faecal matter through the body.
- Eat very slowly. Chew food thoroughly. Digestion starts in the mouth. Bowel elimination is dependent upon good digestion.
- In cases of chronic constipation, use the following nutrients for the first three weeks. Thereafter, you may wish to gradually reduce the amounts. When the constipation clears, you may discontinue this programme. Aloe vera, triphala, wild blue-green algae or spirulina, red chrysanthemum flower essence, flax oil, psyllium, milk thistle, vitamin C with bioflavanoids, vitamin B complex (rice-based), magnesium. *Ongoing Support*: beneficial bacteria in the form of acidophilus; digestive enzyme complex with every meal; linseeds, pumpkin and black sesame seeds.
- Invest in a small stool approximately 10–12 inches high of the ground. Place the stool in front of the toilet. When you sit on the toilet, place your feet on the stool. This positions your body into a simulated squatting position, improving bowel movements. The bowel movement trigger points are released more efficiently causing the ileo-caecal valve between your small intestine and large intestine to function better, preventing the seeping of faecal matter bacteria back up into the small intestine.
- Liquid chlorophyll supplements.

CORNS AND CALLOUSES
Corns and callouses are areas of excessive growth of skin tissue leading to hardening and thickening. Callouses are usually on the feet while corns are usually on or between the toes. These areas can be tender and painful.

CAUSES MAY INCLUDE
- Friction and pressure due to ill-fitting shoes.

- ► Excess wear and tear.
- ► Walking about barefoot.
- ► An infection.
- ► An overly acidic body.

Action plan

You might be surprised at the role that diet can play with the state of your feet. Once you increase those essential fatty acids, you will be well on your way.

⠿ EAT/DRINK

- ► Nuts, seeds, avocados, cold-pressed oil and oily fish for essential fatty acids.
- ► Berries, artichokes and green vegetables for immunity.
- ► Raw fruit and sprouted pulses for alkalinity.
- ► Grains such as quinoa, millet or buckwheat, which are gluten free, easy to digest and strengthening.

⠿ AVOID

- ► Wheat.

⠿ EXTRA TIPS

- ► Soak the feet in water containing cider vinegar or Epsom salts for 20–30 minutes. Dry off then massage as below.
- ► Massage the feet. Add a few drops of lavender or geranium oil to almond or olive oil and use as a massage lotion.
- ► At night, place a piece of lemon over the corn or callous and attach with micropore tape. Repeat each night until it has softened and disappeared.
- ► Dab a cut raw garlic clove over the corn or callous three times a day.
- ► To relieve pressure on the area, use corn pads available from chemists. Place the hole over the corn and attach with micropore tape.

- ► Vitamin E oil can help to soften hardened tissue.
- ► Get to a chiropodist as soon as you can as this kind of pain is draining and can make you tired and grumpy.

CRAMPS

Cramps are painful spasms in the muscles, usually of the legs, toes or feet. The muscle feels knotted and can be very sore.

CAUSES MAY INCLUDE

- ► Mineral deficiency.
- ► Vitamin deficiency.
- ► Poor circulation.
- ► Lack of movement.
- ► Dehydration.
- ► Medication may contribute in some cases.
- ► Pregnancy.
- ► Excessive exercise.

Action plan

Making sure your diet includes foods plentiful in minerals is key.

⠿ EAT/DRINK

- ► Water. You need up to 8 glasses a day. You can count veggie juices and herbal teas as water intake. But alcohol, caffeinated teas and coffee do not count.
- ► Calcium-rich foods such as collards, turnip greens, kale, tahini, broccoli, almonds, amaranth, sesame seeds, sardines, natural yoghurt, dandelion greens.
- ► Magnesium-rich foods such as nuts, legumes, parsley, quinoa, mustard greens, watercress and other dark green leafy vegetables.

▶ Potassium-rich foods such as bananas, canteloupes, peaches, plums and grapes.

⠿ **AVOID**

▶ Fizzy drinks and caffeine which deplete the body of vital minerals and dehydrate you, too.

HERBS AND SUPPLEMENTS

▶ Horse chestnut can be taken in supplement form. This works best in an adult when pain is due to poor circulation.

▶ The herb cayenne is a natural way to improve circulation and avoid spasms.

▶ Fresh ginger-root tea. You can add lemon for extra flavour.

▶ Oatstraw, horsetail or red clover tea.

▶ Take supplements of magnesium as a safety net. If you can get a combination of magnesium, calcium and boron, you should be well on your way to preventing muscle spasms.

GROWING PAINS

Children sometimes complain of pains in their legs when they are little. These are often referred to as 'growing pains'. But I must tell you that if your child is experiencing these pains, then it is a sign of a possible manganese deficiency and possibly other minerals, too, such as zinc, and the vitamin B6.

Deficiencies of these nutrients have now been connected to scoliosis, a curvature of the spine which can be extremely painful as you get older and may affect the kidneys. You need to get your child liquid minerals from a health-food store to rectify such deficiencies if they are complaining of leg pains, or buy powder capsules, open up the contents and blend into smoothies. Also take them to see a nutritionist and a GP.

CROHN'S DISEASE

Crohn's disease is chronic inflammation, ulceration and narrowing of the digestive tract.

Symptoms tend to flare up every few months and then go into remission. It is important to continue eating a healthy diet even when in remission to avoid triggering an attack.

SYMPTOMS

▶ Diarrhoea and constipation.

▶ Pale, bulky stools.

▶ Flatulence and bloating.

▶ Abdominal pain.

▶ Weight loss.

▶ Lack of energy.

CAUSES MAY INCLUDE

▶ Imbalance in bowel bacteria.

▶ Food intolerances.

▶ Infections.

▶ Drugs.

▶ Nutrient deficiencies.

▶ Compromised immune function.

▶ Lack of digestive juices.

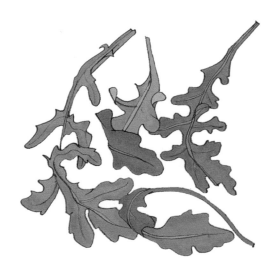

C

Action plan

Keeping a food and mood diary will help you understand how your diet is so closely related to this condition.

⠿ EAT/DRINK

► Vegetable juices. They are full of healing nutrients and the removal of the fibre means they do not irritate the gut wall. Carrot and apple juice is soothing and palatable.

► Fish oils. These are especially healing to the digestive tract.

► Flaxseed and hemp seed oils.

► Fresh pineapple juice for its anti-inflammatory compounds.

⠿ AVOID

► Food to which you may be intolerant. Dairy products, gluten grains, citrus fruits, yeast, corn and tomatoes are common problem foods.

► Salt, spices, pickles, carbonated drinks, caffeine, alcohol, sugar, processed foods and additives. These may all increase inflammation.

HERBS AND SUPPLEMENTS

► Herbal teas such as camomile, fennel, nettle, fenugreek and peppermint, hot water with fresh ginger. All are beneficial to gut function.

► Horsetail tea, high in silica, can aid in the intestinal tissue healing.

► Slippery elm bark tea. This can coat and soothe the digestive tract and reduce irritation.

► Aloe vera juice.

► Take green superfoods such as spirulina or blue green algae. These can aid cleansing and healing of the gut and improve nutrient status.

► Supplement with probiotics such as acidophilus and bifido bacteria. These can help to repopulate the gut with good bacteria and normalize bowel function.

► Supplements of liquid chlorophyll can bring a certain amount of relief.

► Supplement with digestive enzymes to increase absorption of nutrients.

► L-glutamine can aid healing of the gut wall and provide fuel for the intestines.

► Vitamin B complex. This will aid digestion and improve your stool.

⠿ EXTRA TIPS

► Learn to deal with stress. The gut and nervous system are closely linked. Emotional stress can have a huge impact on bowel health. Try meditation and breathing exercises daily.

► If you notice blood in your stools, consult your doctor.

I have had Crohn's disease since the age of 18. For years I was in and out of hospital, on steroids and anti-inflammatories, and even got to the point where the doctors said if I did not have 2ft of my intestine removed then I would not get better. At this stage I was very underweight, in constant pain, and so tired I could hardly walk. But I really did not want the operation, so I decided to take my health into my own hands, changing my diet and my lifestyle, and going on a juice fast for the first few weeks to let my digestive system heal. The doctors were amazed when, a couple of months later, I was in great health with no medication or operation! Now, 18 months later, I follow a wheat-free, dairy-free, sugar-free, organic diet, and do yoga three times a week, and have never felt better.

CYSTITIS

Cystitis is inflammation of the urinary bladder where a bacterial infection takes hold resulting in frequent, painful and burning urination as well as pain in the lower abdomen. The sufferers are mainly women.

CAUSES MAY INCLUDE

► Bacterial infection in the urethra, vagina or sometimes the kidneys. Most infections are caused by *E.coli* (an inhabitant of the lower bowel).

► Thrush can cause pathogens from the vagina to invade the urethra. In chronic cystitis it is worth investigating whether candida (see page 219) is part of the problem.

► Sexual intercourse can irritate the urethral orifice causing 'honeymoon cystitis'. Sex is also a means by which bacteria can enter the urethral orifice.

► Some contraceptive devices can increase the risk of infection due to their detrimental effect on the vaginal microflora.

► In menopausal women irritation may be caused by vaginal dryness or narrowing of the urethra due to low oestrogen.

► In men structural abnormalities or prostate enlargement may be implicated.

► Alkaline urine may be to blame. This can result from excess ammonia and bicarbonate being excreted due to an acid-forming diet.

► Exposure to chemical irritants (soaps, etc.).

► Dehydration caused by insufficient, fluid intake or excess diuretics.

► Substances in the urine that irritate the bladder such as additives, spices, acidic foods (meat, dairy, sugar), coffee, tea, alcohol, fruit juices, colas, food allergens.

Action plan

Conventionally, antibiotics are prescribed; however, this can lead to resistant bacterial strains and a disturbance in the microflora.

⸭ EAT/DRINK

► Sugar-free cranberry and/or blueberry juice to inhibit bacteria. You can add cranberries or blueberries to smoothies.

► Low-protein, high-fibre foods, such as brown rice, millet, oats, fruit and vegetables.

► Barley water to rejuvenate the kidneys.

► Fresh fruit and vegetables.

► Filtered water: two litres a day to increase clearance of urine. Avoid iced water.

⸭ AVOID

► Tea, coffee, fruit juices, soft drinks.

► Processed or allergenic foods.

► Asparagus, spinach, potatoes, tomatoes, citrus fruits and strawberries.

► Red meat.

► Milk and ice cream.

► Chlorinated water.

► Sugar and refined carbohydrates.

► Irritating hot spices like chillies and black pepper.

HERBS AND SUPPLEMENTS

► Cinnamon, garlic, onions, oregano, thyme, ginger, fenugreek, chicory and nettles may all reduce infection and inflammation.

► Golden seal and uva ursi can be supplemented for their antibacterial properties. I use the herb burdock due to its antibiotic properties and diuretic action. Cranberry capsules help too.

► Juniper berries, buchu, burdock, cleavers, parsley and shavegrass are helpful, too.

► Supplement with probiotics to repopulate the gut with good bacteria.

► Vitamin C (magnesium ascorbate) stimulates the immune system and hinders bacterial growth.

► Vitamin A (not in pregnancy) can be good for protecting the bladder wall.

► Vitamin E is protective and enhances the immune response.

► Take bromelain enzyme supplements if you have been on antibiotics.

⁞⁞ EXTRA TIPS

► Add apple cider vinegar to a warm bath with a few drops of eucalyptus, bergamot, lavender or juniper essential oils.

► Wear cotton underwear and avoid perfumed soaps, tight-fitting trousers, deodorants and wipes.

► Use pessaries made from lactobacilli species: Yeastguard (Biocare), Vagillac (Higher Nature).

► Exercise helps the immune system so get active but in moderation. Overdoing it when not well creates stress. Walking, swimming, tai chi and yoga are all suitable.

► Essential oils in the bath such as cedarwood, cypress, fennel, geranium, ginger, juniper, thyme and rosemary all have useful properties. Avoid in pregnancy and check with a medical practitioner before using them.

► If there is no improvement in 48 hours or if symptoms such as fever, nausea or back pain appear or worsen, go to a doctor immediately or a hospital emergency unit; the infection could be spreading up to the kidneys, causing a life-threatening condition, pyelonephritis.

► If you are a regular sufferer of this condition, it's a good idea to keep a food diary to see if any foods or drinks are potential triggers or appear to make it worse.

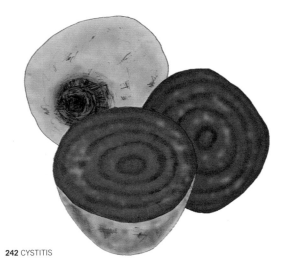

DANDRUFF

Dandruff is characterized by flakes of dead skin accumulating in the scalp and hair.

CAUSES MAY INCLUDE

▶ Imbalance in the oil-secreting glands of the scalp.

▶ Fungal infection.

▶ Deficiency in essential fats or zinc.

▶ Hormonal imbalances.

ACTION PLAN

Using shampoos alone doesn't get to the root of the problem (if you'll pardon the pun).

EAT/DRINK

▶ Foods containing fibres that feed the beneficial bacteria in the gut: chicory, Jerusalem artichokes, sauerkraut, brown rice, quinoa and carrots.

▶ Oily fish. These contain anti-inflammatory essential fats that are often low in people with dandruff.

▶ Hemp, flax, sunflower and pumpkin seeds. The cold-pressed oils of these seeds can be used in salad dressings for extra benefits.

▶ Biotin-rich foods: spinach, Swiss chard, broccoli, soya, edamame, sweet potatoes, brown rice, mushrooms and fish. Biotin helps to stop yeasts (cause of dandruff) budding full cycle.

▶ Raw garlic. Garlic has excellent anti-fungal properties.

▶ Zinc-rich foods, including fish, pumpkin seeds and raw shelled hemp seeds.

▶ Selenium-rich foods for immunity, including Brazil nuts, broccoli, dulse, garlic and kelp.

AVOID

▶ Sugar, alcohol, refined carbohydrates, yeasts and dairy products. These can all adversely affect fungal conditions.

HERBS AND SUPPLEMENTS

▶ Pau d'arco tea can help to combat potential elevation of intestinal yeasts.

▶ Supplement with probiotics. These can help to repopulate the gut with good bacteria and reduce fungal growth.

▶ Biotin supplements.

▶ Zinc supplements are critical as dandruff sufferers usually test deficient.

EXTRA TIPS

▶ To improve the bacterial balance of the scalp, rub in natural yoghurt after washing and rinsing hair. Leave the yoghurt on for 15 minutes then rinse with warm water. Rinsing with warm rosemary tea is also beneficial.

▶ Prior to hair washing, pour two capfuls of flax oil over your head and massage gently.

▶ Use neem or tea tree oil shampoo and conditioner. Both of these have anti-fungal properties. Alternate between the two. Rinse with one cup of cider vinegar and 10 drops of peppermint oil.

DEPRESSION

Depression can manifest itself in many ways: lack of motivation; no pleasure in daily life; feeling low; a deep sadness; despondency; no interest in doing anything; not inspired by anything, mood-swings, crying, lack of self-esteem, no interest in food, self-blame for all kinds of things. There's also a seasonal depression that affects some people due to lack of sunlight which is referred to as SAD (Seasonal Affective Disorder).

D

CAUSES MAY INCLUDE
- Liver stagnation.
- Food sensitivities.
- Vitamin deficiencies, especially the Bs.
- Hereditary factors.
- Personal loss or bereavement.
- Adrenal fatigue.
- Thyroid problems.
- Emotional stress.
- Medications.
- Too much sugar in the diet.
- Poor diet.
- Low levels of tryptophan and serotonin.
- Low blood-sugar levels.
- Low hydrochloric acid.

Action plan

It is essential to talk to your GP if you feel you are suffering from depression. Diet is one piece of the treatment puzzle, but an important one.

⠿ EAT/DRINK
- Water: two litres daily. When your fluid levels are low, the liver cannot detoxify properly and becomes overburdened. Pure juices, especially vegetable juices, are also excellent fluids for the liver.
- Wholefoods high in complex carbohydrates because complex carbs contain serotonin which affects brain chemistry and mood: bananas, tomatoes, walnuts and dates, brown rice, rice pudding, quinoa, buckwheat, millet, yams, potatoes with lentils all contain complex carbs.
- Fish, nuts, avocados and seeds. These contain essential fats, a lack of which can cause depression.

- Low thyroid function can be a catalyst for feeling low, so get this checked by your GP. Eating seaweeds can help to counteract low thyroid.
- Certain fresh fruits help to stimulate energy flow through the liver, especially dark grapes, blackberries, huckleberries, strawberries, blueberries and raspberries.
- Mangoes contain natural mood elevators.
- Foods high in chlorophyll such as spirulina, wild blue-green algae, wheat grass or barley grass will supply your diet with essential fatty acids, in particular the omega-3.
- Vegetables containing sulphur which are high in specific liver-building enzymes: broccoli, Brussels sprouts, cabbage, cauliflower, nuts, seeds (especially flax, sunflower and pumpkin), kohlrabi, turnip roots.

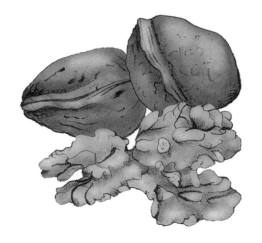

► Green vegetables and leafy greens are good sources of magnesium. Magnesium is very important for preventing low moods and depression. Grains containing magnesium include amaranth, millet, quinoa; legumes: kidney beans, peas, soya beans, tofu.

► Wheat germ (added to smoothies), tofu, beans, lean meats like turkey and chicken, bananas. They contain tyrosine and phenylalanine which tend to make you feel better.

► Brazil nuts, which I call the Good Mood Nut, are a good source of the mood-lifter mineral selenium.

► Eating foods rich in tryptophan naturally boosts serotonin. These include chicken, turkey, brown rice, bananas, eggs, fish, nuts, wheat germ and avocados.

∷ AVOID

► Added sugars, alcohol, caffeine.

► Diet drinks and fizzy colas containing chemical sweeteners and additives which can trigger depression.

HERBS AND SUPPLEMENTS

► Herbs containing magnesium include: basil, bay leaves, black pepper, cardamon, cumin, ginger and rosemary.

► Drink nettle tea and dandelion tea as they are high in minerals and support the liver.

► The herbal plant milk thistle contains flavanoid compounds which are antioxidant plant pigments. It protects the liver from damage, enhances the flow of bile and fats to and from the liver, and improves the detoxification process.

► St John's wort has been proven as an antidepressant.

► If you are suffering from low moods or depression and are going through the menopause, fluid extracts of black cohosh may help.

► Ginkgo biloba, fluid extract. Take the herb gota kola in conjunction with ginkgo for even better effect.

► Kava kava liquid extract has mood-enhancing properties, too.

► Vitamin B complex is a must. B vitamin deficiency can lead to depression. If you get depressed before your period, that is usually hormonal and a sign that you need vitamin B6. So take that supplement 10 days prior to your period.

► Take vitamin B1 alongside your B complex as B1 thiamine is very helpful in cases of depression.

► The supplement 5-hydroxytryptophan (5HTP) has produced good results with depression by increasing the level of the feel-good neurotransmitter, serotonin.

► The supplement s-adenosylmethionine (SAME) has been found to influence brain neurotransmitters.

∷ EXTRA TIPS

► Eat little and often: six meals a day is what you need. Make sure that each meal contains complex carbohydrates to trigger the production or release of serotonin.

► Look at your diet and keep a food and beverage intake diary for 7–10 days so that you can see if there is any connection between what you are eating and your mood. Food affects mood.

► Once you have changed your diet, you will find more inspiration to move and exercise your body. But make a promise

D

to yourself to take up a form of exercise that you enjoy. As soon as you exercise, you will find that your mood improves.

▶ One night a week before bed, mix 1 tablespoon of warm olive oil with the juice of a grapefruit and drink. Lie down on your left side and massage your right side underneath the ribs. This supports liver detox.

▶ Meditation has been shown to improve both psychological and physical wellbeing.

I suffer from depression and had to go on antidepressants after having my first child, Daniel, who's now three and a half years old. I'd been having very low spells through my second pregnancy (I'm 31 weeks pregnant) where I just couldn't bring myself to even get out of bed and just cried for hours. I decided to find the foods that contain serotonin as I thought it was worth a try. I now eat lettuce with every sandwich, four celery sticks a day (love them), drink boiled water with a slice of fresh lemon and make sure I have vegetables with my main meal, and fruit in the evening. I'm by no means strict as I still very much enjoy my naughty foods! But the difference it's made is incredible. My lows are nowhere near as low and I have so much more energy. I'm two stone lighter at this stage in my pregnancy than I was in my last and feel fantastic!

DIABETES

Diabetes mellitus (from the Greek for 'fountain of sweetness') is characterized by a high blood sugar (glucose) level, resulting from a defect in the production of the hormone insulin. What this means is that if you have diabetes, your body is unable to regulate your blood sugar properly.

When we eat carbohydrates or starchy foods, they are broken down in the digestive tract and enter the bloodstream as glucose. In a healthy person, the pancreas produces insulin which helps to transport the glucose from the bloodstream into cells where it is used as energy. However, in people with diabetes, the pancreas does not produce sufficient insulin, so the glucose is not transported from the bloodstream into the cells. If left untreated, raised glucose levels in the blood can damage surrounding tissues, leading to complications such as eye, kidney and heart disease.

SYMPTOMS

▶ Increased thirst.
▶ Frequent urination.
▶ Excessive hunger.
▶ Tiredness and fatigue.
▶ Weight loss.
▶ Irritability.
▶ Blurred vision.
▶ Slow wound healing.
▶ Genital itching.

TYPES OF DIABETES

There are two main types of diabetes: type 1 and type 2. In the UK, approximately two million people have been diagnosed with diabetes, and it's believed there are about a further 750,000 people who have the condition but have yet to be diagnosed. Of those who have diabetes, between 85 and 95 per cent have type 2.

TYPE 1 DIABETES

Type 1 – also known as insulin-dependent diabetes or juvenile-onset diabetes – occurs mostly in children and young adults. In this form of diabetes, the body cannot make insulin due to the destruction of the insulin-producing cells in the pancreas. Treatment includes insulin injections several times a day (for life), along with a monitored diet and exercise regime.

CAUSES MAY INCLUDE

► Genetic predisposition.

► Auto-immune disease.

► Certain viruses.

TYPE 2 DIABETES

Type 2 – also known as non-insulin-dependent or adult-onset diabetes – is the most common form of diabetes, occurring mostly in adults over 40. However, due to dietary and lifestyle changes over the last few decades, this type of diabetes is becoming increasingly common in younger people, and is associated with the growing obesity trend in the west. Statistics show that more than 80 per cent of people diagnosed with type 2 diabetes are overweight.

In type 2 diabetes, the pancreas continues to produce insulin, but either it does not make enough or the body is unable to use it efficiently. This form of diabetes is usually treated with tablets that help the body to make better use of the insulin that is produced and/or a

carefully planned dietary and exercise regime. In some people, insulin injections may also be required.

RISK FACTORS INCLUDE

► A close family member has diabetes.

► You are overweight.

► You have a waist circumference of more than 37 inches (94 cm) for men and 31.5 inches (80 cm) for women.

► You have high blood pressure or high cholesterol.

► You've had a heart attack or a stroke.

► You're a woman with polycystic ovary syndrome and are overweight.

► Your GP has told you that you have impaired glucose tolerance.

► Sedentary lifestyle.

Action plan

If you have been diagnosed with diabetes, your aim should be to try to achieve normal blood glucose levels. This action plan will help you to keep your blood sugar level under control, maintain energy and lose weight.

CAUTION

If you have type 1 diabetes, or you are taking insulin or oral medication for type 2, please check with your GP before following any of the recommendations in this action plan, as they may enhance the effect of your drugs, possibly leading to your blood sugar level dropping too low. Therefore this plan, or any part of it, should be undertaken only under the supervision of a health professional.

⠿ EAT/DRINK

► Wholefoods, choosing complex carbohydrates rather than simple (refined) ones. So opt for brown rice instead of white rice, wholemeal bread instead of white bread. Complex carbohydrates are high in fibre and vitamins and minerals, important factors in helping to regulate blood sugar. Refined carbohydrates have had their fibre and nutrients removed, and act in a similar way to refined sugar when eaten, raising your blood sugar quickly and aggravating diabetic symptoms.

► Fresh raw and steamed vegetables. These are low in calories and fat and high in essential vitamins, minerals and phytonutrients. Some vegetables, such as white potatoes, parsnips, beetroot and carrots, are high in naturally occurring sugars. So always eat these with protein foods such as beans or lentils so that you don't get a blood-sugar rush.

► Fibre-rich foods, as fibre helps to slow the release of glucose into the

bloodstream. It can also help to reduce high cholesterol, common in diabetics, and can help to keep your weight down by making you feel fuller quicker. High-fibre foods include brown rice, oats, beans, lentils, Swiss chard and flax seeds.

► Courgette juice or soup has an anecdotal history of helping blood-sugar imbalances.

► Onions are rich in chromium, important for regulating blood-sugar levels.

► Protein which slows down the digestion of carbohydrates and the rate at which they enter the bloodstream. Choose protein sources that are low in saturated fat such as fish, white meat, tofu, nuts, seeds, quinoa, beans, lentils and whole grains. Mung beans are a great anti-diabetic, slow-release food.

► Apples. When it comes to beating diabetes, there is nothing forbidden about this particular fruit. Apple peel contains quercetin, a flavanoid whose antioxidant effect has been found to reduce diabetes.

► Asparagus which is an excellent source of glutathione, an antioxidant compound that can help to keep your blood-sugar levels stable.

► Soya beans. Not only are these members of the legume family a complete source of protein, they also provide phytoestrogens, isoflavones and saponins that can help to balance your blood sugar.

► Essential fats as these help to improve glucose tolerance, and reduce high triglyceride and cholesterol levels. Good sources of these fats include oily fish, flaxseed oil, dark leafy green vegetables, seeds, nuts and tofu.

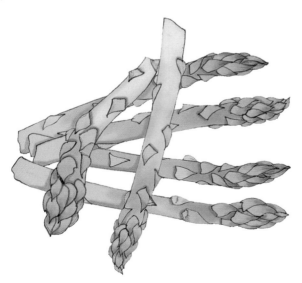

► Garlic (preferably raw) as it can help to lower cholesterol and triglyceride levels in the blood.

► Water. Drink at least 8 glasses of water daily.

► Herbal teas including nettle, peppermint and camomile.

::: **AVOID**

► Sugar and all foods that contain sugar, like biscuits and cakes. If you want something sweet, opt for fresh fruits in moderation. Blackberries, blueberries, raspberries, cherries and grapefruit are good choices as they are not overly sweet.

► Hidden sugar. Sugar comes in many guises including sucrose, dextrose, glucose, maltose, lactose, corn syrup, golden syrup, honey and treacle – to name but a few. So always check the ingredients list on food products – even items like tinned soups and baked beans often contain these.

► Bad fats. Avoid fried foods, saturated fats (red meat and full-fat dairy products) and products that contain trans-fatty acids such as hard margarines and most fast foods. These increase the risk of type 2 diabetes.

► Stimulants such as coffee, tea and cigarettes.

► Alcohol. If you must have a drink, have something to eat first. Organic red wine is probably the best choice as it contains the mineral chromium, which aids blood-sugar balance. Limit your alcohol consumption to no more than one or two drinks twice a week.

► Salt. Use herbs and spices to flavour your food instead.

HERBS AND SUPPLEMENTS

► Prickly-pear cactus pads – a favourite in Mexico – could reduce blood-sugar rises after a meal by up to 50 per cent.

► The following herbs may help to lower high blood-glucose levels in people with type 2 diabetes: aloe vera juice, bitter melon, cinnamon, gymnema, mistletoe.

► Vitamin B complex improves glucose metabolism.

► Antioxidant vitamins A, C and E help to protect against the development of diabetic retinopathy (damage to the retina of the eye).

► Chromium improves blood-glucose levels in type 2 diabetes by increasing insulin sensitivity.

► Magnesium improves insulin production in type 2 diabetes.

► Zinc. Many people with type 2 diabetes have been found to be deficient in this mineral.

► Alpha-lipoic acid. This vitamin-like compound is an antioxidant and improves glucose uptake in type 2 diabetes. It may also aid diabetic nerve damage and reduce pain.

::: **EXTRA TIPS**

► Beware of food claims. Just because the label on a product states 'unsweetened' or 'no added sugar', it may still contain ingredients that are high in naturally occurring sugars (like dried fruit or fruit juice concentrates), or unhealthy artificial sweeteners.

► Do not skip meals. Eating regularly throughout the day will help to balance your blood-sugar level.

► Take moderate exercise at least five times a week as it helps with blood-sugar

D

management and weight control. Good forms of exercise include walking, power walking, swimming, jogging and yoga. However, check with your GP before starting a high-intensity exercise programme.
► Always eat something light before exercising, like a few oatcakes, so that your blood-sugar level doesn't drop too low. Afterwards, top up on water and don't wait too long until your next meal.
► Reduce your waistline. Excess abdominal fat makes the body less sensitive to insulin. Do not try to lose weight quickly. It should be done over a gradual period with the aim of losing one to two pounds a week.
► Get enough sleep. People who get less than six hours sleep per night are less sensitive to insulin than those who get eight hours, which leads to blood-sugar highs and lows.

DIARRHOEA

Diarrhoea is characterized by frequent, loose, watery bowel movements. Diarrhoea that lasts just a day or two is usually caused by an acute infection and is the body's way of ridding itself of the invading organism as quickly as possible. You may hear your stomach make glugging sounds. If you have chronic diarrhoea lasting more than three days, consult your doctor.

CAUSES MAY INCLUDE
► Parasites.
► Bacterial infection.
► Yeast overgrowth (see Candidiasis, page 219).
► Food poisoning.
► Lactose or other food intolerances (see page 178).
► Coeliac disease (see page 231).
► Colitis.
► Diverticulitis (see page 252).
► Crohn's disease (see page 239).
► Weak digestive function.
► Intestinal permeability.
► Poor diet.
► Inflammation of the bowel.
► Liver overload.
► Caffeine.
► Overactive thyroid.
► Too much sugar.
► Stress.
► Intestinal spasm.

Action plan
Identify the cause and deal with it as necessary. If you have blood in the stools, black stools, fever, severe pain or the diarrhoea lasts more than three days, consult your GP.

▦ EAT/DRINK
► Fluids. Diarrhoea can result in serious dehydration. Drink warm, not cold, water as cold water can send the digestive system into spasm.
► Barley or rice water daily. Simmer ½ cup of barley or brown rice in 4 cups of water for 45–60 minutes. Strain and drink.

► Blackberry juice which is reputed to help in combating diarrhoea.

► Freshly pressed vegetable juices which contain minerals. Diarrhoea causes a loss of minerals, particularly sodium and potassium. Include celery, carrots, apples, bananas and cabbage for their nourishing and healing properties.

► Buckwheat which is believed to strengthen the intestines and is useful in the treatment of chronic diarrhoea. Cook it well in plenty of water.

► Garlic and onions if infection is present.

► Well-cooked whole grains; try short-grain brown rice, quinoa, millet or oats.

► The juice of blueberries or blueberries in whole form are a well-known antidote for diarrhoea due to their antibacterial compounds.

► Leeks contain a helpful astringent quality.

⁙ AVOID

► Alcohol, caffeine, tea, soft drinks and carbonated drinks which irritate the bowel.

► Wheat bran, sugar and spices which also irritate the bowel and perpetuate the problem.

► Dairy products as diarrhoea damages the intestinal walls causing temporary lactose intolerance.

► Raw foods.

HERBS AND SUPPLEMENTS

► Peppermint oil will help to calm the bowel and relieve spasm.

► The herb gentiana in liquid form can make a big difference.

► Grapefruit seed extract can help to combat amoebic or parasitic infection.

► Take slippery elm bark to coat and soothe the wall of the colon. It can also be mashed into a ripe banana or stirred into oatmeal porridge.

► Apple pectin can help to reduce the looseness. It absorbs water from the contents of the intestines.

► Astragalus can help to strengthen spleen function which will have a knock-on positive effect on your bowel.

► Cinnamon and ginger can benefit the digestive system.

► Herbal teas such as peppermint, camomile, raspberry leaf and lemon balm are also recommended for their soothing properties. Agrimony tea can also help chronic cases. Drink agrimony for two weeks maximum.

► Supplement with probiotics. These are beneficial bacteria that are needed for normal bowel function and protection from infection. Diarrhoea can lead to a depletion in good bacteria and also be an indication that the good bacteria are not there in sufficient quantities to provide protection and support digestion.

⁙ EXTRA TIPS

► Eat light meals. Just liquids are best to begin with. The more solids you eat, then the more diarrhoea you will probably have. Avoid putting a strain on the digestive system when it is already struggling.

DIVERTICULITIS

The diverticula are small pouches that form in the wall of the bowel. Diverticulitis is inflammation caused by partially digested foods and waste products that have become trapped in the diverticula where they provide food for putrefactive bacteria and yeasts.

It generally affects people over the age of 50. Often there may be a chronic underlying condition with acute flare-ups when the pouches become infected.

The rise of diverticulitis cases throughout the 20th century closely parallels the rise in consumption of processed foods that are stripped of natural fibre. When dietary fibre intake is reduced, the bowels work harder to keep food moving.

SYMPTOMS

► Pain, especially on the left-hand side of the abdomen.
► Constipation.
► Diarrhoea.
► Gas and bloating.
► Cramps.
► Fever.

CAUSES MAY INCLUDE

► Low-fibre diet.
► Insufficient water.
► Smoking.
► Stress.

Action plan

Not all fruits and vegetables are ideal for people with diverticulitis. For instance, the seeds in tomatoes and cucumbers may cause problems for some sufferers. Whole grain products can cause problems, too. Wheat and rye (along with dairy products) can prompt mucus development in the digestive tract. Pressure on the colon wall increases when mucus builds up and solidifies.

▓ EAT/DRINK

► Vegetable juices. The removal of the fibre in the juicing process makes them especially beneficial as fibre can cause irritation and pain in those with diverticulitis. Include carrots, cabbage, celery, parsley, ginger, apples and alfalfa sprouts in your juices.
► Apple purée to soothe and nourish.
► Soups and steamed vegetables. These are nourishing without being irritating.
► Whole grains, once things have started to calm down. Try short-grain brown rice, quinoa and millet cooked in three times the amount of water until all the water has been absorbed. Chew thoroughly before swallowing.
► Papaya between meals. Papaya aids digestion and provides a soft fibre that can help to improve bowel movements.

▓ AVOID

► Coffee, tea and alcohol.
► Dairy products.
► Wheat.
► Sugar and spices.
► Fried and processed foods.
► Nuts and seeds which can get caught in the bowel pockets.
► Raw foods. You may not be able to tolerate raw at all at first. Eat grated carrots and apples once symptoms have started to improve.

HERBS AND SUPPLEMENTS

► Green super-foods such as spirulina, blue-green algae or sprouted barley grass are great for cleansing the colon.

► Camomile, lemon balm, ginger, elderflower, peppermint, fennel and slippery elm teas can all soothe an irritated colon. Slippery elm powder is also very helpful.

► Aloe vera juice can aid the healing of the inflamed areas and can help to prevent constipation.

► Pau d'arco is antibacterial, anti-fungal, antiviral and healing. It can be drunk as a tea or taken as a tincture.

► Flaxseed tea can aid healing and ease bowel movements.

► Supplement with probiotics to improve bowel function and immunity. A lack of beneficial bacteria is often at the root of bowel disorders.

► Take digestive enzymes with meals. These can help to break down food so it can pass through the bowel without becoming trapped.

► Fibre supplements such as psyllium may be helpful in maintaining regularity of bowel movements and cleansing the intestinal tract.

► Echinacea root supports the immune system.

► L-glutamine provides fuel for the colon and aids healing of the mucous membranes.

► Vitamin K deficiency is common in intestinal disorders so may need to be supplemented.

► Vitamins A, C, E, zinc and essential fatty acids can all reduce inflammation, support the immune system and aid healing and protection of the colon lining.

⋮⋮ EXTRA TIPS

► Do not combine animal protein with grains or starchy vegetables such as potatoes. Eat fruit on an empty stomach. This will allow food to pass through the system more quickly so there is less chance of particles becoming trapped and causing pain.

► Keep your stools soft by drinking nettle tea and taking supplements of magnesium citrate.

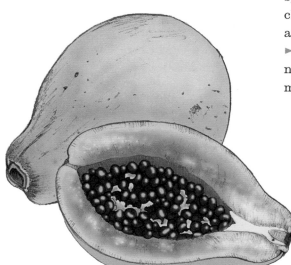

DRY SKIN

Dry skin is due to a slowdown in natural exfoliation, while chapping occurs when dryness has weakened the skin's natural barrier to the extent that irritants creep in, leaving you with rough, chapped, sometimes itchy skin. Skin tends to get worse during winter when colder climates play havoc with the skin's natural oils.

Your skin is the largest organ of the body. It accounts for 16 per cent of your total body weight. Besides protecting delicate internal structures, the skin assists the colon, lungs and kidneys in the elimination of toxic waste. It also regulates your body's thermostat by increasing sweat when you get too hot or producing goose pimples when the temperature falls to the other extreme.

CAUSES MAY INCLUDE
- Age.
- Climate.
- Pollution.
- Stress.
- Fluctuations in hormones.
- Nutritional deficiencies.

Action plan

Good fats provide the foundation of this nutrition plan that will leave you with hydrated, supple skin.

⠿ EAT/DRINK
- Foods rich in antioxidants such as berries, spinach, romaine lettuce and broccoli are especially important. They improve the health of your skin by stimulating oil production, helping in the production of collagen and protecting against cell damage.
- Foods containing essential fatty acids (EFAs), particularly omega-3 fatty acids and mono-unsaturated oils, which help to create moister, softer skin and tissues. These include salmon, tuna, flax seeds, raw pumpkin seeds, raw shelled hemp seeds, olive oil and almonds.
- Apples, pears, cabbage, brown rice, soups, watercress, radishes, pumpkin, millet, seaweeds, peaches, plums, celery juice, cauliflower, chard, chickweed, olives, flax, turnip, daikon and apricots all contain nutrients needed for healthy skin.
- Avocados are a source of good, healthy fats, iron, potassium, magnesium and vitamins A, C, and E. They are also rich in oils that rejuvenate the skin and reduce eye puffiness.
- Fibre. It keeps your intestinal tract regular, and aids the elimination of waste products from your body. Good sources of fibre include brown rice, millet, quinoa, beans, peas, lentils, fresh fruit and vegetables.
- Filtered or mineral water, at least 6–8 glasses daily. Make sure that it is not ice cold, though. This will keep you hydrated and will flush countless toxins from your body as well as helping to keep your skin healthy and fresh.

⠿ AVOID
- Tea, coffee and alcohol.
- Salt. Excess sodium in the system leads to skin puffiness and swelling.
- Spices.
- Red meat, dairy products, refined and fried foods, and foods that contain hydrogenated oils or fats.
- Sugar, chemicals, pesticides, tobacco and drugs which deplete nutrient stores.

HERBS AND SUPPLEMENTS

► Take EFA supplements mainly as omega-3s.

► Take flax oil every day until the skin improves.

► Rotate evening primrose oil supplements and borage oil supplements.

⁙ EXTRA TIPS

► Take up meditation or yoga breathing exercises and learn how to breathe properly.

► Avoid taking long, hot showers or baths. They can strip your skin of its natural moisturizers. Instead, take a short, warm shower or bath. Try to pat your skin almost dry, and apply a moisturizer while your skin is slightly damp.

► Add a few spoonfuls of olive oil to your bath water. It will help to moisturize your skin and leave it feeling soft and smooth.

► Consider your home heating system. If your home is extremely dry, you could get yourself a humidifier to help to prevent your skin from drying out.

► Swap foaming cleansers and soaps for gentler lotion or skin cleansers and instead of vigorous exfoliation (which can remove some of the skin's protective barrier function), use a gentler exfoliant instead. Use a richer moisturizer and you'll notice an immediate difference in the way your skin feels.

► Take exercise. Exercise activates and rejuvenates the skin, improving circulation and blood flow. Also, body sweat triggers the production of sebum, which is the skin's own natural moisturizer.

► Protect your skin when you go outside. Exposed skin suffers in winter so cover up as much as you can. Gloves, scarves, hats and mufflers will keep you warm. Don't forget that your skin is still at risk from sun damage during the winter, so make sure your lip balm has an SPF of at least 15 and use it liberally.

► Get adequate sleep. Sleep helps to maintain oxygen levels and promotes renewal of skin cells, thus delaying the winter degenerative skin ageing that usually sets in during the cold season.

► Apply manuka honey three times a week to your face (or any other part of your skin). Leave the honey on the skin for approximately 30 minutes, then rinse it off with warm water. It will leave your skin soft, supple and youthful.

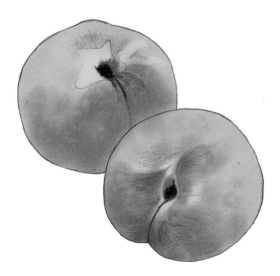

E

ECZEMA

Eczema, or dermatitis as it is sometimes called, is a skin condition which can affect people of all ages. In the UK one in five children and one in 12 adults are affected by it. According to research, 60–70 per cent of children grow out of the condition by the time they reach their mid teens.

Eczema can vary in severity and can develop on any part of the body but typically occurs on the face, neck, scalp and the insides of the elbows, knees and ankles. Mild forms leave the skin dry, itchy and inflamed, whilst in more severe cases the skin can become raw and broken, causing it to weep or bleed. Although eczema may sometimes look nasty, it is not contagious.

SYMPTOMS

▶ Rash.
▶ Itching.
▶ Dry, flaky skin.
▶ Redness and inflammation.
▶ Blisters.
▶ Bleeding or weeping.

CAUSES

The causes of eczema are varied and there are several different types.

Atopic eczema

Atopic eczema is the most common form and is often hereditary. It is a chronic condition thought to be caused by an overactive immune response to environmental allergens such as dust mites and animal hair, or to dietary allergens. It can be exacerbated by stress, emotional upset, nutritional deficiencies or changes in weather. Symptoms include itchiness, dryness, inflammation and scaling. Constant scratching can cause the skin to split and bleed, leaving it susceptible to infection. Individuals who suffer from atopic eczema often tend to have problems with asthma and hayfever as well.

Most people with eczema have food allergies and once these have been identified, avoidance of the trigger foods can lead to a significant improvement. There are two types of food allergies: Type A and Type B. Type A reactions occur immediately after contact with an allergen. Type B reactions can occur between one and 72 hours later.

Allergic contact dermatitis

This type of eczema develops when the body's immune system reacts to a material in contact with the skin. The allergic reaction often comes about over time through recurring contact with a substance to which the person has developed a specific sensitivity. For example, a reaction may occur to nickel, which is found in cheap jewellery, belt buckles and jeans buttons. It arises several hours after contact with the material and settles down again within a few days once the skin is no longer in contact with it.

Irritant contact dermatitis

This type of eczema is caused by regular contact with everyday substances, such as soaps, detergents and other chemical-based products, which are irritating to the skin. Unlike allergic contact dermatitis, the immune system is not involved and it can be prevented by avoiding the irritants.

Other types of eczema

These include infantile seborrhoeic dermatitis (cradle cap) which affects babies under the age of one. Although the precise cause is unknown, this form of eczema often clears up within a few months. Adult seborrhoeic dermatitis, which usually manifests as mild dandruff, can sometimes spread to the face, ears and chest. It is believed to be linked to yeast infections. Discoid eczema is also found in adults and manifests as coin-shaped areas of red skin, normally on the trunk or lower legs.

Action plan

Get tested for food allergies. This can be done either through your GP or via a private laboratory (see www. gillianmckeithinfo.com). As eczema may be linked to both type A and/or type B food allergies it might advisable to be tested for both and then avoid all the foods that you test positive to. Alternatively, eliminate the foods that you think could be problematic – cow's milk, eggs, wheat, soya, nuts and shellfish are common triggers – and see if your eczema symptoms improve.

If you have to avoid certain foods due to food allergy, make sure you do not lose out on any important nutrients as nutritional deficiencies can affect your skin. For example, if you've eliminated dairy produce, ensure you get enough calcium from other sources such as nuts, seeds, tofu and green leafy vegetables. If wheat is a problem, make sure you get sufficient fibre and B vitamins from other whole grains. If you have multiple food allergies, you might want to buy a natural food guide so you can work out what nutrients you might be missing out on and other sources. Taking a general vitamin and mineral supplement or a nutrient-rich food-based supplement like spirulina may also help to prevent nutritional deficiencies.

If you think that your eczema could be linked to a yeast overgrowth such as *Candida albicans*, you may need to follow a strict anti-candida diet. For more about what to eat and avoid on this diet, see page 219.

EAT/DRINK
▶ Whole grains and fresh fruit and vegetables.
▶ Lots of water.
▶ Foods that are rich in essential fatty acids such as oily fish (sardines, mackerel, wild salmon), seeds (flax, pumpkin, sunflower) and tofu as they are important for skin health and have an anti-inflammatory effect.

AVOID
▶ Foods that have a clogging effect on the body such as red meat, dairy products, fried and fatty foods and hydrogenated fats and oils, as they are likely to exacerbate skin problems.
▶ Caffeine and alcohol as these have a dehydrating effect on the skin.

HERBS AND SUPPLEMENTS
▶ Milk thistle is important to strengthen the liver. With all skin problems, there is usually a liver connection.
▶ Nettle and dandelion teas.
▶ Evening primrose oil. It has been reported that eczema sufferers do not

E

have the ability to process a fatty acid in the body called gamma-linolenic acid (GLA). Supplementation with oils that are rich in GLA such as evening primrose oil have been shown to be beneficial in reducing the symptoms of eczema.

► Fish oil. It is thought that the omega-3 fats in fish oil reduce levels of leukotriene B4 in the body, a substance that is involved in the inflammatory process. Vegetarians can take flaxseed oil for its omega-3 fats instead.

► Probiotics may reduce allergic reactions by improving digestion, enhancing bowel health and altering immune system responses.

► Vitamin B complex. Eczema flare-ups can sometimes be stress-related. As the body uses larger than normal amounts of B vitamins during times of stress, taking a B vitamin complex may be helpful.

► Biotin. Increasing biotin levels has been shown to improve seborrhoeic dermatitis in some people.

► Vitamin C may reduce eczema symptoms by boosting the immune system.

► Zinc aids healing and enhances immune function.

EXTRA TIPS

► Topical applications to try include vitamin E oil or evening primrose oil; St John's wort cream; camomile cream; calendula and chickweed.

► Avoid harsh soaps, detergents and chemicals – use natural hypoallergenic toiletries and household products instead.

► Keeping your skin moist is important so use a moisturizing cream or lotion several times a day. Choose an organic, alcohol-free moisturizer for sensitive skin.

► Learn how to deal with stress effectively as it may aggravate eczema conditions. Regular exercise and mind-relaxing techniques such as meditation or yoga might help.

EMPHYSEMA

Emphysema is one type of chronic obstructive pulmonary disease (COPD).

The lungs of those with emphysema have lost their elasticity. They do not expand and contract on inhalation and exhalation as they should, but tend to remain expanded. This prevents proper exhalation and impedes full inhalation. Carbon dioxide and stale air remain in the lungs and oxygen cannot get to the tissues.

The main symptoms are breathlessness, particularly on exertion, often accompanied by coughing. The lack of oxygen affects all body parts and fatigue is common.

CAUSES MAY INCLUDE

► Chronic smoking is by far the most common cause of emphysema.

► Deficiency of anti-trypsin in the blood, but this is relatively rare.

Action plan

Give up smoking! There is no debate about this. Your lungs cannot heal fully while you continue to smoke. Seek help if necessary. Also avoid being in smoky atmospheres.

EAT/DRINK

▶ Flaxseed and hemp-seed oils in salad dressings. These oils contain anti-inflammatory essential fats as well as vitamin E. Vitamin E aids in healing of the mucous membranes and is a powerful antioxidant.

▶ Fruit and vegetables, particularly apples, contain compounds that are protective of the lungs.

▶ Cruciferous vegetables, such as broccoli, cauliflower, cabbage, Brussels sprouts and kale.

▶ Green foods which contain chlorophyll and magnesium. Chlorophyll can help to improve lung function and magnesium is a natural muscle and nerve relaxant. Good sources include kale, broccoli, savoy cabbage, spinach, chard, salad leaves, pak choi and alfalfa sprouts.

▶ Warm water. Water is needed to thin the mucus so that the body can eliminate it.

▶ Betacarotene-rich foods. Betacarotene is the precursor to vitamin A, which is needed for healing the mucous membranes in the lungs. Good sources include carrots, apricots, papaya, squash, pumpkins, spinach, watercress and broccoli.

AVOID

▶ Dairy products, fried foods, red meat and processed meats, eggs, refined white carbohydrates, processed foods and junk foods. These can all lead to mucus building up in the respiratory tract which can reduce breathing capacity and cause irritation in the lungs.

▶ Cold foods and drinks. These can create spasms and coughing fits.

HERBS AND SUPPLEMENTS

▶ Take co-enzyme Q10. This can improve oxygenation to the tissues.

▶ Take vitamin C with bioflavanoids. Vitamin C can help to heal inflamed tissue and prevent infection.

▶ Astragalus may help to strengthen lung function.

▶ Mullein can help release mucus from the lungs.

EXTRA TIPS

▶ Avoid chemicals and pollution as much as possible. Use only natural household products in your home as chemicals in most household products can irritate the lungs.

▶ Avoid perfume and scented lotions.

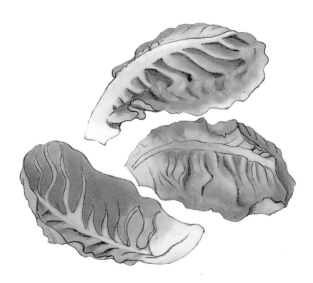

► Apply castor oil packs to the front and back of the chest for one hour three times a week. Castor oil packs with a hot-water bottle over them can help to clear mucus.

► Learn to relax. Stress has a great impact on our breathing. If you feel stressed, inhale so that you feel your abdomen rise and exhale as much as you can. Do this for five minutes but do not strain. Just go back to normal breathing if it becomes difficult.

► Once you have given up smoking and things have started to improve, gradually increase your daily exercise. Walk for 10 minutes a day and increase by one minute a day. Go back to previous levels if you get really breathless or exhausted and start to build up slowly again. Walk in a park or by the sea rather than by a road if possible.

ENDOMETRIOSIS

Endometriosis is a chronic condition whereby tissues that are supposed to develop inside the inner layer of the uterus wall end up outside it, in other parts of the body. This rogue tissue can migrate into the ovaries and fallopian tubes and can even move to the bladder, vagina, colon and lungs. The biggest problem of all is that the rogue tissue, even though it is outside the uterus, behaves as it would inside the uterus and follows the rhythm of the menstrual cycle. So that means that the escaped tissue fills with blood and bleeds every month. Normal bleeding will shed through the vagina. In women suffering from this condition, the blood accumulates in the pelvic cavity (bowels, bladder, ovaries) forming cysts. These cysts can become very large over time; large enough to affect organs, possibly causing them to stick to one another. Most cysts are on the ovaries but they could be in other places, too.

SYMPTOMS

► The most common symptoms include painful periods, heavy periods, lower back pain during menstruation, pelvic pain, pain during sex, bleeding between periods, difficulty becoming pregnant, fatigue and lower backache. If the endometriosis is affecting the bowel symptoms such as bleeding from the rectum, painful bowel movements and bowel blockages may occur.

CAUSES MAY INCLUDE

► Menstrual tissue reflux along fallopian tube.

► Genetic predisposition, embryonic defect.

► High oestrogen and low progesterone.

► Liver weakness.

► *Candida albicans* (see page 219).

► Environmental toxins and oestrogens.

► Menstrual tissue reflux.

► Over-consumption of caffeine.

► Stress.

► Immune damage from dioxin.

► Iodine deficiency.

Action plan

The following plan will help reduce inflammation and improve hormonal balance.

EAT/DRINK

► Wholefoods: soya beans, lentils, tofu, beans, legumes, vegetables, seaweeds (for the iodine which if deficient may trigger the condition), seeds, nuts, brown rice, quinoa, oats, millet, fruits.

► Foods rich in betacarotene: pumpkins, squash, yams, sweet potatoes, carrots, apricots.

► Oily fish such as salmon, mackerel and tuna; linseeds, nuts, raw shelled hemp seeds, all of which contain essential fatty acids.

► Liver-building foods such as artichokes, sauerkraut, cherries, cauliflower, cabbage, Brussels sprouts, broccoli, apples.

► Pineapple for its anti-inflammatory property, bromelain.

► Vitamin C-rich foods: lots of berries including blueberries, raspberries, strawberries and gooseberries.

► Zinc-rich foods: fish, kelp, brown rice, wheat germ, pulses, pumpkin seeds, peas, chicken. Use ginger in your cooking to help improve your body's nutrient-uptake of zinc from foods.

► Magnesium-rich foods: dark green leafies, parsley, prunes, figs, dates, nuts, seeds, apples, alfalfa, mullein (i.e. tea), wheat germ, seaweeds (dulse and nori), dandelion greens, kelp, almonds, Brazil nuts, lemons, watercress, millet, artichokes, avocados, cashews, celery, oatmeal, black-eyed peas, lentils, lima beans, brown rice, kale, spinach.

AVOID

► Alcohol, red meat and dairy products.

► Sugary baked goods and sugar as they will create inflammation in the body.

► Coffee as it inhibits mineral absorption.

Mineral depletion will make the symptoms worse.

HERBS AND SUPPLEMENTS

► Supplement with kelp tablets if you are not a fan of seaweed. But try the food first as you can enjoy veggie sushi, stews and soups with seaweed as one ingredient.

► Add lots of fresh green herbs to your cooking as well as gentle anti-inflammatory spices turmeric and ginger.

► Flaxseed oil.

► The herbal extract agnus castus to balance hormones.

► The herbal extract motherwort to ease pain.

► Wild yam extract has also been found to alleviate some symptoms.

► The herb dong quai can help to relieve symptoms by reducing inflammatory compounds.

► Dandelion tea to help the liver and also nettle tea to keep your iron levels up.

► Siberian ginseng tea if you are feeling stressed.

► Vitamin B complex.

► Magnesium in the week leading up to your period.

► Zinc citrate as there is often a zinc deficiency associated with this condition.

EXTRA TIPS

► Do not dry-clean your clothes. Women suffering from this condition may be sensitive to the solvents used in this process.

► Regular abdominal massage can help to increase lymph movement and break adhesions of tissues. Use oils of lavender and marjoram.

► Get good bacteria into the gut to keep your colon healthy to deal with excess oestrogen.

► If you are overweight you will suffer more. It has a negative effect on hormonal balance.

► Take sitz baths. These involve sitting in a tub of hot water covering only your hips and buttocks for up to 20 minutes (you can also alternate between a tub of hot water and a tub of cold every three minutes). Sitz baths are thought to help improve blood circulation and reduce inflammation and may be taken up to three times a week, but should not be taken during menstruation or pregnancy.

► Exercise can help immensely. So find something you like that will keep you fit.

EPILEPSY

An epileptic fit is a spasmodic disturbance of electrical energy in the brain causing a seizure. Loss of consciousness, heavy breathing, spells of staring and upturned eyes are common symptoms.

Fits can be classified according to type, including grand mal, temporal lobe and petit mal. Petit mal fits are most common in children and are usually indicated by staring into space and being unaware of what's going on. They tend to last for less than a minute. Triggers include becoming too warm, flickering television or computer screens, flash photography, stress, lack of sleep and hypoglycaemia.

Action plan

Conventional treatment for fits includes drugs such as phenytoin that help to reduce their frequency. However, the following nutritional pointers may help.

EAT/DRINK

► Oatmeal. Oats are relaxing to the central nervous system and contain slow-releasing carbohydrates that keep blood-glucose levels stable. This is important for proper brain function as the brain cannot function without glucose.

► Fruit, vegetables and pulses. These are a great source of potassium needed to balance sodium for proper signalling in the central nervous system.

► Green vegetables for their magnesium content. Magnesium is relaxing to the nervous system.

► Raw, unsalted nuts and seeds. These are a great source of vitamin E that has been found to reduce the incidence and severity of epileptic fits.

► Olive oil and cold-pressed seed oils in salad dressings are a good way of increasing vitamin E levels.

AVOID

► Alcohol, caffeine, sugar, refined and fried foods, artificial sweeteners, pesticides, cigarettes and anything to which you may be intolerant. These can all interfere with body chemistry in a negative way and create stress for the central nervous system.

► Salt. Sodium and potassium play a big role in electrical impulses in the central nervous system. Often there is an excess of sodium relative to potassium.

HERBS AND SUPPLEMENTS

▶ Herbal teas such as passionflower, skullcap, hops, lobelia and camomile can relax the central nervous system.

▶ Take vitamin B complex. The B vitamins are vital for normal brain and central nervous system function.

▶ Magnesium calms the muscles and nerves.

▶ Co-enzyme Q10 improves oxygen flow to the brain.

▶ Vitamin E can reduce the severity and incidence of seizures.

▶ Chromium keeps blood- and brain-glucose levels stable.

⠿ EXTRA TIPS

▶ Use stainless-steel, glass or ceramic cookware. Avoid aluminium as it can leach into food and affect brain function.

▶ Have Epsom salts baths three times a week. Epsom salts are basically magnesium sulphate and are a great way of increasing magnesium levels in the body.

▶ Take regular but moderate exercise. Exercise improves circulation and oxygen flow to the brain.

▶ Learn to meditate and practise daily. Meditation is one of the best ways of calming the central nervous system.

EYE PROBLEMS

BLEPHARITIS

Blepharitis refers to inflammation of the outer eyelids. Symptoms include redness, burning, itching, swelling, watery eyes and pain. There may be secretions that form crusts making the eyes stick together.

CAUSES MAY INCLUDE

▶ An infection.

▶ Measles.

▶ Straining the eyes.

▶ Allergies.

▶ Poor hygiene.

▶ Poor nutrition and lifestyle habits.

▶ Being run down.

▶ Seborrhoea of the face or scalp and other skin diseases may also be contributory factors.

Action plan

It is important to treat the underlying cause as well the condition itself.

⠿ EAT/DRINK

▶ Fruit and vegetables as these contain antioxidants needed for the immune system. They have healing, anti-inflammatory and anti-infectious properties.

▶ Freshly pressed vegetable juice to support the immune system. Good vegetables to include are carrots, apples, celery, fennel, beetroot, ginger, parsley, spinach and lettuce.

▶ Foods rich in betacarotene as this converts to vitamin A in the body. Vitamin A is vital for eye health and immune function. Carrots, apricots, squash, pumpkin, spinach, watercress, broccoli and goji berries are all rich in betacarotene.

► Water. Water is vital for cleansing, immune function and eye health.

⠿ AVOID

► Sugar, refined carbohydrates, coffee, alcohol, processed foods and fast foods. These may suppress the immune system and deplete the body of nutrients.

HERBS AND SUPPLEMENTS

► Drink echinacea tea to support the immune system.

► Supplement with vitamin A (but not if you are pregnant or trying to become pregnant). Vitamin A is vital for eye health and immune function.

⠿ EXTRA TIPS

► Avoid eye strain or spending too much time staring at a computer screen or television as this can dry out the eyes and slow healing.

► Wash your hands before touching your eyes in order to apply anything.

► Herbal compresses are great for reducing inflammation and infection. Make a tea of eyebright, calendula, fennel, elderflowers, raspberry leaves or camomile by steeping the herbs in hot water for 10–15 minutes. Once the tea is cool enough soak some sterile cotton or muslin in the water and apply this to the eyes for 20 minutes. Dip a fresh piece of cotton in the tea and wipe along the eyelids and lashes to remove any flaking skin or secretions.

► Apply cold slices of potato to the eyes for 10–15 minutes to reduce inflammation.

BLOODSHOT EYES

The little vessels on the eye surface become inflamed giving a red, tired-out appearance to the eyes. The eyes feel irritated.

CAUSES MAY INCLUDE

► Too much alcohol.
► Hangover.
► Allergies.
► Pollens.
► Pollution.
► Overwork.
► Stress.
► B vitamin deficiencies.
► High cholesterol.
► High blood pressure.
► Eye strain.
► Diabetes.

Action plan

Give your eyes the nutritional version of a rest.

► It's a sign that the blood system is overheated, so drink nettle tea and eat seaweeds twice weekly to help to cool the system down.

► Eat plenty of berries.

► Drink cooling vegetable juices of cucumber and celery.

► The herbal remedy kudzu is a traditional remedy for bloodshot eyes. Drink 10 drops in water twice daily.

► Bilberry capsules or powder can help but you need to take them for a three-month period to help to improve the strength of the blood vessel linings.

► Take a 20-minute break every day to lie down and rest your eyes.

CATARACTS

Cataracts are one of the major causes of blindness. You might find that you cannot see well at night even in a well-lit room. You may have difficulty distinguishing different colours. There is a definite loss of vision clarity and images appear blurry. The eye lens which is supposed to be clear becomes clouded over, leaving an opaque layer on the eye.

CAUSES MAY INCLUDE

► Hereditary problems.
► Ageing.
► Liver weaknesses.
► Deficiency of vitamin B2.
► Steroidal use.
► Reading in poor light.
► Poor diet.
► Lack of antioxidants.
► Diabetes.
► Smoking.
► Too much direct sunlight exposure and not wearing UV filtering sunglasses.

Action plan

See your optometrist on a regular basis for this serious condition. The following may help as a support to conventional treatment.

⋮⋮ EAT/DRINK

► Fresh fruits and vegetables.
► Bioflavanoid-rich foods such as goji berries, strawberries, gooseberries, blueberries and raspberries.
► Carotenoid-rich foods such as squashes, pumpkins, sweet potatoes, carrots, apricots, tomatoes, melons and watermelons.
► Leafy greens such as spinach and peas for the eye protector lutein.

⋮⋮ AVOID

► Dairy products. Many cataract sufferers do not break down milk proteins/sugars properly.

HERBS AND SUPPLEMENTS

► Turmeric.
► Studies have shown that the herb bilberry has eye-protecting qualities and may lower the risk of cataract formation.
► Studies have shown that vitamins E and C together may help to prevent cataracts.
► Drink ginkgo tea to help to improve circulation in the eye.

CONJUNCTIVITIS

Conjunctivitis is an unpleasant swelling of the membrane that lines the eye and eyelid, causing it to become inflamed. The eyelid feels gritty, heated. It blurs your vision and there might be a yellow discharge.

CAUSES MAY INCLUDE

► Poor immune system.
► Allergies.
► Bacterial infection.
► Viral infection.
► Vitamin deficiencies.

Action plan

There is a real need to strengthen the immune system here. Poor eating and a junk-food diet sets you up for these kinds of infections. It is imperative to eat a healthy wholefood diet and to take a multivitamin/mineral complex daily to cover possible nutrient deficiencies.

⋮⋮ EAT/DRINK

► Plenty of fruits and vegetables, including vegetable juices to aid immune function.

► Shitake mushrooms, sprouted seeds and sprouted pulses plus lots of raw foods for the immune system.
► Zinc-rich foods, including seeds, chickpeas and tahini.

⠿ AVOID
► Any possible allergenic foods.
► Sugar and refined carbohydrates, which are not helpful to the immune system.

HERBS AND SUPPLEMENTS
► The herb astragalus is a fantastic immune supporter.
► Sage tea is recommended as an immune booster.
► An eye bath of the herbs eyebright or camomile can really soothe and help the inflamed eyelids.
► Take capsules of betacarotene for a week to help fight infection.
► Zinc citrate. Liquid algae and slippery elm are also sources of zinc.

⠿ EXTRA TIPS
► An old-fashioned remedy is to place a slice of cold bread over your eye.
► Colloidal silver drops in the eye can help too.

DARK CIRCLES UNDER THE EYES
These usually indicate food allergies and weak kidney energy.

Action plan
The primary goal is to improve kidney function and lymphatic flow.

⠿ EAT/DRINK
► Unsweetened cranberry juice.
► Kidney-building foods. Quinoa, barley, aduki beans, kidney beans, black beans, mung beans, salmon, trout, water

chestnuts, black sesame seeds, walnuts, cloves, cinnamon, ginger, garlic, fenugreek, fennel, onions, chives, beetroot, parsley, celery, blackberries, blueberries, seaweeds.

⠿ AVOID
► Salt and salted processed food.

HERBS AND SUPPLEMENTS
► Take magnesium.
► Take the herbal adaptogen Siberian ginseng in liquid or tea form.

⠿ EXTRA TIPS
► Get to bed at a decent time so that the liver and gallbladder can do their best job.
► Rotate your foods; in other words, do not eat the same foods every day.

EYE FLOATERS
Floaters are black flecks and spots that appear in your line of vision. They are caused when cells in the eye fluid clump together. They tend to be more common in short-sighted people and the elderly as well as those with food intolerances (see page 178), candidiasis (see page 219) and diabetes (see page 246).

CAUSES MAY INCLUDE
► Elevation of yeast in the body.
► *Candida albicans*.
► Lack of beneficial bacteria in the gut.

Action plan
The aim is to improve the overall health of the body, particularly the liver and digestive system, making sure levels of yeast are in check.

⠿ EAT/DRINK
► Carrots, goji berries, apricots, blueberries, blackberries, raspberries and strawberries

which are good sources of vitamins and bioflavanoids.

▶ Brazil nuts, hemp seeds, sunflower seeds, pumpkin seeds, linseeds and oily fish which contain essential fats, zinc and selenium. These may all help to prevent damage to the eye and its fluids.

▶ Eye floaters are often an indication that the liver is struggling with its load. Helpful foods include artichokes, lecithin and green vegetables.

▶ Dandelion coffee, another liver supporter.

AVOID
▶ Dairy products, fatty meats, yeast, margarines, processed foods, sugar and refined carbohydrates.

HERBS AND SUPPLEMENTS
▶ Herbs that can help with liver function and clearing of congestion include milk thistle, dandelion root, burdock, ginkgo biloba and liquorice root.

▶ Probiotics such as acidophilus are also recommended to support digestion and restore bacterial balance in the intestines. This can help to reduce candida and aid the digestion of foods generally.

MACULAR DEGENERATION

This is the main cause of blindness today. People who suffer from this have a blind spot in the centre of their vision. The small blood vessels supplying the back part of the eye, known as the macula, begin to leak, swell and cause scarring that leads to blurred vision. Typically, treatment is geared towards sealing off the leaking blood vessels, usually with the use of lasers. The problem with such treatment, however, is that a laser also destroys some of the healthy retinal cells. That's why prevention of macular degeneration is so important.

Action plan

The aim is to help protect your eyes and prevent the development of macular degeneration.

EAT/DRINK
▶ Plenty of green leafy vegetables. These contain carotenoids that are present in the macular and have a protective effect on the eyes.

▶ Bilberries and blueberries are high in flavanoids that are protective for the eyes.

▶ Oily fish that contain protective omega-3 fats.

▶ Pumpkin seeds, rich in zinc.

AVOID
▶ High blood pressure can increase the risk of developing macular degeneration. Reducing caffeine, saturated fats and alcohol are all recommended.

HERBS AND SUPPLEMENTS
▶ Taurine.

▶ Luteine, lyopene and xeaxanthin.

▶ Ginkgo.

▶ Bilberry.

F

FIBROCYSTIC BREAST DISEASE

Fibrocystic Breast disease (FBD) is characterized by small lumps on the breasts under the skin. The lumps can easily move and may change in size. They are not usually considered to be precursors to cancer. FBD is extremely common in menstruating women. The breasts may feel more tender and lumpy prior to menstruation. FBD can be diagnosed by a doctor who will insert a needle into a lump. If the lump contains fluid it is a cyst and FBD is diagnosed.

CAUSES MAY INCLUDE
► Excess oestrogen relative to progesterone.
► A diet high in sugar and refined foods with high levels of insulin.
► Underactive thyroid or iodine deficiency.

Action plan

If you discover any kind of lump in your breast, you must see your GP immediately. Fibrocystic breasts can indicate that liver function is compromised. Usually the liver breaks down and eliminates oestrogen from the body, but if the liver is struggling with its load then a condition of oestrogen dominance can occur. This can lead to fibrocystic breasts. Our aim, therefore, is to support the liver and improve hormone balance to help give the body a chance to break down the cysts.

✜ EAT/DRINK
► Dandelion tea daily to relieve water retention and support liver function.
► Oily fish, shelled hemp, flax, pumpkin and sunflower seeds plus the cold-pressed oils of these seeds are all good sources of essential fats for their beneficial effect on hormones. These also contain vitamin E, an important antioxidant and breast tissue protector.
► Fresh fruit and vegetables for their cleansing effects.
► Sea vegetables such as kelp, nori, arame and dulse. These are high in iodine needed for ovarian and thyroid function.

⋯ AVOID
► Sugar, refined carbohydrates, alcohol and caffeine. These can all increase blood sugar and insulin levels. Caffeine in particular has been implicated in FBD.
► Salt to reduce fluid retention. This means avoiding processed and packaged foods as these generally contain salt to increase their shelf life and as a cheap form of flavouring.
► Dairy products, non-organic meat, poultry and eggs, heated or refined vegetable oils and fried or fatty foods. These can all interfere with hormone balance.

HERBS AND SUPPLEMENTS
► Take evening primrose oil which contains essential fats needed for hormone balance.
► Take magnesium citrate and vitamin B6 (pyridoxine) for hormonal balance. If supplementing with single B vitamins in the long term it is advisable to take a B complex so as not to cause imbalances.
► Poke root has been shown to reduce the size of lumps.
► Agnus castus is great for helping to balance oestrogen and progesterone.

❖ EXTRA TIPS
► Eat small, regular meals and snacks and avoid large meals. Large meals raise insulin and put a strain on the body.

► Check your breasts regularly so that you know what is normal for you. Consult your doctor if new lumps are felt.

► Take regular, moderate exercise. This helps to keep blood-sugar levels stable and gets the lymph moving.

► Dry skin brush daily. This gets the lymph moving and aids clearance of toxins. Do not brush any areas that are tender. Follow with hot and cold showers, concentrating the water over the breasts.

FIBROIDS

Fibroids are non-malignant growths of muscle tissue on the internal or external wall of the uterus or cervix. They can vary in size from a pea to a melon. It is possible to have fibroids without experiencing any symptoms. However, they frequently do cause problems such as heavy and/or frequent periods, sometimes with blood clots, pain during sexual intercourse, vaginal discharges, pain due to pressure exerted on the bowel or bladder and frequent urination or constipation. The heavy bleeding can lead to anaemia and fatigue. Fibroids may even be a factor in cases of infertility. Sometimes surgery is recommended to remove the fibroids. This is known as a myomectomy.

Fibroids are common in women in their thirties and forties. They often shrink when oestrogen levels fall after the menopause.

CAUSES
Fibroids are thought to be caused by high oestrogen levels relative to progesterone.

The contraceptive pill may increase the risk of fibroids because of its oestrogen content.

Action plan
If you suffer from any of the symptoms above, consult your GP.

⠿ EAT/DRINK
► Sea vegetables which are useful for breaking down growths such as fibroids. Try kelp, nori, dulse, kombu and arame. Kelp and nori may be the easiest to use as they can be bought as flakes that can be sprinkled onto soups and salads. Use just a small amount at a time as they are very concentrated foods.

► Fibre to aid removal of old hormones. Fruit, vegetables, whole grains, pulses and flax seeds are all useful.

► Oily fish, hemp seeds, flax seeds, pumpkin seeds and sunflower seeds and the cold-pressed oils of these seeds are all good sources of essential fats which have an anti-inflammatory effect and are essential for hormone balance.

► Drink nettle tea to replace lost minerals if bleeding is heavy.

⠿ AVOID
► Coffee, tea, chocolate, dairy products and non-organic meat and eggs. These may all have an oestrogenic effect.

HERBS AND SUPPLEMENTS
► Take agnus castus every morning to balance oestrogen and progesterone.

► Use castor oil packs to break down lumps and growths.

► Take milk thistle tincture and drink dandelion-root coffee.

► Take evening primrose oil which can help to balance oestrogen levels and can be anti-inflammatory.

► Take magnesium which is vital for female hormone balance.

⁙ EXTRA TIPS

► Lose weight if you need to. More fat generally means more oestrogen.

► Have a series of colonics if bowel congestion is an underlying factor. After this, supplement with probiotics and ensure the bowels are moving at least twice a day.

► Improve circulation to the area; hot and cold showers, dry skin brushing, massage and exercise can all aid circulation and remove congestion.

FIBROMYALGIA

Fibromyalgia is a chronic condition with a number of symptoms. Widespread muscular pain (with no obvious physical cause) and fatigue are the most common. The muscular pain is characterized by a number of tender points in specific muscles throughout the body and is often worst first thing in the morning. Aching and stiffness of the muscles of the back, neck, shoulders, chest, thighs, arms and legs are common. There are usually certain points known as tender points. Other symptoms that sufferers often experience include headaches, poor sleep patterns, digestive problems, PMS, anxiety, palpitations, brain fog, food intolerances, depression and dizzy

spells. The condition is strongly linked with chronic fatigue syndrome (also known as CFS or ME) (see page 227). It is a surprisingly common condition that is estimated to affect about 4 per cent of the general population and affects 10 times as many women as men.

CAUSES

Fibromyalgia does not seem to have a specific cause. It is likely that there are several contributory factors for each individual with the syndrome. Candidiasis, parasites, leaky gut, food intolerances, viral infections, stress, compromised immune function, heavy metal toxicity, acidity, nutrient deficiencies, imbalances in brain chemistry, blood-sugar problems and low thyroid function may all play a part.

The condition is most common in females in their 20s and 30s. It can be brought on and exacerbated by periods of stress, infections, trauma and over-exertion. It is generally chronic but may go into remission intermittently.

Many sufferers have been found to have low levels of magnesium. Magnesium is needed to aid muscle relaxation and energy production in cells and a deficiency could account for muscle tenderness and fatigue. Fibromyalgia is also often accompanied by low serotonin levels. Serotonin is a chemical responsible for transmitting communication between nerve cells and plays an important part in controlling pain and regulating sleep. Low serotonin can account for increased pain and disrupted sleep patterns.

Action plan

It is important to address as many of the underlying causes that are relevant to an individual as possible. The treatment plan may not be the same for each sufferer but the following may well help many.

Toxins, which can accumulate in the body over a period of time, may also exacerbate the symptoms of fibromyalgia and are found in many disorders of a rheumatic nature. Food allergies are also a significant trigger.

⠿ EAT/DRINK

▸ Vegetables, fruits, whole grains, nuts, seeds, lean white meat and fish. These high-quality foods will supply essential nutrients that renew energy and build immunity.

▸ Eat something green every day. Green foods, such as kale, broccoli, Brussels sprouts, lettuce and sea vegetables, are high in magnesium needed for muscle and nerve function. Other sources of magnesium include nuts, seeds, brown rice, millet, quinoa, alfalfa and apricots.

▸ Increase your intake of essential fats or omega-3s. These have anti-inflammatory properties and are needed for nerve function. Food sources include oily fish, hemp seeds, pumpkin seeds, sunflower seeds, flax seeds, cold-pressed oils and avocados.

▸ Raw foods. I have seen a lot of improvement with this condition when the intake of raw, not cooked, foods is increased. You can make raw soups, pâtés, dips, smoothies, juices, salads and more.

▸ Fresh juices are an excellent way to supply vitamins and minerals. For a fruit juice rich in magnesium, juice a couple of apples and a punnet of berries. Or juice a couple of carrots and celery sticks with a handful of spinach and a couple of broccoli florets for a magnesium-rich vegetable juice (add an apple if it is too bitter).

▸ Include figs in your diet to ensure your bowels are regular.

▸ Serotonin is derived from tryptophan, and foods rich in this amino acid include milk, bananas, eggs and turkey. Use ground turkey in place of minced beef to make a bolognaise sauce and eat with complex carbohydrates such as brown rice or sweet potatoes as complex carbs can also help to raise serotonin levels.

⠿ AVOID

▸ Sugar, refined carbohydrates, salt and additives. These can all put a strain on the digestive and immune systems and provide little in the way of nutrients.

▸ Anything to which you are intolerant or allergic. Certain foods may challenge your immune system. Common culprits are wheat and other gluten grains (oats, rye, barley, kamut and spelt), dairy products, eggs, soya, tomatoes and citrus fruits. Try eliminating any foods that you eat every day or have a food intolerance test (www.gillianmckeith.info).

▸ Processed, damaged and saturated fats. These are found in red meat, processed meats, margarines, dairy products, heated vegetable oils and burnt or fried foods. These can have a pro-inflammatory effect and can interfere with your body's use of the essential fats.

▸ Caffeine and alcohol, as these add toxicity as well as being stimulants which can disrupt sleep patterns.

► Fizzy drinks containing aspartame.

► Foods with MSG (monosodium glutamate).

► Green peppers, aubergines, tomatoes and white potatoes, as they contain solanine, which interferes with enzymes in the muscles and may cause pain and discomfort.

HERBS AND SUPPLEMENTS

► Use ginger root in your cooking to help clear mucus.

► To improve immunity, rotate the following herbal supplements: Siberian ginseng, echinacea and astragalus.

► Drink herbal teas such as nettle, dandelion, camomile or echinacea.

► Milk thistle is an important herb to include in your regime to help liver detoxification.

► Valerian can also be useful at bedtime to aid relaxation and sleep.

► Look for magnesium malate and magnesium citrate which seem to relieve muscle pain.

► The supplement 5-hydroxy tryptophan (5HTP) has also been shown to be of benefit, as it raises the levels of serotonin in the brain.

► Taking acetyl carnitine in between meals may help to reduce muscular pain.

► Supplement with fish oils twice a day. These have anti-inflammatory properties and can help to relieve muscle and joint pain.

► Take a really good-quality multivitamin containing all the B vitamins daily.

► Enhance your digestion to help relieve any symptoms of IBS by taking a probiotic supplement, such as acidophilus. Improving your digestion will also ensure that you absorb the vitamins and minerals from your food more efficiently.

► If digestive problems are present, supplement with probiotics and digestive enzymes. These will improve digestion, absorption and immune health.

⸭ EXTRA TIPS

► Detoxify your body. Drink 2 litres of water a day to help flush out toxins. Consume just fruit, vegetables and vegetable juices and broths for a couple of days once a month.

► Reduce fatigue by stabilizing blood-sugar levels. Reduce blood-sugar dips (hypoglycaemia) by removing sugar and other white, refined foods from your diet and replacing them with brown, wholewheat varieties.

► Regularly consume small meals and healthy snacks to keep a steady supply of protein and carbohydrate available for proper muscle function and energy.

► Reduce your stress levels and learn how to relax, particularly as stress depletes magnesium in the body.

► Take low-intensity, regular exercise. This can be a daily walk and gentle stretching, which will keep muscles and joints flexible. Yoga is a good form of exercise and may aid relaxation.

► Ensure you get enough rest, even if sleep eludes you.

► Lavender oil can be useful in helping to induce relaxation and sleep.

► Take up meditation.

► Further help is available at www.gillianmckeith.info/fibromyalgia.

FRACTURES

A fracture is a crack or break in a bone. An open fracture is when the skin is pierced, while a closed fracture is when the skin is not broken.

There is likely to be extreme pain and swelling and sometimes tingling or numbness around the fracture. Fractures are more common as we grow older as bones become more brittle.

CAUSES MAY INCLUDE
► Accident and injury.
► Osteoporosis.

Action plan

There is much that can be done by natural means to reduce the risk of fracture and to aid healing. If you suspect that you have a fracture, visit your GP or local hospital.

EAT/DRINK
► Sea vegetables such as arame and hijiki. These are full of minerals needed for bone health.
► Freshly pressed vegetable juices. These are a great way to increase intake of nutrients needed for bone health. Include carrots, celery, parsley, lettuce, fennel, ginger and cabbage.
► Fresh, raw pineapple between meals. The core of pineapple contains bromelain, which has anti-inflammatory effects.
► Cinnamon which can aid the healing of fractures.

AVOID
► Soft drinks and red meats. These are high in phosphorous which interferes with the utilization of calcium.

► Tea, coffee, alcohol, sugar, refined carbohydrates, salt and processed foods. These can all act as anti-nutrients at a time when you need maximum nutritional intake to speed healing.

HERBS AND SUPPLEMENTS
► Herbs to aid healing include horsetail, nettle, comfrey, fenugreek, alfalfa and mullein. They can be taken as teas or tinctures.
► Take a bone-supportive supplement containing magnesium, calcium, boron, zinc, vitamins A, D and K.
► Take vitamin C with bioflavanoids. Vitamin C is important for bone health and repair.
► Take glucosamine sulphate. This has anti-inflammatory properties and stimulates the repair of joints.

EXTRA TIPS
► Apply a comfrey poultice daily for three hours to speed healing. Mash some fresh or dried comfrey leaves with apple cider vinegar to form a paste. Spread a thick layer of the mash on the wound and hold it in place with a cotton cloth. The poultice can also be applied at bedtime and left on overnight.
► Take regular, weight-bearing exercise. Exercise is one of the best ways of building strong bones and preventing fractures. It is also necessary after healing has taken place to rebuild bone and muscle strength.

GALLBLADDER REMOVAL (CHOLECYSTECTOMY)

The gallbladder receives bile from the liver. Its main role is to concentrate the bile and to secrete it into the digestive tract when food is eaten to aid the digestion of fats. Once the gallbladder is removed, a continuous trickle of unconcentrated bile from the liver goes directly into the small intestine. So, difficulties with fat digestion are not uncommon. Bile also acts as a natural laxative so changes in bowel habits may also result after surgery. Bloating and abdominal discomfort are not uncommon. This may be due to the constant trickle of bile into the intestines or from post-surgical adhesions or intra-abdominal scars.

Action plan

To support the liver and digestive system after gallbladder removal.

EAT/DRINK

▶ High-fibre foods such as whole grains and pulses. Fibre is needed to remove toxins and excess cholesterol from the body and to keep the bowels healthy.
▶ Fresh fruits and vegetables. These are easy to digest and packed full of nutrients needed for healthy liver function. Apples are particularly useful for their pectin content. Pectin is a soluble fibre that can remove excess cholesterol and can slow transit time where diarrhoea is present.
▶ Freshly pressed organic vegetable juices. Include carrot, beetroot, celery and apple juices which are especially rich in the nutrients needed for healing

after surgery and will not tax the digestive system or liver.
▶ Beetroot which is great for the liver. Combine it with a mixture of lemon juice and flaxseed or hemp-seed oils.
▶ Artichokes which contain cynarine which has liver-regenerating properties.

AVOID

▶ Saturated fats from margarines, crisps, pastries, fatty meats and dairy products.
▶ Alcohol, caffeine, sugar and refined carbohydrates as these all put an extra strain on the liver and can irritate the digestive tract.

HERBS AND SUPPLEMENTS

▶ Drink dandelion coffee which can support liver function and has a slight laxative effect so can be helpful if the bowels become sluggish after surgery.
▶ Drink nettle tea which is great for cleansing and toning the bowel.
▶ Add turmeric to casseroles at the end of cooking as it has excellent liver cleansing and healing properties.
▶ Take a digestive enzyme containing lipase. Lipase is the enzyme that breaks down fat.
▶ Sprinkle lecithin granules onto meals twice a day. Lecithin is a component of bile that helps to emulsify fats and thus makes them more usable for the body.

EXTRA TIP

▶ Eat small meals and snacks and avoid large meals as these can put a strain on the liver and digestive system.

GLANDULAR FEVER

Glandular fever is a viral infection caused by the Epstein-Barr virus. It affects the blood, glands, lymph nodes, spleen and especially liver. Fever, sore throat, swollen glands, debilitating fatigue and muscle aches are symptoms.

Action plan

You must get lots of rest and also focus on strengthening the blood, liver function and immunity. This will be the key to a successful recovery. It is common to have problems with candidiasis after contracting glandular fever (see page 219). You may not feel like eating much, but nourishment is essential.

EAT/DRINK

► Veggie juices and soups for easy digestion.
► Fruits and smoothies for your immune system.
► Tofu, seeds, peaches, strawberries, leeks, onions, quinoa grain, sprouted broccoli seeds, aduki beans, parsley, dandelion, chicory and cruciferous veggies including cabbage, kale, and Brussels sprouts.

AVOID

► Sugar, alcohol, soft drinks with additives and overly processed foods.

HERBS AND SUPPLEMENTS

► Mix the superfood, blue-green algae into smoothies.
► Drink aloe vera juice before meals.
► The herb milk thistle is an absolute must along with the herbal plant astragalus.
► Vitamin C requirements are super high during a gland infection.
► Pau d'arco tea can help to clear the dampness from the body that comes with this illness.
► Drink nettle tea at least three times daily for a mineral boost.
► Take a reishi mushroom supplement, co-enzyme Q10, acidophilus powder and triphala powder every night to help in the removal of liver toxins.

EXTRA TIP

► In severe cases, intravenous vitamin therapy can really help.

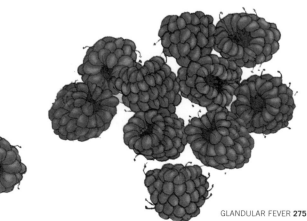

GOUT

Gout refers to the deposition of uric acid crystals around joints caused by a disturbance in protein metabolism. The uric acid should be excreted in the urine but sometimes this elimination does not occur and crystals can form. The fingers and toes are the most likely joints to be affected. They can become red, hot, shiny, swollen and painful. Urine may be scanty and strong smelling.

CAUSES MAY INCLUDE

► Genetic predisposition.
► High alcohol consumption.
► High meat intake.
► Insufficient water.
► Insufficient fibre, fresh fruit and vegetables.
► Obesity.
► Crash dieting.
► Nutrient deficiencies.
► Chemotherapy.
► Surgery.

Action plan

Gout is very much affected by diet so the following guidelines should help.

⣿ EAT/DRINK

► At least 8 glasses of water a day. This is necessary for ensuring proper elimination through the kidneys and bladder.
► Vegetable juices. Gout indicates that the body is in an acidic state (see acid–alkaline balance, page 169). Vegetable juices are a great way to alkalize the body. They are also rich in anti-inflammatory antioxidants.
► Raw fruit and vegetables. Gout is often a sign of too much rich food and insufficient fruit and vegetables. Include something green every day; green foods contain chlorophyll that can aid cleansing of the tissues and magnesium that can alkalize the tissues.
► Fresh pineapple. The core of raw pineapple contains the enzyme bromelain, which has an anti-inflammatory effect.
► Cherries and strawberries. These can help to neutralize uric acid.
► Aduki beans are useful for reducing the swelling and heat of gout.
► Sprinkle celery seeds onto your salads. These are great for aiding kidney function.
► Artichokes are a powerful food for the liver.
► Sprinkle flax seeds on salads for omega-3 essential fatty acids which will help to reduce inflammation.

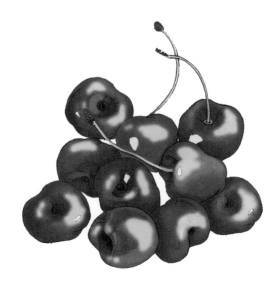

AVOID

► Diets high in red meat and processed meats have been shown to increase the risk of developing gout. These foods are high in prurines which can increase the build up of uric acid in the blood. When there is more uric acid in the body than the kidneys can filter, crystals of uric acid may be deposited in the joints, leading to gout.

► Products containing yeast as high in prurines.

► Alcohol. It increases the levels of uric acid in the body and can predispose you to crystal formation.

► Fried foods and saturated fats may increase inflammation and pain.

► Salt, sugar and refined carbohydrates. Gout is caused by sodium urate crystals building up in the joints, so it is very important to avoid salt.

► Anchovies, herrings, mussels and sardines are high in prurines.

► Tomatoes, peppers, aubergines, potatoes, mushrooms and chillies.

► Tobacco. Its solanine content can increase inflammation.

HERBS AND SUPPLEMENTS

► Every morning, drink ¼ glass of aloe vera juice.

► The herb devil's claw, taken 3 times daily for 6 months will help to dissolve compounds which trigger gout symptoms.

► Nettle tea which can help to improve kidney function.

► Take the green supplement spirulina.

► Fish oils can help to reduce inflammation because of their essential fat content.

► Supplement with vitamin C and bioflavanoids. Vitamin C has anti-inflammatory properties and can reduce uric acid levels.

► Take digestive enzymes with meals to aid proper digestion and absorption of nutrients.

► Take bromelain and quercetin.

► Take folic acid which helps to lower uric acid levels by inhibiting the enzyme essential for uric acid.

EXTRA TIPS

► Take Epsom salts baths. Epsom salts are rich in magnesium which is needed for alkalizing the tissues.

► Apply apple cider vinegar to the affected areas. This can help to reduce the swelling.

► Take moderate, daily exercise. Start gently with walking and build up gradually.

► Lose weight slowly if you are overweight.

► Take hot and cold showers to improve circulation and elimination of crystals. After a warm shower switch the water to cold and direct it particularly to the affected areas. Go back to hot, then cold, three times in all.

HAEMOPHILIA

Haemophilia is an hereditary disease transmitted to their sons by mothers who carry the recessive gene. It only affects males. It is characterized by a failure of blood to clot. This is caused by an impairment in the production of clotting factors leading to excessive bleeding from minor injuries. There may also be blood in the urine. External bleeding is less of a problem than internal bleeding as blood can leak into joints, muscles, air passages, the brain and other organs. The severity of the disease varies, depending on how impaired the clotting mechanism is.

Action plan

Internal bleeding requires immediate medical treatment. Signs and symptoms include a blow to the body or a fall, bubbling sensations, tingling, feelings of warmth, stiffness, headaches, confusion, drowsiness, difficulty using the limbs, excessive bruising and swelling.

EAT/DRINK

▶ Alfalfa sprouts, kale, asparagus, oatmeal, Brussels sprouts, broccoli, cauliflower and soya beans, which all contain vitamin K, needed for blood clotting.

▶ Vegetable juices daily. Include carrots, celery, beetroot, Brussels sprouts, broccoli, cauliflower, kale and asparagus.

▶ Buckwheat, which contains rutin, which can strengthen capillary walls and reduce the likelihood of bleeding.

▶ Raw peanuts which can be helpful to stop bleeding. Make sure they are organic and very fresh.

▶ Fruit and vegetables which are rich in vitamin C and bioflavanoids. These are vital for strong capillary walls and blood coagulation. Good sources include the pith of citrus fruits, kiwis, peppers, blackcurrants, apricots, cherries, prunes and rose hips.

▶ Green vegetables, almonds, sesame seeds, tahini, figs, quinoa, Brazil nuts, hazelnuts, oats, sea vegetables and haricot beans which are all good sources of calcium and magnesium needed for blood clotting.

AVOID

▶ It may be advisable to avoid taking fish oil or vitamin E supplements as these can thin the blood, as can garlic. Check any supplements you are taking with your GP.

HERBS AND SUPPLEMENTS

▶ Drink nettle tea. Nettles can strengthen the vascular system and contain vitamin K, iron, calcium and magnesium.

▶ Supplement with calcium and magnesium. These are needed for blood clotting.

▶ Supplement with vitamin C with bioflavanoids. These are needed for blood coagulation and to strengthen capillary walls.

▶ Supplement with vitamin B complex. The B vitamins are also needed for proper blood clotting.

▶ Take goldenseal extract which has been found to be helpful for haemophiliacs.

HAEMORRHOIDS

Haemorrhoids or piles are swollen bluish, reddish or purple, often large, inflamed veins and capillaries sticking out of the rectum. They are a bit like varicose veins in the legs and range in size from a pea to a grapefruit. They can be sore, itchy, even bleed at times.

Haemorrhoids usually occur because the system, which brings blood from the stomach and intestines, backs up if the liver is too congested to receive the blood. So when the liver is congested, you end up with haemorrhoids, fissures and rectal inflammation.

CAUSES MAY INCLUDE

► Straining on the toilet.
► Bad eating habits.
► Lack of fibre.
► Too much sugar.
► Too much coffee.
► Too much alcohol.
► Laxative use.
► Constipation.
► Lack of exercise.

Action plan

Improving liver function can help enormously with this condition.

⠿ EAT/DRINK

► Berries and cherries as they contain proanthocyanidins which can help to strengthen the capillary walls. You can use berries in juices, too.
► Foods that nourish the liver: cabbage, cauliflower, kale, broccoli, sprouted seeds and figs.
► Natural yoghurt.
► Dark green leafy vegetables and alfalfa, sources of vitamin K, a good preventative.

⠿ AVOID

► Coffee and alcohol. Both will make the situation worse.
► Junk food and sugar.

HERBS AND SUPPLEMENTS

► Drink dandelion and nettle teas.
► Add the herb bilberry to your dietary regimen. It is high in bioflavanoids which are anti-inflammatory compounds. Bioflavanoids help to relieve haemorrhoids and the distended veins of haemorrhoids.
► Drink aloe vera juice before meals.
► Take milk thistle to help soften stools and cleanse the liver.
► The herb butcher's broom can improve vein tone by reducing the inflammation of the tissue surrounding the haemorrhoid.
► The herb plantain can help to soften the stools and make them easier to pass.
► B vitamins are essential for liver health and haemorrhoid-prone individuals are often low in the vital Bs. So take vitamin B with extra vitamin B6.

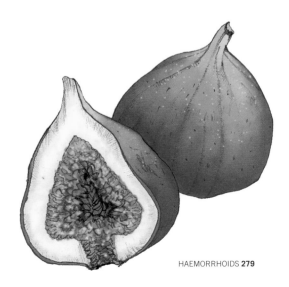

EXTRA TIPS

► Sit in a small basin of cold water to reduce inflammation and ease the engorged blood vessels.

► Apply green clay. Mix it with water. It's messy, but may relieve the swelling and pain. To remove the clay, take a bath or shower.

► Don't strain on the toilet. This will only make matters worse. Put your feet on a stool that is about 12 inches from the floor so your body is in a simulated squatting position and makes straining impossible.

► Mineral salts added to a bath are soothing. Add some oil of Cyprus, too.

► Take sitz baths. These involve sitting in a tub of hot water covering only your hips and buttocks for up to 20 minutes (you can also alternate between a tub of hot water and a tub of cold every three minutes). Sitz baths are thought to help improve blood circulation and reduce inflammation and may be taken up to three times a week, but should not be taken during menstruation or pregnancy.

► Take a food sensitivity test.

► If you have recently given birth, apply calendula ointment and gently try to push the protruding haemorrhoids back into the rectum.

NATURAL HAEMORRHOID CREAMS

Try a rotation of the following natural herbal creams. Start with the first cream and continue use until the haemorrhoid disappears, or until the cream runs out. If the cream runs out and you still have the haemorrhoids, start on the second herbal cream and so on.

► *Hamamelis virginica* (witch hazel), especially if the haemorrhoid is painful to touch. Witch hazel compresses can help to constrict and shrink the veins.

► Pilewort ointment.

► Horsechestnut ointment.

► Plantain and yarrow ointment.

HALITOSIS

Halitosis basically means bad breath. As soon as I smell bad breath on someone, I think poor internal plumbing and bad gut health.

CAUSES MAY INCLUDE

► Poor dental hygiene, tooth decay and gum disease.

► Nose and throat infections.

► Constipation.

► Breathing with your mouth open.

► Digestive problems such as lack of digestive juices.

► Bacterial imbalance in the digestive tract.

► Poor gut health.

► Smoking.

► Diabetes.

► Dehydration.

► Liver toxicity.

Action plan

These tips will help improve the state of your digestion.

EAT/DRINK

► Raw food and juices. Bad breath can be a sign of toxicity and imbalances in the digestive tract.

► Millet which can help to reduce bacterial overgrowth in the mouth. Add parsley or fennel for extra beneficial effects.

► Watercress which contains chlorophyll which is cleansing and hot so aids digestive function generally.

► Alfalfa sprouts. These can help to cleanse the system and sweeten the breath.

⠿ AVOID

► Sugar and refined carbohydrates. These cause tooth decay and encourage yeasts and unhelpful organisms in the gut.

HERBS AND SUPPLEMENTS

► Liquid cholorophyll can help gut health and keep you regular. It comes in liquid or capsules but I suggest the liquid for best results.

► Chew parsley after meals to freshen the breath.

► Take digestive enzymes with meals. These can help to improve breakdown of foods that would otherwise putrefy and cause bad odours.

► Take acidophilus capsules morning and evening. These can help to re-establish the balance of good bacteria in the gut.

⠿ EXTRA TIPS

► Visit your dentist and oral hygienist.

► Brush your teeth at least 3 times a day. Also brush your tongue every morning.

► Use a natural mouthwash. You can make your own by putting 2–3 drops of tea tree or myrrh oils in a small glass of water.

► Make digestion easier by eating fruit alone, never for dessert. Try not to mix dense proteins such as chicken or fish with dense carbs such as potatoes or rice.

HANGOVER

That awful morning-after feeling where your mouth feels like sandpaper, your head is pounding, you are dehydrated and feel as if you have been run over by a double-decker bus. It is all a result of drinking too much alcohol.

Alcohol contains toxins, upsets blood-sugar levels, depletes the body of nutrients and causes dehydration. It is the toxic load on the liver, low blood sugar and dehydration that lead to symptoms such as headaches, tiredness, grouchiness, depression and poor brain function.

Greasy foods that are high in saturated fat, sugar, salt and empty calories are typically craved after excessive alcohol consumption because alcohol causes abrupt blood-sugar highs followed by troublesome blood-sugar lows, leaving you starved for energy and nutrients and looking for a quick fix. Excessive alcohol consumption also contributes to lowered levels of the feel-good brain chemical serotonin and a kebab binge is the equivalent of self-medicating to get a fatty, carbohydrate high that temporarily boosts serotonin. Don't go there. If you do go the greasy route, you will end up feeling worse at the end of the day instead of better.

Action plan

To overcome a hangover, you absolutely must support the liver in its work of detoxification, to stabilize blood sugar levels and to replenish lost body fluids and nutrients.

ANTI-HANGOVER STEPS

► Before drinking, eat some wholemeal bread, whole grain crackers or vegetable crudités. A bowl of brown rice or quinoa will fill up your stomach and complex carbohydrates will delay alcohol absorption.

► Take evening primrose oil, olive oil or flax oil to coat your stomach.

► Take milk thistle seed extract before you go out and again when you come home.

⁙ EAT/DRINK

► Fluids in the form of water, herbal teas, dandelion coffee and vegetable juices. Aim for at least 2 litres a day.

► Fruit and vegetables which are some of the best sources of antioxidants, vitamins and minerals that the body needs in order to repair the damage.

► Berries for their high antioxidant content and good effect on the liver. Blueberries, blackberries and raspberries are all ideal.

► Oats which are a great source of slow-releasing carbohydrates with good amounts of soluble fibre needed for bowel and cardio-vascular health. A bowl of porridge or sugar-free muesli with rice or oat milk would be great. Sprinkle some ground seeds onto the porridge as these will provide essential fatty acids needed by the brain which often functions poorly during a hangover.

► Beetroot which is particularly good for the liver; celery which is cleansing; carrots which are a great source of the antioxidant betacarotene; and apples which add sweetness.

► Sprouted seeds and sprouted nuts which are cleansing and will not tax the digestive system. Make a dressing of olive oil and lemon juice to sprinkle on your salad. Both are good for the liver.

► Green vegetables containing magnesium and chlorophyll both of which can help with energy and cleansing. Add some spirulina or blue-green algae for extra benefits.

► Raw cabbage to dissipate a headache.

► Asparagus to support the liver.

⁙ AVOID

► Consumables that upset blood sugar, challenge the liver and digestive system, provide empty calories and deplete the body further. These include sugar, refined carbohydrates, caffeine, alcohol, fatty meats, dairy products, salt, crisps, processed foods and soft drinks.

HERBS AND SUPPLEMENTS

► Nettle tea will help to support liver and kidney function and supply minerals and chlorophyll needed for detoxification.

► Ginger will aid circulation thus helping to get the nutrients to the cells.

► Take the amino acid L-glutamine; this will help to prevent brain fog.

⁙ EXTRA TIPS

► Eating small, regular meals and snacks will help to stabilize blood-sugar levels and prevent cravings for more stimulants and sugar.

► Go for a brisk walk in the fresh air to re-oxygenate the tissues and help to get the circulation going.

► Have an early night and continue to eat lots of fresh fruit and vegetables the next day with plenty of water and herbal teas.

HEART DISEASE

Heart disease is still one of the leading causes of death in this country. Unfortunately, the majority of heart attacks occur with little or no warning, making it essential to focus on preventive measures.

Cardio-vascular disease is the general term for heart problems which may include conditions such as coronary heart disease, congestive heart failure, cardiomyopathy, cerebral vascular disease, stroke, carotid artery disease and peripheral vascular disease. Cardio-vascular disease is generally caused by a lack of blood flow to the arteries supplying either the heart, carotid arteries, brain or legs. This can result from a condition known as atherosclerosis (see page 193) or a build-up of plaque which leads to a lack of oxygen supplying the vascular tissue. Common symptoms can include chest pain, skipped or irregular heart beats, shortness of breath, high blood pressure, dizzy spells and pain in the jaw or legs.

CAUSES MAY INCLUDE

- Poor diet.
- Genetic predisposition.
- Atherosclerosis.
- High blood pressure.
- High cholesterol.
- Smoking.
- Diabetes.
- Being overweight/obese.
- Sedentary lifestyle.
- Bad fat, trans-fats and saturated fat diet.
- Hormone weaknesses.
- Gum disease.
- High levels of the inflammatory marker CRP (ask your GP about this).
- Bacterias.

Action plan

There is a great deal you can do to help by looking at your diet, and you know what I'm going to say: if you are a smoker, STOP. If you are being treated with any medication consult your GP.

EAT/DRINK

- Fatty, cold-water fish such as salmon, haddock and sardines. They contain omega-3 fatty acids which have been found to prevent the naturally occurring substance prostaglandin E2 from contributing to inflammation in the blood vessels and the formation of plaque.
- Fibre. Diets high in soluble fibre have been shown in some studies to lower total cholesterol and LDL cholesterol by as much as 30 per cent. The soluble fibre used in these studies included oat bran and beans. Some additional excellent food sources of fibre include raspberries, mustard greens, cauliflower, collard greens, broccoli, chard and turnip greens.
- Whole grains such as quinoa and oats which are a good source of B vitamins, in particular B3 and B6 and folic acid. These B-complex-related vitamins make significant contributions to the normal function of the innermost layer of the blood vessels, which is necessary for maintaining normal blood pressure. They also help the body to excrete homocysteine, which can accumulate and damage the blood vessels. Folic acid is so important for cardio-vascular function that a major 1995 study concluded that 400

micrograms per day of folic acid could prevent 28,000 cardio-vascular deaths per year.

▶ Asparagus. Rich in niacin, also known as vitamin B3, it helps to decrease the body's production of cholesterol. Other excellent food sources of niacin include crimini mushrooms, tuna, chicken, halibut and salmon.

▶ Soy. Cultures in which soy foods constitute a major portion of the diet typically have much lower rates of heart disease than cultures with a low consumption of soy. Soy is a good source of the co-enzyme Q10 which has been shown to lower blood pressure by lowering cholesterol levels and stabilizing the vascular system via its antioxidant properties. These actions reduce resistance to blood flow through the arteries.

▶ Garlic. A member of the lily or allium family which includes onions, garlic is rich in a variety of powerful sulphur-containing compounds. Numerous studies have demonstrated that regular consumption of garlic lowers blood pressure. Garlic's positive cardio-vascular effects are due not only to its sulphur compounds, but its vitamin C, selenium and manganese and also its vitamin B6. Vitamin B6 helps to lower blood pressure by lowering levels of homocysteine. An intermediate product of an important cellular biochemical process called the methylation cycle, homocysteine can directly damage blood vessel walls.

▶ Bananas which are a good source of potassium. Excessive consumption of dietary sodium (from table salt) coupled with diminished dietary potassium is a common cause of high blood pressure. Numerous studies have shown that sodium restriction alone does not improve blood pressure control in most people, but must also be accompanied by a high potassium intake. Why is sodium such a big issue? Because too much of the mineral can cause the body to retain extra fluid. This extra fluid makes the heart work faster which in turn causes blood pressure to rise. Why is potassium important for lowering blood pressure? Because potassium has a diuretic effect on the body's fluid levels, it helps to excrete salt and keep sodium levels in balance.

▶ Cranberries. It has recently been shown that drinking cranberry juice can cause a significant increase in HDL (good) cholesterol levels. While the mechanism by which cranberry juice changes cholesterol levels has not been clearly established, the researchers have concluded that the effect is due to the fruit's high levels of polyphenols, potent antioxidants.

▶ Sunflower seeds which are rich in magnesium. Population studies provide considerable evidence that a high intake of magnesium is associated with lower blood pressure.

▶ Blackcurrants which are an excellent source of vitamin C and flavanoids. Studies have shown that the higher the intake of vitamin C the lower the blood pressure. Flavanoids (which co-occur naturally with vitamin C in many colourful fruits and vegetables) support the antioxidant actions of vitamin C and help to strengthen and protect the inner lining of blood vessels.

► Lima beans have been found to have heart-protective benefits.

► Olive oil which is much more resistant to oxidation than oils that contain high levels of poly-unsaturated fats, such as corn or safflower oil. In addition, the substitution of mono-unsaturated fats for saturated fats in the diet has been shown to decrease total cholesterol and to decrease LDL (bad) cholesterol.

► Carrots which are a good source of beta-carotene. Betacarotene, like vitamin C, is also able to increase vessel dilation and reduce vessel spasm.

► Almonds which, along with sunflower and safflower oils, are a good source of vitamin E. Of all the antioxidants, the fat-soluble antioxidant vitamin E not only reduces LDL (bad) cholesterol but also increases HDL (good) cholesterol levels, and increases the breakdown of fibrin, a clot-forming protein.

► Walnuts and hazelnuts. These nuts

contain high levels of folic acid and arginine and have been found to significantly reduce total cholesterol and LDL cholesterol, as well as increasing the elasticity of the arteries.

⠿ AVOID

► Saturated fats, trans-fats, burnt (including chargrilled) foods and fried foods.

► Alcohol.

► Cigarettes.

► Refined foods, processed foods and added sugars.

HERBS AND SUPPLEMENTS

► Hawthorn leaf extracts may help to strengthen the heart muscle. In general, the leaf has a higher concentration of the active constituents than the berry.

► Ginkgo biloba tea is another powerful heart helper.

► Motherwort herbal extracts.

► Supplemental niacin has been found not only to help in reducing LDL levels, but also to raise levels of protective HDL; however, it is important that you check with your medical practitioner before taking supplemental niacin for this purpose. Good food sources of niacin include sunflower seeds and nuts.

► Omega-3 fish oils are an option if you do not want to eat oily fish. Many studies have demonstrated that either fish oil supplements or flaxseed oil, two great sources of omega-3 essential fats, are very effective in lowering blood pressure.

► Red yeast rice extract can lower total cholesterol, LDL and triglycerides as well as inflammation in the blood vessels.

► Take a supplement of co-enzyme Q10.

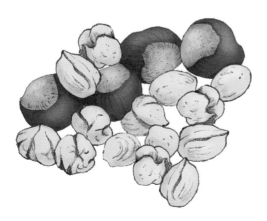

⠿ EXTRA TIPS

► Each morning, drink a cup of warm water with some grated tangerine peel or lemon peel. A class of compounds found in citrus fruit peels called polymethoxylated flavones (PMFs) have the potential to lower cholesterol.

► Add peel to meals as a heart helper, too. Grate the peel of lemon or tangerine into salads, salad dressings, soups, oatmeal, buckwheat or brown rice.

► Get to the dentist. Studies have shown that people with gum disease are at a greater risk of heart disease. Such harmful bacterial components in the blood can travel to other organs such as the heart, leading to atherosclerosis and heart attacks.

► Get chelated. EDTA chelation should be strongly considered for patients with all forms of cardio-vascular disease. Chelation therapy is a medical treatment shown to reverse heart disease and atherosclerosis (see page 193). Chelation is the intravenous infusion of vitamins, magnesium and a chelating agent known as EDTA. This mixture serves to chelate, or bind, toxic heavy metals, calcium deposits and free radicals in blood-vessel walls, which are then excreted in the urine. As a result, blood vessels become more pliable and circulation improves, which leads to the reduction or elimination of chest pain and other symptoms of vascular disease.

► Take up relaxation techniques and meditation.

HEARTBURN

Heartburn is a sensation of burning pain above the tummy button or under the breastbone, possibly accompanied by nausea. The pain can move along the body, radiating down the arms and neck. These symptoms are similar to an angina attack. It is the stomach acid moving into the oesophagus that causes the burning sensation. Chronic heartburn is usually due to a weakened lower oesophageal sphincter valve.

CAUSES MAY INCLUDE

► Obesity.
► Overeating.
► Too many different types of food at one meal.
► Large, heavy, rich meals.
► Sensitivities to citrus or spicy foods.
► Pregnancy.
► Smoking.
► Aspirin.
► Alcohol consumption.
► Eating on the move.
► Exercising straight after eating.
► Bending down after eating.
► Emotional upset.
► Stress.
► Poor digestion.
► Gastrointestinal reflux.
► Hiatus hernia.

Action plan

A change of diet, watching how you combine foods and slowing down when you eat will make all the difference.

⠿ EAT/DRINK

► Eating a banana can help to reduce the effects of rising acid and is soothing.

⠿ AVOID

▶ Saturated fats, fried foods and red meats. These foods stay in the stomach too long and may also lead to the weakening of the sphincter valve.

▶ Caffeine. It will only make it worse.

HERBS AND SUPPLEMENTS

▶ Drink aloe vera juice before meals.

▶ My favourite remedy for heartburn is the herb slippery elm.

▶ For stress-related heartburn, coptis herbal tincture can help but it tastes awful so you need to find a way to disguise the taste.

▶ Goldenseal tincture is a nicer-tasting option to the coptis.

▶ Sounds disgusting but raw potato juice is an age-old remedy for heartburn.

▶ Adding turmeric to meals can be beneficial.

⠿ EXTRA TIPS

▶ Do not jump around or bend down after eating. This weakens the sphincter muscle so acid residue comes back up into the oesophagus. End result: heartburn.

▶ Eat fruit by itself and never for dessert. Separate dense proteins from dense carbs. So, instead of chicken with potatoes, eat chicken with salad and vegetables.

▶ Eat small meals instead of big ones.

▶ Chew and chew and chew your food really well. Do not be a food inhaler.

▶ Drink before you eat. Avoid slurping down copious amounts of liquid when eating.

▶ Do not lie down after a meal. You would be much better going for a gentle stroll. Lying down may cause stomach acids to wash back up.

▶ Don't chew gum. It won't help!

HEPATITIS

There are several different types of hepatitis, including hepatitis A, B, non A, non B and C. All types of hepatitis involve some degree of inflammation of the liver, usually triggered by a viral infection. The liver generally becomes enlarged and tender. Digestion, absorption of nutrients and detoxification all suffer. All types of hepatitis are contagious and can become chronic.

General symptoms include fatigue, fever, nausea, vomiting, dark urine, headaches, poor appetite, aches and pains, light-coloured stools, abdominal pain and jaundice (yellowing of the skin and whites of eyes due to increased bilirubin in the blood). Diagnosis usually involves a blood test for increased liver enzymes followed by measurement of antibodies to the viruses in the blood. The causes and symptoms of each type may differ slightly.

Hepatitis A, sometimes referred to as acute infectious hepatitis, is usually transmitted by the faecal-oral route. It is caused by a virus that can be contracted by eating contaminated shellfish that have been living in polluted waters. It can also be spread through contact with infected persons and sharing of food, clothing, towels, etc. The virus grows in the intestines and can be passed out via the bowel.

Hepatitis A is contagious up to four weeks before symptoms appear and for a week or two afterwards. Once you have had it, you are immune to it. Many people may have it without symptoms.

Hepatitis B is spread through contact with infected blood or body fluids. It can, thus, be transmitted by sexual contact, blood transfusions and contaminated needles. The symptoms include aches, pains, fatigue, jaundice and general malaise. However, it is possible to have hepatitis B and be asymptomatic.

Hepatitis B can become chronic and liver damage and death can occur. It has an incubation period of up to six months. Hepatitis C can also be transmitted via the blood in the same ways that hepatitis B is spread. It is commonly transmitted via blood transfusions, although testing for infected blood is improving.

Those with hepatitis are more susceptible to other liver diseases later in life.

Action plan

The aims of treatment should be to inhibit viral reproduction, repair the liver, improve bile flow and improve immune function.

⠿ EAT/DRINK

► All vegetable juices will be beneficial in healing and nourishing the liver. A good combination would be chard, carrot, beetroot and fennel. Celery, kale, radish, cabbage and parsley can also be included in juices.

► Grape juice. Grapes contain blood-purifying and anti-inflammatory properties. The juice is particularly useful for liver disorders such as hepatitis as the properties are released from the fibrous skins that can be hard for the digestive system to break down.

► Well-cooked oats. These are particularly beneficial for those who are frail and have a poor appetite.

► Fruit and vegetables. A one-to-three-day cleanse where only fruit, vegetables, fresh juices, herbal teas and potassium broth are eaten can speed recovery.

► Artichokes. Globe artichokes can improve bile flow and relieve liver congestion.

⠿ AVOID

► Saturated fats found in red meat, processed meats, margarines, processed foods and dairy products. These put a strain on the liver and bowel and slow recovery.

► Caffeine, alcohol, sugar, salt and refined carbohydrates. Again these can all give the liver extra work without supplying nutrients needed for recovery.

► Hot spices such as chillies.

HERBS AND SUPPLEMENTS

► Sprinkle lecithin granules on your food. Lecithin aids fat digestion and absorption and supplies some essential fats.

► Use turmeric in your stews, casseroles and vegetable dishes. Turmeric has excellent liver-enhancing properties as well as being anti-inflammatory.

► Other useful culinary aids include mint and oregano leaves.

► Take milk thistle extract. Milk thistle is famous for its liver protective and regenerative properties. It is a useful remedy in all types of hepatitis.

► Take gentian root before meals to stimulate appetite and aid digestion.

► Other useful liver herbs include yellow dock, burdock, goldenseal, wild yam, liquorice, barberry and blue flag.

► Drink dandelion coffee. Make sure you buy the roasted dandelion root rather than the instant kind. Dandelion is great for protecting and stimulating the liver and improving bile flow.

► Take vitamin C which has antiviral and anti-inflammatory effects.

► Take vitamin B complex daily. The B vitamins are all vital for liver function. Look for a complex that contains choline and inositol as these are particularly important for liver function.

⠿ EXTRA TIPS

► Lie down and apply castor oil packs to the liver area for up to two hours a day between three and six days a week. Castor oil packs can stimulate the liver to heal. It is important to make sure that the bowels are moving two to three times a day if using castor oil packs as elimination is important.

HERPES

There are various types of herpes virus including genital herpes, herpes simplex and herpes zoster. Herpes simplex virus type 1 is responsible for cold sores (see page 232) while herpes simplex virus type 2 is responsible for genital herpes. Herpes simplex can also develop into herpes keratitis which affects the cornea of the eye. This can lead to scarring of the eye tissue and can affect eyesight. Herpes zoster is responsible for chickenpox and shingles (see page 369).

Here we will focus on herpes simplex type 2. Initial symptoms include soreness and a tingling or burning sensation in the genital area. This may be followed by the development of blisters around the genital area. There may be discharge from the urethra and pain on urination. Pus may erupt from the blisters and

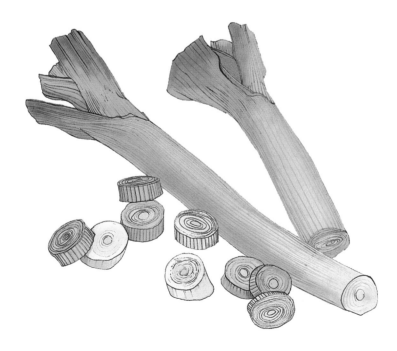

ulceration may develop. Fever, headaches and general flu-like feelings may also be part of the picture.

Symptoms usually last a few days after exposure to the virus. They may be so mild that they are not noticed. Once the herpes virus has entered the body it never leaves. It can lie dormant in nerve cells for years but may be reactivated by stress, illness or nutrient depletion.

Action plan

The key is to strengthen your immune system to prevent recurring outbreaks. That means a really good diet and a balanced lifestyle that includes getting to bed at a decent time. Lack of quality sleep weakens immunity.

EAT/DRINK

► Water: 2 litres a day. Fluids are vital for cleansing the body and for the white blood cells to function.

► Fresh fruit and vegetables. These contain the antioxidants needed by the immune system to fight the virus.

► Apples, pears and beetroot which all have a good L-lysine to L-arginine ratio so can be eaten freely.

► Chicken, turkey and fish also have good amounts of L-lysine relative to L-arginine.

► Spinach and chard. These both contain sulphur which aids cleansing and are cooling. Both these properties can help to relieve herpes.

► Freshly pressed vegetable juices. This is one of the best ways of giving the body the nutrients it needs to overcome the virus and to speed healing. Beetroot, apples, carrots, celery, radishes, parsley,

ginger and cabbage can all be included.

► Garlic and onions. These have antiviral and anti-infective properties.

► Olive oil, flaxseed oil and hemp-seed oil. These are high in vitamin E which can speed healing of lesions.

AVOID

► Sugar, refined carbohydrates, soft drinks, alcohol, caffeine and salt. These can all suppress the immune system and deplete the body of nutrients.

► Foods high in the amino acid L-arginine. Arginine suppresses the amino acid L-lysine which is one of the body's main lines of defence against viral growth. Arginine is found in pecans, sesame seeds, walnuts, citrus fruits, wheat, chocolate, dairy products, corn and peanuts. These are best avoided or eaten in moderation during an attack.

HERBS AND SUPPLEMENTS

► Nettle, lemon balm, liquorice, rose hip, fennel and echinacea teas.

► Supplement with L-lysine which has well known antiviral effects.

► Supplement with vitamin C and bioflavanoids. Vitamin C also has anti-viral and immune supportive properties. You can take it with the L-lysine as it can enhance the effectiveness of the lysine.

► The herb echinacea can be taken to increase the body's general resistance and help to fight infection.

► Supplement with zinc which is an important nutrient for the immune system and is often depleted.

EXTRA TIPS

► Topically, you can apply black walnut extract. This has antiviral effects.

L-lysine or zinc creams can also be applied topically for their antiviral effects.

► Aloe vera gel is soothing and can be applied locally to relieve symptoms.

HIGH BLOOD PRESSURE

When we talk about blood pressure, we are referring to the pressure of the blood against the artery and blood-vessel walls. According to the World Health Organization (WHO), high blood pressure, also referred to as hypertension, is when the pressure of the blood pumping round the body is higher than 160/90. Normal blood pressure would be considered to be between 100/70–140/90. Anything above this should lead to further investigation and dietary and lifestyle changes.

The higher number is the systolic reading, which indicates the pressure of the blood when the heart contracts (pumps) and pressure is at its highest. The lower figure is the diastolic pressure and this refers to the pressure when the heart relaxes between pumps. This is when pressure is at its lowest.

The pressure of the blood depends on a number of factors: the power of the heart, the amount of blood in the body and the health of the blood-vessel walls. For example, if the blood vessels are clogged up with plaque and cholesterol, they will be narrower and the pressure of the blood will be greater. In turn, high blood pressure can cause damage to the artery walls. This can lead to the deposition of cholesterol and plaque in order to patch up the damage.

Those with high blood pressure may have no particular symptoms. However, some people present with headaches, nosebleeds, palpitations, visual disturbances, dizziness, chest pains, fatigue and breathlessness. Having high blood pressure puts you at increased risk of heart disease and suffering a heart attack or stroke. Other associated conditions include obesity, diabetes, arteriosclerosis, atherosclerosis, kidney problems and hyperthyroidism.

Essential or primary hypertension refers to high blood pressure with no apparent physical cause. Secondary hypertension refers to high blood pressure that has been caused by another disease. For example, the narrowing of the blood vessels, as in atherosclerosis (see page 193) and arteriosclerosis, will increase the pressure of the blood. Poor kidney function can increase the amount of fluid in the blood and this can also lead to high blood pressure.

CAUSES

There are many possible contributory factors to high blood pressure. These include:

► Genetic predisposition.

► Stress.

► Being overweight.

► Nutrient deficiencies, particularly the essential fats, magnesium, B vitamins and vitamin C.

► Diet high in salt, saturated fat and sugar.

- High cholesterol.
- Kidney disorders.
- High caffeine and alcohol consumption.
- Smoking.
- Hyperactive thyroid.
- Food intolerances.
- Damaged arteries.

Action plan

It is really important to add nutrient-rich foods to your diet as well as cutting out salt. Make any changes in consultation with your GP.

⁝⁝ EAT/DRINK

- Garlic and onions. These have been found to be especially beneficial for cardio-vascular health.
- Fruit and vegetables: 8 servings daily. Fruit and vegetables are rich in potassium and magnesium. These are both vital for cardio-vascular health.
- Kiwi fruit are easy on the digestion and a good source of potassium.
- Lentils and beans which are good sources of potassium.
- Green vegetables, nuts, seeds and whole grains such as brown rice and quinoa which are good sources of magnesium.
- Bananas: two a day of this potassium-rich fruit can help to control high blood pressure.
- Oily fish, hemp seeds, pumpkin seeds, flax seeds and sunflower seeds and the cold-pressed oils of these seeds. They contain essential fats needed for healthy capillary walls.
- Whole grains, such as buckwheat. Not only do these provide magnesium and B vitamins, both essential for heart health, they are also a great source of fibre. Fibre is also needed for the removal of excess cholesterol from the body. High cholesterol can lead to high blood pressure and vice versa.
- Vegetable juices. These are great for giving your body a burst of potassium and magnesium along with other nutrients in a readily available form. Include carrots, beetroot, radish, ginger, cabbage, chard and celery.

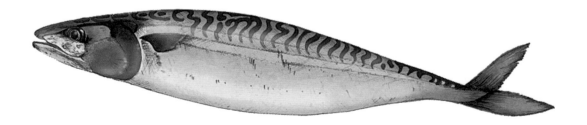

AVOID

▶ Salt. This is not just a matter of not adding salt to your food but of avoiding all processed and packaged foods. They all contain salt to give them shelf life and flavour. It is found in bread, cheese, ham, bacon and all processed meats, soups, tinned foods, biscuits, cereals, cakes, pastries and soy sauce. Read all labels and get into the habit of cooking from scratch using whole natural foods.

▶ Caffeine, alcohol, nicotine, sugar, refined carbohydrates, processed foods, saturated fats, processed fats, fried foods and dairy products. These can all have a negative impact on cardio-vascular health and this, in turn, can raise blood pressure.

HERBS AND SUPPLEMENTS

▶ Flavour your food with herbs and mild spices. These generally have health-giving properties and will give your taste buds a variety of flavours to enjoy. Try parsley, thyme, rosemary, basil, coriander, mint, chervil, fennel, dill, cumin, ginger, garlic, turmeric and cinnamon.

▶ Drink nettle tea and dandelion root coffee. These can both help to remove excess fluids from the body and can replace lost potassium. Other useful herbal teas include camomile, lemon balm, peppermint, yarrow and lime flowers. Hawthorn tea or tincture is also useful for heart health.

▶ Take magnesium supplements. They have been shown to lower blood pressure.

▶ Fish oils can improve circulation and aid healing of the blood-vessel walls. Do not take if you are on blood-thinning medications.

▶ Take vitamin C with bioflavanoids. Vitamin C is important for healing the blood-vessel walls and is used up in stress.

▶ Take vitamin B complex. B vitamins are important for cardio-vascular health and the stress response. Look for one containing choline and inositol.

▶ Co-enzyme Q10 is a potent antioxidant supplement that may help lower high blood pressure. You need to take it for at least six months.

EXTRA TIPS

▶ Moderate exercise daily is essential. Walking is a good place to start if you don't currently do any exercise. Start with 20 minutes a day; swing your arms naturally and aim to get your heart rate up without actually panting when you finish.

▶ Learn to manage stress. High blood pressure is often linked to stress, so review your life and see what is stressing you. Yoga, tai chi, meditation and breathing exercises are all techniques that can help.

▶ When you get up in the morning, before you jump out of bed and start your day, take five minutes to just be still. Sit on the end of your bed, close your eyes, place your right hand on your stomach and simply breathe in through your nose and out through your mouth very slowly. Feel the breath in your stomach. Do this 20 times.

▶ Monitor your blood pressure. It is important to monitor your blood pressure to see how you are getting on. Do not be alarmed if your blood pressure rises initially. This can be a result of sodium being released from the cells as you replace it with magnesium and potassium. Do not give up on the diet because you think it is not working. This is a sure sign that your body is restoring balance. Stick with it and you should start to see the readings coming down and overall health improving.

► Treat yourself to essential oil massages. Essential oils are absorbed through the skin and can have a calming effect on the nervous system which controls blood pressure and stress reactions.

HIGH CHOLESTEROL

Cholesterol is a fat soluble substance that is made in the liver, as well as being derived from the diet. It is only found in animal products. There is no cholesterol in plant foods. Despite its reputation, cholesterol is essential for health; it is needed for healthy cell membranes and is a precursor to the steroid hormones (including testosterone, progesterone and oestrogen).

Cholesterol is carried in the bloodstream from the liver to the cells by lipoproteins. Low-density lipoproteins, or LDLs, carry cholesterol to the cells. High-density lipoproteins, or HDLs, carry cholesterol from the cells back to the liver so that it can be reused or eliminated. The reason LDLs are called bad cholesterol and HDLs are called good cholesterol is because if there is too much LDL or not enough HDL, cholesterol can build up in

the body and be deposited on the artery walls. This can then contribute to many diseases of the cardio-vascular system.

There may be no symptoms of high cholesterol but related disorders include obesity, atherosclerosis, arteriosclerosis, high blood pressure, heart attacks, strokes and gallstones.

When cholesterol levels are tested, results are usually given for total cholesterol as well as LDL, HDL and triglycerides (blood fats). Total cholesterol should not be more than 5mmol/l. LDL cholesterol levels should be no more than 3mmol/l while HDL cholesterol should be above 1mmol/l.

CAUSES

The cholesterol we get from food accounts for only about 20 per cent of our total cholesterol. The rest is made in the liver. For vegans, 100 per cent of their cholesterol will be made by the liver. So, while it is wise not to eat too many high-cholesterol foods, it is actually more important to avoid the foods that increase the liver's production of cholesterol. These are saturated fats, mainly from red meat and dairy products, sugar, alcohol and refined carbohydrates.

Action plan

The aim is to normalize the balance between LDL and HDL cholesterol and reduce the oxidation of cholesterol. If you are being treated with any medication consult your GP.

⠿ EAT/DRINK
► Fibre which is needed for the removal of excess cholesterol from the body.

Good sources include whole grains, fruit, vegetables, black-eye peas and pulses.

► In the case of cholesterol it is true that an apple a day keeps the doctor away. Apples contain pectin, a fibre that can help to lower cholesterol.

► Olive oil, garlic, onions, apples, fish, artichokes, beetroot, carrots, oats and lentils, all of which have proven cholesterol-lowering properties.

► Walnuts and/or almonds. They are excellent sources of cholesterol-lowering nutrients. Soak your almonds overnight for easy digestion.

► Fresh fruit and vegetables. These contain antioxidants needed for repairing the artery and blood-vessel walls. Aim to eat a range of colours as this will give you wide-ranging protection.

► Complex carbohydrates found in brown rice, millet, buckwheat, oats, quinoa and barley.

► Pecans can help to reduce bad (LDL) cholesterol and are high in antioxidants.

► Essential fats found in oily fish, raw nuts, seeds and cold-pressed oils. These are needed for healthy circulation.

► Mono-unsaturated fats found in olive oil, olives and avocados. These have been shown to lower blood cholesterol levels.

► Whole soya beans which contain plant sterols which have been shown to inhibit absorption of dietary cholesterol.

⠿ AVOID

► Margarines, heated fats, junk foods, processed foods, palm oil and fried foods. These can all increase total cholesterol and negatively affect cardio-vascular health.

► Sugar, white flour, white bread, white rice and white pasta.

► Fatty meats, processed meats, dairy products,

► Alcohol, coffee and fizzy drinks.

HERBS AND SUPPLEMENTS

► Drink fenugreek seed tea. This can reduce cholesterol levels and aid fat metabolism.

► Sprinkle lecithin granules on your food. Lecithin aids in fat metabolism and is a source of essential fats.

► Include turmeric, ginger and cayenne pepper in your diet. Turmeric aids liver function and ginger and cayenne pepper are good for the circulation.

► Supplement with B vitamins. These are important in controlling cholesterol levels and fat metabolism. Look for those that contain choline and inositol.

► Take vitamin C with bioflavanoids. Vitamin C can help to lower cholesterol and repair damaged artery walls.

► Take fish oils. These contain fats that are important for blood circulation and heart health. Do not take if you are on blood-thinning medication.

► Take vitamin E daily. Vitamin E can help to repair damaged artery walls and prevent the oxidation of cholesterol. Do not take if you are on blood-thinning medication.

► Supplement with probiotics such as acidophilus. These are important for the metabolism of cholesterol in the bowel and can help to lower cholesterol.

⠿ EXTRA TIPS

► Take daily, moderate exercise. Exercise can improve heart function, lower blood pressure and cholesterol and reduce weight. Start with a brisk 20-minute walk every day and build up gradually.

► Learn to relax. Stress is heavily implicated in high cholesterol and heart disease generally. Review your life and see if you can avoid the causes of stress or change your response to them. Stop worrying about the past and future and live in the present; that is all you can influence. Take some time out each day for relaxation. Meditation, breathing exercises, yoga and tai chi are all tried and tested techniques. Even having a warm bath with some lavender oil in the evening is a good way to wind down.

I have been eating organic porridge oats made with filtered water and topped up with fresh strawberries and banana or frozen unsweetened fruit / berry mix for the last year and my cholesterol has dropped from 5.2 to 4.8. I also eat a huge mixed green salad every day with mung beans, lentils, alfalfa and the more I eat fresh, the more I love it!

HIGH HOMOCYSTEINE

Homocysteine is an amino acid that is naturally produced in the body during the breakdown of methionine, another amino acid present in many foods. While methionine is a beneficial amino acid, homocysteine is extremely damaging. For this reason, it should be present in the blood for only a split second before being converted to S-adenosyl methionine (SAMe) and glutathione, both of which

are beneficial to health. SAMe is a natural antidepressant and is helpful for reducing arthritis and other inflammatory disorders. Glutathione is vital for detoxification and has anti-ageing properties.

Having high homocysteine levels increases your risk of developing Alzheimer's (see page 183), heart disease (see page 283), strokes, dementia, pre-eclampsia and multiple sclerosis (see page 329) among other diseases.

Homocysteine levels can be tested by a simple pin-prick blood test. Ideally, levels should be lower than 7mmol/1.

CAUSES

Certain nutrients are needed for the conversion of homocysteine to SAMe and glutathione. These include vitamins B6, B12, zinc, folic acid and tri-methlyglycine (TMG). A diet low in these nutrients can therefore lead to homocysteine levels building up in the blood. Other factors that can increase homocysteine levels include some pharmaceutical drugs, poor absorption of nutrients, ageing, smoking, excessive alcohol consumption, menopause, hypothyroidism, kidney failure and genetics. Some people have a genetic tendency to levels of homocysteine building up in the body; this is called homocysteinuria.

Action plan

The main aims for those with high homocysteine levels are to increase the nutrients needed for the breakdown of homocysteine and to reduce or avoid the factors that can lead to a build-up of homocysteine in the body. The following plan addresses both of these. If you are being treated with any medication consult your GP.

⠿ EAT/DRINK

► Whole grains, such as brown rice, quinoa, buckwheat and oats which all contain good amounts of B vitamins as well as the minerals zinc and magnesium needed for the chemical breakdown of homocysteine.

► Spinach, which is a great source of vitamin B6 and folic acid, both of which are needed to reduce levels of homocysteine.

► Broccoli, cauliflower, asparagus, Brussels sprouts, tomato juice, beans and lentils which are all good sources of folic acid.

► Bananas, chicken, turkey, salmon, halibut, spinach, peppers, turnip greens and broccoli which contain vitamin B6.

► Fish, meat, poultry and eggs which are the best sources of vitamin B12. However, many people do not absorb vitamin B12 particularly well, especially the elderly or those with compromised digestive function so supplements may be useful (see below).

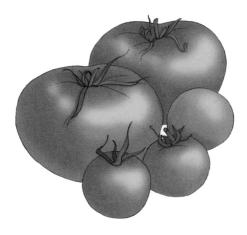

► Beetroot, a good source of tri-methylglycine (TMG) which is also valuable in the conversion of homocysteine into safer substances. Juiced beetroot may be one of the best ways to get dietary TMG but supplements may be needed initially to bring down homocysteine if levels are too high.

⠿ AVOID

► Alcohol. It interferes with the absorption of many nutrients including vitamin B6, folic acid and vitamin B12. It can also increase the elimination of these in the urine so the body ends up depleted.

► Sugar and refined carbohydrates which are low in nutrients and can deplete the body of precious B vitamins needed for lowering homocysteine.

► Tea and coffee strip the body of the nutrients needed to reduce homocysteine.

HERBS AND SUPPLEMENTS

► Take TMG or betaine, folic acid and vitamins B12 and B6.

► Other useful nutrients are choline, inositol, zinc and magnesium.

► If you suffer from digestive symptoms with poor absorption of nutrients, supplement with digestive enzymes. These can aid absorption and nutrient status and therefore overall body functioning.

► To get tested for homocysteine levels, go to www.gillianmckeith.info.

⠿ EXTRA TIPS

► If you smoke, stop now. Smoking depletes the body of the nutrients needed for the proper breakdown of homocysteine in the body and puts you at increased risk of disease.

► Exercise daily. People who engage in regular, strenuous exercise have lower homocysteine levels than those who are sedentary. Exercise can also reduce your risk of developing many of the diseases associated with high homocysteine levels. Do 30 minutes a day of walking, jogging, swimming, dancing or cycling to a level at which your heart rate is raised.

HIVES

Hives, also known as urticaria, are characterized by a red, raised, itchy or prickly rash. Often there is whiteness in the centre or around the redness.

CAUSES

The rash is caused by a histamine released in the skin by the immune system in response to a perceived threat (an allergen). The following are common culprits:

► Peanuts.

► Eggs.

► Sesame seeds.

► Strawberries.

► Celery.

► Shellfish.

► Some citrus fruits.

► Processed and cured meats.

► Alcohol.

► Chemicals.

► Plants.

Action plan

Hives indicate that the immune system has reacted to something that it sees as a threat to the body. Our aims are to support the immune system and reduce the histamine and inflammation.

EAT/DRINK

► Apples and red onions. These contain quercetin which has an antihistamine effect.

AVOID

► In addition to avoiding any foods to which you are intolerant, don't eat the same foods day in, day out.

► Foods that contain any chemicals.

HERBS AND SUPPLEMENTS

► Nettle, burdock, juniper berries and lobelia teas or tinctures. They contain natural anti-histamines.

► Take vitamin C with bioflavanoids. Vitamin C has powerful antihistamine effects.

► Take L-glutamine powder before main meals. This can sometimes help to prevent reacting to some foods. It also helps to nutrify the liver.

► Apply cooled camomile or elderflower tea to the area. These both have a soothing effect.

► Aloe vera gel or pulp can be applied for its anti-inflammatory effect.

EXTRA TIPS

► Identify and avoid the irritant where possible. You can always try one potentially offending food at a time at a later date once your immune system is stronger.

HYPERTHYROIDISM

Hyperthyroidism refers to overactivity of the thyroid gland, usually involving an overproduction of the thyroid hormones. The thyroid hormones control our metabolic rate (the rate at which we burn up calories for energy). Thus an excessive amount of thyroid hormones leads to a faster metabolism and speeding up of all body processes. Severe hyperthyroidism is called Grave's disease. It can also be referred to as thyrotoxicosis.

CAUSES

It is not really known what causes hyperthyroidism. It may be an abnormal immune response or lumps on the thyroid that stimulate excessive hormone production. Symptoms include feeling hot, sweating, insomnia, fatigue, diarrhoea, hand tremors, rapid heart beat and irritability. Changes in the menstrual pattern may also occur.

Action plan

Many people are recommended radioactive iodine or surgery as treatment options. It may well be worth changing your diet and lifestyle.

⠿ EAT/DRINK

► Raw cruciferous vegetables (broccoli, cabbage, kale and cauliflower, swede), soya and millet. These can help to slow down thyroid function.
► Water and calming herbal teas. Camomile, lemon balm, peppermint, fennel and hops are all recommended.
► Oats and lettuce. Both of these have calming effects.

⠿ AVOID

► Stimulants. Tea, coffee, alcohol, drugs, chocolate, salt, colas and nicotine can all speed up the metabolic rate so are not recommended.
► Sea vegetables. These are rich in iodine and can increase the production of thyroid hormones so are best avoided until thyroid function returns to normal.
► Sugar, refined carbohydrates and processed foods and dairy.

HERBS AND SUPPLEMENTS

► Take green superfoods daily such as spirulina, blue-green algae or barley grass. Those with an overactive thyroid have a higher need for nutrients and these foods are a good way of increasing nutrient intake without taxing the system.
► Take magnesium citrate. Magnesium is calming to the nervous system.

EXTRA TIP

► Keep blood-sugar levels stable. This will help to keep energy levels stable. Eat small, regular meals and snacks.

HYPOGLYCAEMIA

This means low blood-sugar levels. When blood-sugar levels drop too low, this causes an overwhelming craving for refined carbohydrates. To satisfy that craving more and more sugary foods are devoured, causing a see-saw effect of soaring and plummeting sugar levels. This is why if you start to eat just one chocolate bar, you crave another one.

The sugar gives you the rush but the drop is not far behind it. Excess insulin is produced with this condition. This will cause trouble for the pancreas as time goes on and that's when hypoglycaemia can end up as type 2 diabetes. There should be up to two teaspoons of sugar in the blood at any time for physical function and brain function. If your blood sugar is low you may feel tired, emotional, irritable, shaky and you may have headaches and crave sweet foods or carbohydrates. This is hypoglycaemia.

CAUSES MAY INCLUDE
▸ Glucose imbalance.
▸ Poor diet of too many refined simple carbohydrates.
▸ Malabsorption.
▸ Low hydrochloric acid.
▸ Stress.
▸ Childbirth.
▸ Breastfeeding.
▸ Over-sugarization of the body.
▸ Alcohol.
▸ *Candida albicans* (see page 219).
▸ Food allergies/sensitivities.

Action plan
Learn how to keep your blood-sugar levels balanced through diet, exercise and lifestyle and you will notice an amazing difference.

EAT/DRINK
▸ Whole grains such as brown rice and quinoa, slow-releasing carbohydrates which break down into sugar slowly, releasing a steady trickle into the blood stream that keeps your energy stable.
▸ Wholefoods such as pulses, nuts, seeds, fish, lean meat, vegetables and fruit.
▸ Liver-friendly foods, such as cabbage, sauerkraut, sprouted seeds, broccoli, kohlrabi and Jerusalem artichokes.
▸ Green vegetables, root vegetables, avocados, beans, legumes, tofu, fish, sea vegetables and white lean meats.
▸ Almonds and Brazil nuts.
▸ Raw shelled hemp seeds or sesame seeds.
▸ Low glycaemic foods help to regulate blood-sugar levels and tame sugar cravings. Whole grains and fresh veggies are great choices.

AVOID
▸ Sweets, sugar, refined white bread, sodas, tea, coffee, alcohol and chocolate. These can further stimulate blood-sugar imbalances and strain organs.

HERBS AND SUPPLEMENTS
▸ Take spirulina or wild blue-green algae for their high mineral content and protein source. These greens can help to tame fluctuating blood-sugar swings.
▸ Take a vitamin B complex supplement. Royal jelly is another option.
▸ Start taking the following nutrients on a daily basis with food until the hypoglycaemia regulates:
* GTF chromium.
* Zinc.
* Manganese.
* Digestive enzyme complex.
* Amino acid complex or protein.
* Biotin.
* Pantothenic acid.
▸ I generally recommend a rotation of the following herbs until the hypoglycaemic symptoms subside. Start with one herb and use until the entire bottle is finished.

If symptoms persist, start the next herb and complete the course before moving on to the next.

* Barberry.
* Ginseng.
* Yellow dock.
* Goldenseal.
* Oregon grape root.

⁞⁞ EXTRA TIPS

► Get to bed early to let the liver and gallbladder do their detox work. Do not burn the candle at both ends.

► Eat breakfast. Running out of the door on an empty stomach is a recipe for disaster, energy slumps and low blood-sugar levels.

► Eat regularly, six meals a day should do it. Breakfast, snack, lunch, snack, dinner, snack. You must adhere to my eat-often rule. It works.

► Combine proteins and carbs together at the same meal until you stabilize the condition. So, eat chicken and fish

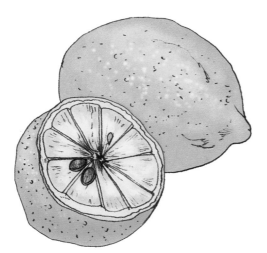

together with salad and veggies. If you are vegetarian, make sure that you are getting enough sprouted seeds, tofu, sesame seeds, almonds, beans and eggs.

HYPOTHYROIDISM

Hypothyroidism refers to an underactive thyroid meaning the thyroid does not produce sufficient quantities of thyroid hormones. As the thyroid hormones control our metabolic rate (the rate at which we burn up calories for energy) a deficiency of them can result in fatigue, weight gain, low appetite, feeling cold, slow heart rate, weakness, constipation and depression. Other symptoms often associated with hypothyroidism include dry, yellowy-coloured skin, goitre (an enlargement of the thyroid), hair loss, loss of the outer third of the eyebrows and brain fog.

CAUSES

In hypothyroidism there may be a lack of thyroid hormones or there may be a problem with the conversion of thyroid hormones into their active form. Another contributory factor may be the presence of thyroid antibodies that suppress thyroid function. It is not known why any of the above would happen. Lack of certain nutrients needed for thyroid hormone production is one contributory factor. Lack of exercise, food intolerances and disturbances in the rest of the endocrine system may also be involved.

Action plan

If you suffer from the above symptoms, ask your GP to test your thyroid function. The following may help those with symptoms of an underactive thyroid.

⠿ EAT/DRINK

► Sea vegetables which contain iodine needed for the production of thyroid hormones. Kelp and nori are particularly useful.

► Brazil nuts as they are one of the best sources of selenium which is also needed for thyroid function.

► Fresh fruit, vegetables, nuts, seeds, whole grains, pulses and fish contain the essential fats, B vitamins, zinc, vitamin C and magnesium. Thyroid malfunction is often the result of chronic adrenal stress which leads to deficiencies in the above.

► Water: at least 8 glasses daily. Fluid levels are vital for the whole endocrine system, including the thyroid.

⠿ AVOID

► Wheat. The gliadin in wheat can be toxic to the thyroid so is best avoided. Some people do best without the other gluten grains as well (oats, rye, barley, kamut and spelt).

► Raw cruciferous vegetables (broccoli, cabbage, kale, cauliflower, swede), soya and millet. These can all be goitregenic (suppress thyroid function). The cruciferous vegetables are fine if cooked, and fermented soya in moderation is fine (natto, miso, tempeh and tamari).

► I have observed that avoiding challenging products like salt, caffeine and dairy for a while helps.

► Sugar, refined carbohydrates, processed foods and alcohol are all empty calories and can lead to easy weight gain.

► Fluorine and chlorine. These are both chemically similar to iodine and can displace iodine in the thyroid. Fluorine is found in many toothpastes, tap water and tea. Chlorine is found in tap water and swimming pools. It is best to filter your water and use fluoride-free toothpaste.

HERBS AND SUPPLEMENTS

► Take L-tyrosine. This amino acid is needed for normal thyroid function.

⠿ EXTRA TIPS

► Exercise every day. Exercise stimulates the metabolism and gets the blood circulating to all areas. Yoga is particularly good as the inverted postures get the blood circulating to the thyroid gland in the neck.

► Take the thyroid temperature test. Put a thermometer by your bed. When you wake in the morning, put the thermometer under your arm and lie still with it there for 10 minutes. Record your temperature in this way for five consecutive days. If it is consistently below 36.5C, then your thyroid may be somewhat underactive.

HYSTERECTOMY-RELATED DISORDERS

Hysterectomy refers to the removal of the uterus by surgical procedures. In a total hysterectomy, the cervix and the ovaries are removed. In a partial hysterectomy, only the uterus is removed.

The most dramatic effects are felt if the ovaries are removed as well as the uterus. Menopausal symptoms such as hot flushes and insomnia can arise, menstruation ceases and conception is no longer possible. Oestrogen production is dramatically reduced. Even when the ovaries remain intact oestrogen production is reduced and the menopause is often earlier than it might have been. Many women complain of a complete plummet in libido and report little or no sexual desire.

Other effects include a greater risk of osteoporosis as the protective effects of oestrogen and progesterone are reduced, and increased risk of heart disease.

CAUSES
► Cysts and fibroids.
► Prolapse of the uterus.
► Endometriosis.
► Persistent and heavy bleeding.

Action plan

This may be an important time to support the adrenal glands as once ovarian production of oestrogen ceases or diminishes, adrenal production should increase.

EAT/DRINK
► Essential fatty acids. Good sources include mackerel, salmon, trout, sardines, herrings, flax seeds, hemp seeds, pumpkin seeds and sunflower seeds. These also contain vitamin E. Both vitamin E and essential fats are needed for healing after surgery and hormone balancing.
► Green vegetables. These are high in both calcium and magnesium needed for bone health. Other foods that contain both calcium and magnesium include oats, chickpeas, hazelnuts, Brazil nuts, almonds, sesame seeds, tahini, amaranth and quinoa.
► Dandelion-root coffee for liver and bowel health. The liver is responsible for breaking down old hormones and removing them from the body via the bowel.
► Carrots and beetroot. Both can help with hormone regulation during the menopause. Beetroot is especially good for building the blood which may be necessary after surgery.

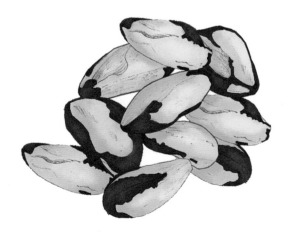

► Soya for its oestrogenic effect. Tempeh, tofu, miso, natto and soya yoghurt are all good. Avoid processed soya as in textured vegetable protein (TVP) or soya isolates and many processed foods.

► Include wheat germ (if wheat is tolerated). Wheat germ is rich in vitamin E, B vitamins and magnesium, all of which are important for hormone balancing and the function of the adrenal glands.

► Ground flax seeds which contain precursors to lignans that have an oestrogenic effect. They also supply essential fatty acids needed for hormonal balance.

► Sea vegetables such as hijiki, wakame, kelp and kombu deserve a special mention for their incredibly high mineral content, including abundant calcium.

⠿ AVOID

► Sugar, refined foods, alcohol, caffeine, salt and artificial additives. These can all upset blood-sugar levels and trigger menopausal symptoms.

HERBS AND SUPPLEMENTS

► Drink oestrogenic herbs as teas. Fenugreek, liquorice, red clover, fennel and sage are all useful. Dandelion and nettle teas are also useful.

► Take evening primrose oil which has an oestrogenic effect and can help to keep skin well hydrated.

► Supplement with vitamin E which has been found to reduce hot flushes, stimulate oestrogen production and aid healing of scar tissue. It can be applied directly to scar tissue; just pierce the capsule and massage in the oil.

► Take probiotic supplements. Surgery can disrupt the balance of bacteria in the bowel. Good digestion and nutrient absorption is dependent on good bowel health.

► Herbs such as dong quai and black cohosh can be used to relieve menopausal symptoms (see page 138 for further information).

► Take a bone-supportive formula including magnesium, calcium, boron, vitamins D, K and E.

EXTRA TIP

► Take regular, weight-bearing exercise. This is the best way to ensure strong bones. Walking, aerobics, dancing, lifting weights, skipping, re-bounding and yoga can all help to build muscle and bones.

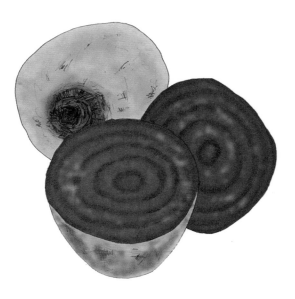

IMPOTENCE

Sometimes referred to as erectile dysfunction, impotence refers to a lack of desire for sex or an inability to maintain an erection either partially and/or fully. More often than not, this problem is stress related. And then it can become psychological.

CAUSES AND RISK FACTORS

- Stress.
- Emotional problems.
- Too much alcohol.
- Smoking.
- Diabetes.
- Overweight.
- Inflammation.
- Heart problems.
- Medications.
- Hormonal imbalances.
- B vitamin deficiency.
- Recreational drug use.

Action plan

It is important to talk to your GP if you suffer from impotence to find the cause. The following dietary advice may help.

❖ EAT/DRINK

- A wholefoods diet of fruits, vegetables, nuts, seeds, legumes (all types of beans, peas, lentils), seaweeds, sprouted seeds and whole grains, particularly quinoa.
- Oily fish such as mackerel, tuna or sardines, which contain anti-inflammatory omega-3 fats, 2–3 times a week.
- Apples contain quercetin, a flavanoid that has been shown to prevent the growth of libido-reducing prostate cancer cells.

- Avocados contain high levels of folic acid, which helps to metabolize proteins, thus giving you more energy. They also contain vitamin B6, a nutrient that increases male and female hormone production, and vitamin E, both of which are vital for overall sexual function.
- Bananas which contain an alkaloid compound called bufotenine which acts on the brain to improve mood, self-confidence and possibly sex drive. Bananas are also rich in vitamin B6 which is important in the manufacture of sex hormones.
- Beetroot. Well known for its immune-boosting and blood-building properties, beetroot contains nutrients that help to support the liver which is where sexual hormones are conjugated. It is also rich in iron, calcium and potassium needed to promote healthy circulation to the reproductive organs.
- Berries, such as strawberries, blueberries and blackberries, are sources of zinc, needed for a healthy reproductive system. Seeds, particularly pumpkin, are also a great source of zinc.
- Celery which contains androstenone, a biochemical cousin of the male hormone testosterone and believed to be the principal chemical of attraction or pheromone. The Romans dedicated celery to Pluto, their god of sex and the underworld, and crushed celery seeds (easily added to salads or breads) are said to be particularly potent.
- Chillies which may heat up your sex life, due to capsaicin – the substance that gives a kick to peppers, curries and other spicy foods. Capsaicin stimulates nerve

endings to release chemicals, raising the heart rate and possibly triggering the release of endorphins giving you the pleasurable feeling of a natural high.

► Cinnamon. According to Chinese medicine, cinnamon is thought to tone the kidneys and produce a strong flow of energy and it is linked to virile sexuality. Studies have also shown that the smell of cinnamon can also boost concentration and alertness.

► Raw cacao, nibs and powders – the emperor Montezuma used to drink chocolate before entering his harem, which gave rise to the belief that chocolate is an aphrodisiac. But the best thing you can do is to eat raw cacao before the cacao is cooked and the sugar added to turn it into chocolate.

► Garlic, which contains allicin, an ingredient that may help increase blood flow to the penis.

► Ginger, which is one of the oldest medicinal spices in the world; it allegedly increases the blood flow to the genitals and therefore acts as an aphrodisiac.

► Spinach, which is a source of iron and calcium. Muscles need calcium to spasm and contract.

AVOID
► Alcohol creates blood sugar highs and lows that will not help performance.

► Coffee. It contains caffeine which can raise blood-sugar levels, disturb sleeping patterns and deplete the body of essential nutrients. Substitute with dandelion coffee or tea which is delicious, caffeine-free and can aid relaxation.

► Sugar – use cinnamon or agave syrup instead.

► White processed foods such as white pasta, white rice and white bread. These are refined carbohydrates, high in sugar, that convert quickly into glucose, making your blood-sugar levels soar within minutes.

► Tinned food with added salt and sugar as salt increases the risk of water retention and high blood pressure while sugar is calorie-rich and nutrient-free, so check soups and canned beans to make sure that they are sugar- and salt-free.

HERBS AND SUPPLEMENTS
► Saw palmetto acts like a tonic for men and has been used for centuries to treat an enlarged prostate (see page 351).

► The herbal extract ginkgo biloba may help with erectile dysfunction.

► The African herb yohimbine may also help but as with all herbal supplements take only on the advice of your GP.

► The amino acid L-arginine has been found to help impotence. (If you suffer from cold sores, avoid this amino acid.)

EXTRA TIPS
► Reduce stress. Take up relaxation exercises like yoga or meditation.

► Work safely, away from radiation and chemicals.

► Exercise regularly and lightly. Stay trim.

► Ask your GP about testosterone creams.

INCONTINENCE

Incontinence refers to an inability to fully control the emptying of the bladder. Anxiety, emotions, heavy lifting, coughing and sneezing may all trigger the release of a few drops or more of urine from the bladder.

CAUSES
► Weak pelvic-floor muscles.
► Prostate problems.
► Gynaecological problems.
► Chronic constipation.
► Obesity.
► Strokes.
► Smoking.
► Old age.
► Stress.
► Spinal injuries.

Action plan

It is necessary to address the underlying causes so investigations may be necessary.

⠿ EAT/DRINK
► Green vegetables. These are high in calcium and magnesium needed for proper muscle and nerve contraction and relaxation. Other good sources include almonds, hazelnuts, Brazil nuts, sesame seeds, sea vegetables, parsley, quinoa and oats.
► Barley water. Grated ginger and lemon juice can be added for extra flavour. This is beneficial to the urinary system generally.

⠿ AVOID
► Salt, alcohol, caffeine and chocolate. These can all put a strain on the kidneys.
► Eat foods rich in oxalic acid in moderation only as they may irritate the bladder. Spinach, chard, rhubarb, eggs, asparagus, beet greens and sorrel are all sources.

HERBS AND SUPPLEMENTS
► Higher intakes of vitamin D, protein and potassium have all been associated with decreased risk of an overactive bladder.
► There is some evidence that vitamins B3 and B6 have a protective effect.
► Calcium hydroxylapaptite has been shown to be effective with stress urinary incontinence.

⠿ EXTRA TIPS
► Practise pelvic-floor exercises daily. These involve isolating and contracting the muscles that control the flow of urine. They are best taught by a health professional so ask your GP for information.
► If you smoke, stop! Incontinence is one of the many problems that are associated with smoking.
► Alternate between hot and cold showers. Direct the flow of water to the lower abdomen to help to tighten the muscles in the area.
► Perform a daily massage. Mix cypress oil with a carrier of almond oil and massage into the lower abdominal area.
► Apply heat to the kidney area either via a hot-water bottle or hot compress.

INDIGESTION

Indigestion is not a single condition but the word is used to describe discomfort caused by eating. Excessive burping, flatulence and heartburn are all signs of indigestion.

CAUSES
▶ Overeating.
▶ Eating foods high in fat.
▶ Excess or deficient stomach acid.
▶ Eating too quickly and not chewing properly.

Action plan

Improve what you eat and the way that you eat it! The following plan should help to prevent indigestion.

▦ EAT/DRINK
▶ Pear and peach juice.
▶ Powdered ginger with a squeeze of lime.
▶ Banana blended with pear or mango juice.
▶ Apple cider vinegar which is a wonderful digestive tonic. Add to a little warm water and sip slowly before meals.
▶ Miso soup, whole grains, fresh veggies and fruits to reduce wind.

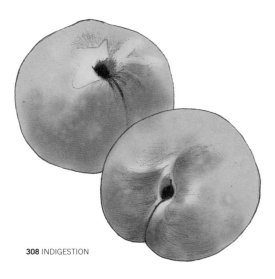

▶ Asparagus, celery, watermelon, and parsley (the parsley will help to freshen your breath as well!). These diuretic 'superfoods' will help to flush the rubbish out of your gut. Coriander also has a reputation for freshening breath.
▶ Umeboshi plums are know as the Japanese Alka-Seltzer.
▶ Pineapple contains bromelain, an enzyme that can aid digestion.

▦ AVOID
▶ Heavily spiced foods, junk foods and fried foods.
▶ Caffeine, alcohol and fizzy drinks.
▶ Rich, creamy foods, full-fat cheeses, wheat-based foods which all increase stomach gas.

HERBS AND SUPPLEMENTS
▶ Slippery elm, peppermint, camomile and thyme teas all help.
▶ Fennel tea which tastes like liquorice and has anti-gas as well as anti-spasmodic properties, making it especially helpful for bloating.
▶ Drink a small glass of aloe vera juice before every meal.
▶ L-glutamine.
▶ Gentiana root for general digestive disorders.
▶ Betaine hydrochloric acid for acid reflux.

▦ EXTRA TIPS
▶ A strip of kombu seaweed cooked with beans helps to pre-digest them.
▶ Eat small, regular meals. Do not overeat but don't starve yourself either. If you leave your stomach empty for long periods of time, the secretion of digestive enzymes slows down which triggers, you guessed it, bloating.

▶ Taking in excess air will cause gas bubbles to form, so when you eat, take small bites and chew carefully, with your mouth closed. And don't drink from a straw.

▶ Get some fresh air. Go for a quick 10-minute walk after eating. Exercise helps gas to pass through the digestive tract more quickly, so you feel better faster.

▶ Eat fruit by itself, and never for dessert. If you eat fruit straight after a high protein food such as turkey, fish or meat, you're guaranteed to expel noxious fumes. The same applies when you eat fruit at the same time as bread, rice or potatoes.

▶ Drink only warm liquids and no ice whatsoever. Drink these liquids before you eat, not with your meals. Drinking a lot of liquid with meals can make you bloated.

▶ Commercial antacids neutralize stomach acid but, over the long term, end up causing the stomach to produce even more.

I developed digestive trouble after the stress in my life spiralled out of control, I was at the end of my tether searching for answers to why I felt so wretched all of the time, and after several frustrating visits to the doctor's surgery and a few sessions with a local nutritionist, things started to become clear: the junky, high carbohydrate food I was eating, coupled with the stress, was the problem! A friend then recommended Gillian's book *You Are What You Eat*, and I haven't looked back since; I'm more aware of my body, I'm eating a sensible diet, cutting out too many naughties and managing stress.

INFLAMMATION

Inflammation is a self-protective mechanism of the body in response to injury, infection or invasion with a potentially harmful substance (e.g., from a bite, sting or pollen). Symptoms of inflammation include reddening, swelling, heat, soreness and restricted range of movement, depending on the function of the afflicted area. Any area of the body can potentially become inflamed. Inflammation can be internal and external.

As a rule of thumb, if you have a condition that ends with 'itis', it means you have inflammation of that area, e.g., tonsillitis = inflammation of the tonsils.

CAUSES INCLUDE

▶ Viruses.

▶ Bacteria.

▶ Allergies or intolerances.

▶ Stings.

▶ Bites.

Action plan

It is important to ascertain and address the source of the inflammation, rather than just suppressing it. If it is a one-off injury, bite or sting that may be easy enough. However, much inflammation is from ongoing wear and tear, food intolerances and imbalances in body function caused by unhealthy dietary and lifestyle habits. These must be addressed so that the body can deal with the perceived threat or heal the damaged tissue.

EAT/DRINK

▶ Fruit and vegetables which contain antioxidants that can reduce inflammation and aid healing. In particular eat blueberries and blackberries for their anti-inflammatory effects.

► Fresh pineapple between meals. The core of pineapple contains the anti-inflammatory enzyme bromelain. This has best effect if eaten away from other foods.

► Anti-inflammatory essential fats. Good sources include oily fish, hemp seeds, flax seeds, pumpkin seeds, sunflower seeds and cold-pressed oils.

► Water: 8 glasses a day. Fluids take healing nutrients to the cells where they are needed and remove waste products.

⠿ AVOID
► Inflammatory foods. These include sugar, refined carbohydrates, additives, dairy products, fatty or processed meats and anything to which you are intolerant.

HERBS AND SUPPLEMENTS
► Anti-inflammatory herbs include camomile, meadowsweet, white willow bark, fennel and yellow dock.

► Vitamin C with bioflavanoids has anti-inflammatory properties and can aid healing.

► Zinc is also vital for proper immune function and healing.

⠿ EXTRA TIPS
► Elevate the inflamed area, apply a cold compress and rest it. This can help to reduce inflammation and speed healing.

INFLUENZA

Influenza or 'flu is caused by a viral infection. Symptoms include fever, fatigue, headaches, aches and pains, feeling hot and cold, coughing and sneezing and general weakness.

CAUSES
The 'flu virus can be spread by being in contact with an infected person. Susceptibility may be increased by having a compromised immune system, stress and lack of sleep. The very old and very young may also be more susceptible.

Action plan
Take the time to take care of yourself and focus on getting back to full strength.

⠿ EAT/DRINK
► Fluids. Warm drinks are better than cold as cold drinks will need to be warmed up to body temperature by the digestive system and this can use up vital energy reserves. Warm water, freshly pressed fruit and vegetable juices, herbal teas and broths are all recommended to replace fluids lost through sweating. Avoid orange juice as it can increase mucus production.

► Vegetable juices and broths, soups and fresh fruit.

⠿ AVOID
► Sugar, refined carbohydrates, dairy products, meat, alcohol, caffeine, salt and additives. These may challenge the digestive system or suppress the immune system.

HERBS AND SUPPLEMENTS
► Herbal teas including ginger, nettle, dandelion, slippery elm, echinacea and pau d'arco. These can all be sipped throughout the day.

► Avoid suppressing the fever if possible. The body raises its temperature in order to burn off toxins and the infection so it is best to let it run its course. A cool flannel can be applied to the forehead if necessary to cool the head.

INSOMNIA

Insomnia is characterized by a general inability to sleep through the night. It can be divided into two categories: the inability to fall asleep and waking up after a short amount of sleep. Some people have a combination of both.

Sleep is one of the most important factors to affect our overall health and wellbeing. Much repair and rejuvenation takes place in our bodies when we sleep. Lack of sleep can lead to slow wound healing and increased susceptibility to infections. Concentration and brain function decline if we do not get adequate sleep. Blood-sugar imbalances and overeating are both more likely if we are sleep deprived.

CAUSES

There are many potential underlying factors that may lead to insomnia, including:
► Blood-sugar imbalance – if blood-sugar levels drop at night the adrenal glands release stress hormones which in turn raise blood-sugar levels. The stress hormones often lead to interrupted sleep.
► Nutrient deficiencies, particularly magnesium, vitamins B6, B3 and the essential fats. Magnesium is needed for muscle and nerve relaxation. Vitamin B6 and the essential fats are needed for brain chemicals involved in relaxation.
► Amino acid deficiencies, particularly tryptophan. Tryptophan gets converted to serotonin and melatonin. Melatonin is the sleep hormone, levels of which should be raised at night. If vitamin B3 levels are low, tryptophan may be converted to B3 instead of melatonin so it is important to keep levels of vitamin B3 up.
► Stress, which affects adrenal release of adrenalin and cortisol. Imbalances in these can lead to an inability to get to sleep and can cause waking in the night or early morning.
► Hyperthyroidism – an excess of thyroid hormones – can lead to nervousness and an inability to completely relax.
► Caffeine, alcohol and nicotine usage as well as other drugs. These are all stimulants that can raise adrenal hormones. Caffeine is found in tea, coffee, chocolate, colas and many medications, such as painkillers.
► Pain and cramps. Both can lead to waking in the night and difficulty with getting to sleep.
► Indigestion, breathing difficulties, snoring, being too hot or too cold, depression, jet lag, restless leg syndrome and anxiety can all affect sleep.
► Many medications can also affect the ability to sleep and the quality of the sleep.

Action plan

It is important to address the underlying causes behind the insomnia so check out other entries in this book if necessary.

⣿ EAT/DRINK

▶ Lettuce in the evening. The milky sap in lettuce contains an opium-like substance called lactucin that can help to induce sleep and relaxation. Try lettuce soup.

▶ Camomile tea before going to bed each evening. Camomile has natural sedative properties that can relax nervous tension.

▶ Green vegetables which contain magnesium, an important mineral involved in the relaxation of muscles and nerves. Good vegetables to include are kale, broccoli, Brussels sprouts, cavolo nero, chicory and pak choi. Other sources of magnesium include whole grains, nuts and seeds.

▶ Tryptophan-rich foods in your evening meal. Tryptophan is converted to the sleep hormone melatonin in the brain. Foods that contain tryptophan include chicken, turkey, brown rice, peas, fish, pumpkin seeds, oats, tuna, figs, natural yoghurt and bananas.

▶ Complex carbohydrates with your evening meal. Eating carbohydrates leads to the release of insulin which is needed to carry tryptophan into the brain where it can be converted into melatonin. Good carbohydrates to include are brown rice, quinoa, buckwheat, oats, millet, barley and sweet potatoes.

▶ Oatmeal in the evening. Oats have tranquillizing and nerve-restorative properties. Simmer 1–2 tbsp of oat flakes or oat meal in a mug of water for 10–20 minutes and sip.

▶ B-vitamin-rich whole grains. The B vitamins are needed for energy over the day and for nervous system function. Whole grains such as brown rice, quinoa, oats, millet and buckwheat are all good sources.

▶ As tryptophan may be converted to vitamin B3 (niacin) instead of serotonin if dietary intake is insufficient, niacin-rich foods are particularly important. These include fish, chicken, eggs, soya beans, peas and fenugreek.

▶ Fish oils found in oily fish such as salmon, mackerel, sardines, pilchards, herrings and trout. Essential fats are so important for brain chemistry and the neurotransmitters required for chemicals involved in sleep.

⣿ AVOID

▶ Sugar, refined carbohydrates, tea, coffee, alcohol, additives, nicotine and any other drugs or stimulants. These can all stimulate the adrenal glands to produce stress hormones and can upset blood-sugar levels.

▶ High-fat, heavy foods. These can increase body temperature meaning sleep becomes difficult. They can also sit in the stomach and cause indigestion which can also interfere with restful sleep.

HERBS AND SUPPLEMENTS

▶ Take a herbal supplement containing relaxing herbs 30–60 minutes before going to bed. Passion flower, hops, skullcap, lime flowers and Californian poppy are all relaxing herbs.

▶ Jujube seeds or powder (open up capsule).

▶ 5-HTP half an hour before bed increases serotonin, which is a precursor to the sleep hormone melatonin.

► The herb valerian may help for some of the short term, but acts as a stimulant for others.

► Supplement with magnesium citrate. Magnesium is needed for muscle and nerve relaxation and is often deficient in our diets. Amino acid complex may help.

⁙ EXTRA TIPS

► To keep blood-sugar levels stable, always have breakfast and eat small, regular meals and snacks during the day. Don't have your last meal too late in the evening but have a small snack before you go to bed. A few hazelnuts or almonds work well.

► Avoid eating a large meal in the evening.

► If you are overweight then aim to lose weight. Being overweight increases your risk of snoring and sleep apnoea, which can interfere with a good night's sleep.

► Avoid strenuous exercise within three hours of going to bed. Exercise raises stress hormones and testosterone, both of which can interfere with sleep patterns.

► However, exercising during the day is great for aiding restful sleep. Try brisk walking, jogging, skipping, dancing, cycling or aerobics.

► Establish a regular bedtime routine. Avoid watching television or using the computer late at night as these are not relaxing activities for the brain. Instead, have a warm bath with some lavender essential oil, listen to relaxing music and light some candles.

► Do not expose yourself to bright lights in the evening or if you wake in the night. Light reduces levels of melatonin, the sleep hormone, making sleep less likely to occur. Use lamps instead.

► Get up at the same time every morning in order to establish a routine. Even if you have taken a long time to get to sleep or have woken in the night, do not be tempted to lie in. This will just perpetuate the problem. Avoid lying in at weekends as this can disrupt the rhythm.

► Learn relaxation techniques or visualizations. These can involve relaxing each part of the body one by one or visualizing peaceful scenes. They can be great for getting the body into a relaxed state. Meditation and playing 'white noise' can also be useful. There are many CDs and tapes around that have white noise such as rainfall or waves crashing on the shore that can induce a state of relaxation.

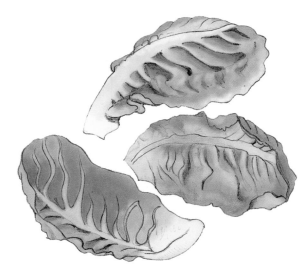

IRRITABLE BOWEL SYNDROME

Symptoms are unpleasant and varied but usually a combination of stomach pain, bloating, cramping, constipation and diarrhoea. A tell-tale sign is also mucus in your stools. What's happening is that the muscular contractions of the gut tract are irregular. Food and waste movement is badly affected as a result.

Many people say it is caused by stress (see page 373). Certainly, stress can induce gastrointestinal spasms but the main cause is what I call the 'body plumbing back up'. Your digestive system is shot and your intestines do not work properly. There is an erratic quality to the strength of contractions which move your food waste through the intestinal tract. When the contractions are too fast and strong, you get diarrhoea; when they are too slow, you become constipated. You end up quite depleted nutritionally as this condition interferes with the absorption of nutrients.

Sometimes IBS can be mistaken for a more serious condition such as ulcerative colitis, diverticulitis or Crohn's disease, so do get checked out by your GP.

CAUSES MAY INCLUDE
► Food sensitivities (see page 178).
► Imbalances in bacteria in the gut.
► Stress.
► Magnesium deficiency.
► Lack of digestive enzymes.
► Low stomach acid.
► Poor diet.
► *Candida albicans* (see page 219).
► Itchy anus or nose.

Action plan

The key is to cut out irritants and add plenty of gut-friendly foods to your diet.

EAT/DRINK
► Veggie juices to boost nutrition because most sufferers will be nutritionally depleted.
► Whole grains, vegetables, legumes and sprouted seeds. These fibre-rich foods pass smoothly through the intestinal tract. However, go easy on broccoli, cauliflower, onions and cabbage which may aggravate this condition.
► Dried figs that have been soaked in water.
► Artichoke soup.

AVOID
► Wheat and dairy products as these are common gut irritants. You might be OK with almond or hemp milks but cow's milk is a trigger so avoid it for now.
► Corn, processed foods, sugars, sweeteners, margarine, red meat, alcohol and coffee for two months and monitor the results. Do not replace sugars with artificial sweeteners.
► Spicy foods, tomatoes, citrus fruits and anything else to which you may be intolerant (consider a food intolerance test, www.gillianmckeith.info).

HERBS AND SUPPLEMENTS
► The best herb for this condition is gentiana root. You may want to disguise its unpleasant taste in some apple purée or mashed banana.
► Two peppermint capsules or peppermint oil in between meals may be enough to reduce gas and intestinal spasms.
► Artichoke extract.
► Use turmeric and ginger in your cooking.

▶ Drink slippery elm tea between meals to help soothe the gut. Camomile, peppermint and fennel teas are also good digestive aids.

▶ Drink pau d'arco tea for its anti-inflammatory properties and its ability to keep yeasts at bay.

▶ Drink flaxseed tea.

▶ Sprinkle linseeds over salads.

▶ Evening primrose oil.

▶ Slippery elm powder to calm down inflammation in the gut. Mix the powder with the oatmeal, apple sauce or a cup of warm water.

▶ Take L-glutamine powder or capsules. Glutamine is used up in large amounts with those who have IBS. One of its jobs is to carry ammonia to the kidneys for excretion.

▶ Triphala tablets and milk thistle tincture help, too.

▶ Supplement with probiotics to help to re-establish good bacterial balance in the intestines. As well as the probiotic, make sure that you take a low-potency B complex once daily to help intestinal tract.

▶ Take digestive enzymes with meals and a tablespoon of apple cider vinegar before meals. Do not take protein digestive enzymes if you have stomach ulcers. You could try papaya enzymes instead.

▶ Betaine with HCL may dramatically improve symptoms if digestive enzymes are not improving your symptoms. Start out slowly with low dosages before meals.

▶ Make sure that you are getting enough magnesium which can act as a gut relaxant.

▶ Take vitamin B complex to help you break down your foods.

▶ A good six months on an intestinal probiotic powder or capsule is beneficial.

▶ Rice bran oil is very helpful for IBS. Ask your health food store for gamma oryzenol.

⁙ EXTRA TIPS

▶ Have a stool analysis done. There are so many conditions that can be similar to IBS.

▶ Do not overeat and chew your food really well. Only swallow it once it has become liquid.

▶ Learn to manage stress and engage in daily relaxation; yoga, tai chi, meditation and breathing exercises are all good. In particular relax before, during and after meals to allow digestion to take place.

▶ Have several treatments of reflexology.

▶ Massage stomach with peppermint oil and almond oil together.

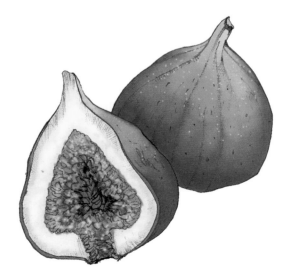

J

JET LAG

Jet lag is caused by travelling across time zones – which upsets the body's circadian rhythm – as well as by the reduced oxygen levels on board planes. The recycled air can also lead to dehydration and the risk of picking up a bug.

Action plan

▶ Before you board the plane, set your watch to the time in your new destination. Aim to eat and sleep according to the new time zone while on the plane.

▶ Avoid alcohol and caffeine both the day before and during the flight. These are dehydrating and stimulating and will prevent good-quality sleep or rest.

▶ Make sure your immune system is in tip-top condition before you fly. Aeroplanes can be breeding grounds for bugs and bacteria so drink a vegetable juice daily for a week before travel and eat plenty of fruit and vegetables.

▶ Get some exercise before you fly. This can help you to feel calm during the flight.

▶ Eat lightly during the flight. Particularly avoid foods high in sugar, salt, refined carbohydrates and fat as these will tax the body, increase dehydration and leave you feeling more tired. Take your own snacks of fruit, nuts and seeds.

▶ Drink plenty of water throughout the flight. Sip it regularly to avoid becoming dehydrated which can cause tiredness and headaches.

▶ Walk around and stretch regularly to keep the circulation going. This helps the tissues remain oxygenated and reduces the chances of developing muscle cramps or deep vein thrombosis (DVT).

▶ If you are travelling overnight, invest in an eye mask and ear plugs. These are inexpensive ways of helping you get some sleep during the journey.

▶ Avoid planning to do too much as soon as you arrive at your destination. Take time to adjust and rest if necessary. However, if you arrive in the morning or during the day, avoid going to bed until the early evening if possible. Try to get into the day-night routine of the place you are in. Exposing yourself to daylight will help you stay awake, so have a wander around and get the feel of the new place.

▶ Drink calming teas to aid sleep on the plane or in the evening before you go to bed when you reach your destination. Camomile, lemon balm and lime flowers are all calming. Other herbs, such as passionflower, skull cap and hops can also be taken as tinctures or capsules to aid sleep and relaxation.

▶ Include high tryptophan foods in your evening meal when you arrive. Tryptophan is an amino acid that can be converted into melatonin (the sleep hormone) in the brain. Tryptophan-rich foods include chicken, turkey, brown rice, soya, fish, bananas and eggs. Oats are also a relaxing food.

▶ Supplement with melatonin before you go to bed when you arrive at your destination. Melatonin is a brain chemical that is released during darkness to aid sleep. The dose is between 2–5mg, depending on your weight and needs. However, while melatonin is available over the counter in America, it is only available on prescription in the UK.

► Alternatively, supplement with 5-HTP – this can be converted into melatonin in the brain and is available from health-food stores.

► Take the supplements magnesium to help aid relaxation if you find travel stressful and/or B vitamin complex if travel tires you out.

► To make your own pick-me-up, add a few drops of astragalus and Siberian ginseng to powdered vitamin C dissolved in warm water.

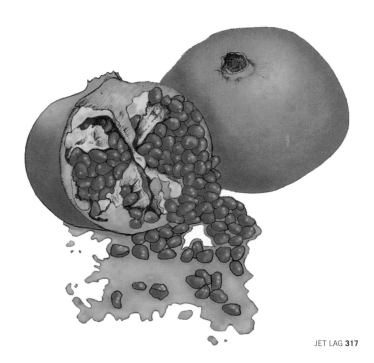

K

KIDNEY STONES

Kidney stones can cause terrible pain in the middle back, travelling even to the stomach area. You can end up in agony. They are almost always made up of calcium oxalate which is created when oxalic acid binds with calcium to form stones instead of coming out in the urine. It's really crystallized calcium. One side effect is that you may find blood in the urine. Fever, nausea and vomiting may occur, too.

CAUSES MAY INCLUDE

- Poor diet.
- Calcium oxalate build-up.
- Uric acid build-up.
- Too much coffee.
- Overly refined diet.
- Too much meat.
- High sodium intake.
- Lack of dietary fibre.

Action plan

This plan will help prevent kidney stones and is not designed to help pass them. It is essential you are monitored by your GP if you have kidney stones.

EAT/DRINK

- A cup of warm water in the morning when you wake up and another one before you go to bed at night. Squeeze a few drops of lemon into the water as that helps to cut down on uric acid, a contributory factor with kidney stones.
- Dark green leafy vegetables, seaweeds, tofu, buckwheat, lima beans, pumpkin seeds, raw shelled hemp seeds and fish which all contain the mineral magnesium. Magnesium makes the oxalate calcium

more soluble so it can leave the body when you urinate.
- Rice bran has been shown in studies to reduce urinary calcium.
- Brown rice, buckwheat, avocados, sunflower seeds, blackstrap molasses and legumes contain potassium, to balance sodium, and magnesium, for the proper utilization of calcium.
- Quinoa, mung beans, water chestnuts, aduki beans and kidney beans are all thought to be beneficial to the kidneys.
- Fibre to slow the movement of food and to bind calcium to the digestive tract. A lack of fibre will send more calcium into the blood stream.
- Grated radish.
- Watermelon juice. Juice the rind, too.
- Black bean juice before you eat.
- Cranberry juice. This will help to reduce urinary calcium.

AVOID

- Fizzy drinks. The phosphoric acid in them could increase kidney-stone formation.
- Salt. Too much salt increases urinary calcium and you are then at greater risk of kidney stones.
- Overly spicy foods, foods with added sugar or red meats as these all put added pressure on the kidneys.
- Dairy products, chocolate and black tea as they contain oxalic acid.
- Spinach and rhubarb are high in oxalates, which may combine with calcium to form insoluble crystals in the kidneys, a common form of kidney stones.
- Peppers, aubergines, tomatoes and white potatoes may promote congestion in the kidneys due to the release of solanine.

HERBS AND SUPPLEMENTS

▶ Drink dandelion-root tea.

▶ Parsley is helpful for kidney complaints.

▶ The herb uva ursi has been traditionally used for kidney stones.

▶ Spirulina and chlorella.

▶ Take digestive enzymes with meals to aid digestion and therefore ease pressure on the kidneys.

⠿ EXTRA TIPS

▶ Eat early in the evening. Don't go to bed on a full stomach or you will overwork your kidneys.

▶ Avoid antacids.

▶ In severe cases, Chelation Therapy may help.

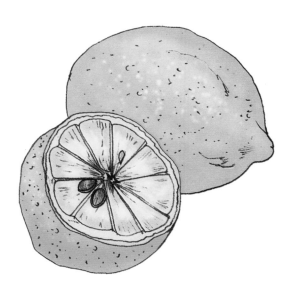

L

LACTOSE INTOLERANCE

Individuals who are lactose intolerant are unable to digest the milk sugar lactose. Digestion of lactose requires the enzyme lactase. Lactase may be deficient or absent in those with lactose intolerance.

Lactose intolerance usually results in unpleasant digestive symptoms when products containing lactose are eaten. Diarrhoea, bloating, flatulence and discomfort are common. Children with lactose intolerance may also suffer from vomiting and failure to gain weight. Caucasians are the least likely group to suffer from lactose intolerance. It is common in adults of all other racial groups.

While most dairy products contain lactose, fermented products, such as yoghurt and kefir, have had most of their lactose digested by the bacteria during the fermentation process.

CAUSES MAY INCLUDE
▶ Genetics.
▶ Damage to the digestive tract caused by other digestive problems such as coeliac disease, gastroenteritis or colitis.

Action plan

Add plenty of non-dairy calcium-rich foods to your diet. There are lots to choose from.

❖ EAT/DRINK
▶ Kale, pak choi, broccoli, romaine lettuce, savoy cabbage, cavolo nero, almonds, hazelnuts, figs, sesame seeds, tahini, chickpeas, alfalfa, oats, fish and soya which are all good sources of bio-available calcium.

▶ Add the seaweeds dulse and wakame, also good sources of vitamin C, to soups, stews and casseroles.
▶ Eat magnesium-rich foods to ensure correct uptake of calcium: Swiss chard, dark green leafies, white beans, broccoli, tofu, pumpkin seeds, avocados, bananas, brown rice, seaweeds dulse and kelp, millet, almonds, hazelnuts and alfalfa sprouts.
▶ Rice, oat and soya milks and soya yoghurts.

⋯ AVOID
▶ Dairy products except fermented ones. Cheese, milk and cream should all be avoided. Butter may be tolerated as it is purely the fat of the milk without the sugar content. Beware low-fat yoghurts as often skimmed-milk powder is added to the yoghurt to thicken it. These yoghurts, therefore, contain lactose and would not be recommended.

SUPPLEMENTS
▶ You could take a magnesium supplement as it mobilizes calcium and people are often deficient in this essential mineral.
▶ It should be possible to include enough calcium in your diet, but if you decide to take a supplement choose an absorbable form such as citrate, rather than carbonates which are not well used by the body.
▶ The enzyme lactase can be added to dairy products before consuming them to aid the breakdown of lactose. Avoidance of dairy products is preferable. Probiotics such as lactobacillus acidophilus may also help.

► Check all labels carefully; dairy products and lactose are found in many products.
► If you have eaten some lactose and are suffering from the symptoms, drink plenty of water and take some acidophilus capsules. Acidophilus can aid the digestion of lactose.

LUNG CANCER

Lung cancer is the second most common cancer in the UK with around 38,300 people being diagnosed every year. Nine out of 10 cases are caused by cigarette smoking and it accounts for approximately 33,500 deaths per annum in Britain alone. Lung cancer is usually fatal, except for the small percentage of patients diagnosed at the early stages of the disease.

The more cigarettes a person smokes, the more likely they are to develop lung cancer, although the length of time as a smoker also matters. For example, if a person has smoked 20 cigarettes a day for 40 years, the risk of lung cancer is about eight times greater than if they have smoked 40 cigarettes a day for 20 years. The good news is as soon as smoking is stopped, the risk of lung cancer begins to decrease, and 15 years after giving up smoking, lung cancer risk is almost the same as a non-smokers.

CAUSES AND RISK FACTORS INCLUDE
► Cigarette smoking.
► Pipe and cigar smoking.
► Passive smoking.
► A family history of lung cancer.
► Scarring from previous lung disease such as tuberculosis (TB).
► Air pollution.
► Exposure to radon gas (the second biggest cause of lung cancer), a naturally occurring radioactive gas that can seep out of the soil into basements. The West Country and the Peak District are areas of higher radon exposure.
► Frequent exposure to certain inhalent chemicals including asbestos, metal dust and fumes, paints, herbicides and insecticides.
► Previous cancer treatment.

SYMPTOMS INCLUDE
► A permanent cough.
► Wheezing.
► Shortness of breath.
► Coughing up phlegm with blood in it.
► An ache or pain when breathing or coughing.
► Loss of appetite.
► Fatigue.
► Unexplained weight loss.

Action plan

The most important factor is not to smoke. Although changing your diet won't reduce your risk of lung cancer much if you continue to smoke, my holistic Action Plan in conjunction with quitting smoking can help increase your chances of protection. If you are being treated for lung cancer, make sure you check with your GP before taking any of the suggested supplements.

EAT/DRINK

► Fresh fruit and vegetables, a minimum of five portions a day. These foods are packed with phytonutrients – potent cancer-fighting compounds. Studies have found that as the intake of fruit and vegetables increases, the risk of lung cancer decreases.

► Foods rich in betacarotene including carrots, sweet potatoes, kale, mustard greens, spinach and winter squash. Betacarotene is an antioxidant and immune booster. In addition, the body is able to convert it into vitamin A, which helps cells reproduce normally.

► Onions and apples. These foods contain a flavanoid antioxidant called quercetin that has been associated with a reduced risk of lung cancer.

► Tomato-based foods. Tomatoes contain a phytonutrient called lycopene, consumption of which has been associated with a reduced risk of lung cancer. Lycopene is better

absorbed when tomatoes are cooked. Lycopene supplements are also an option.

► The antioxidants in peaches are helpful.

► High-fibre foods such as brown rice, whole grain cereals, beans and pulses. Fibre is an essential component of a healthy diet.

► Oily fish such as salmon, mackerel and trout, two to three times a week. Fish eaters have been reported to have a low risk of lung cancer which is thought to be linked with its omega-3 fatty acid content. Vegetarians can obtain omega-3 fats from plant-derived sources including flaxseed, soya, walnuts and dark green leafy vegetables.

► Freshly pressed fruit and vegetable juices. These are concentrated in anti-cancer compounds and help to cleanse the body of toxins and boost energy levels.

► Water, to help keep the cells cleansed and hydrated. Drink at least 8 glasses of bottled or filtered water daily.

AVOID

► Meat. A higher consumption of well-done meat, fried meat and red meat in general has all been linked to an elevated risk of lung cancer. People with the disease are best to get their protein from non-meat sources such as tofu, beans, whole grains, quinoa, nuts, seeds, eggs (no more than five a week) and natural live yoghurt.

► Saturated fat and cholesterol. Lung cancer risk appears directly related to the consumption of foods containing saturated fat (red meat, lard, full-fat dairy products). Other studies have

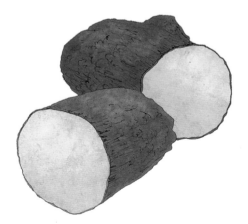

shown that as dietary cholesterol increases, so does the risk of lung cancer.

► Foods that contain toxic trans-fatty acids such as hard margarine, biscuits and anything that has been deep-fried.

► Refined sugar as several studies have found it increases lung cancer risk. Choose naturally sweet foods such as fresh and dried fruit (unsulphured) instead.

► Processed foods. These add toxicity to the body and weaken the immune system.

► Alcohol as it increases the body's toxic load and robs the system of important health-giving nutrients.

► Coffee and black tea. Instead, drink grain coffee substitutes, green tea which has anti-cancer properties, and herbal teas such as nettle, fennel, camomile, peppermint, ginger and rooibosch.

HERBS AND SUPPLEMENTS

► Panax ginseng. Preliminary trials have found that this herb improves immune function in people with lung cancer who have been treated with conventional cancer treatment (chemotherapy and radiation).

► Mullein tea or tincture.

► Lobelia has been reported to help reduce cigarette cravings but you will need to see a herbalist about that.

► A general multivitamin and mineral supplement. In a preliminary trial, lung cancer patients who took vitamin supplements survived almost four times as long as those who did not. This suggests that a good, all-round multi-nutrient formula is beneficial in the treatment of lung cancer.

► Folic acid and vitamin B12. These two B vitamins are required for normal cell replication. In a double-blind trial, smokers with precancerous changes to the lungs who supplemented a combination of these vitamins for four months had a significant reversal of precancerous cellular changes compared to those who received a placebo.

► Vitamin E. As high dietary and blood levels of this nutrient have been linked with reduced lung cancer risk, its supplementation is recommended.

► Selenium. Blood levels of this antioxidant nutrient appear to be low in lung cancer patients. In one study that involved selenium supplementation over a six and a half year period, results showed that there was a 46 per cent decrease in lung cancer incidence and a 53 per cent decrease in deaths from lung cancer, compared to those taking a placebo.

► Salvestrols. These natural plant compounds indirectly target cancer cells and help to destroy them. Cells affected by cancer contain an enzyme called CYP1B1. Salvestrols get converted by this enzyme into chemicals which can kill the diseased cells. Because the CYP1B1 enzyme is not present in healthy cells, salvestrols exert no effects there.

EXTRA TIPS

► Avoid exposure to passive smoke.

► Minimize exposure to air pollution.

► Avoid exposure to radon and other inhalant pollutants associated with lung cancer.

LUPUS

Lupus is an inflammatory disease that is poorly understood. It is an auto-immune disease, in which the immune system makes antibodies that attack body tissues. This creates pain and inflammation. The two main types of lupus are discoid lupus erythematosus (DLE) and systemic lupus erythematosus (SLE).

DLE is mainly a disease of the skin. Symptoms include a red butterfly rash over the nose and cheeks with patches of yellowish lumps on the skin and ears.

SLE can affect many body parts. Symptoms may include weakness, loss of appetite, susceptibility to infection, a red butterfly-shaped rash on the face and sometimes scalp, and joint pains. In severe cases the lungs, kidneys, spleen and brain can be affected.

Those with lupus often have flare-ups with intermittent periods of remission.

CAUSES

Lupus is a complex condition that may be triggered by chronic stress, drugs, viral infections, environmental pollutants, food intolerances and extreme fatigue.

Action plan

It would be advisable to consult a medical practitioner for extra guidance. In the meantime, the aims are to reduce inflammation, aid healing, alkalize the body and support the liver, kidneys and bowel in their work of detoxification and elimination.

EAT/DRINK

► Whole grains and pulses for their B vitamins, magnesium and fibre for internal cleansing.
► Sea vegetables are rich in minerals needed for normal immune function.
► Oily fish. These contain anti-inflammatory oils. Try sardines, mackerel, salmon (wild or organic), herrings and trout.
► Fruit and vegetables which are the best source of nutrients needed for proper immune function and pH balance. Eat at least 8 portions a day. Try to have a large glass of freshly pressed organic vegetable juice daily as well.

AVOID

► Tomatoes, potatoes, peppers, chillies, aubergines, alfalfa and tobacco because they can aggravate inflammatory conditions.
► Alcohol, caffeine, sugar, refined carbohydrates, salt, meat, processed foods and additives are all inflammatory.

HERBS AND SUPPLEMENTS

► Drink dandelion coffee to support the liver and to supply potassium. Potassium helps to alkalize the system.
► Take magnesium citrate. Magnesium is needed to alkalize the system and support bone health.
► Take fish oil supplements. Fish oils contain beneficial anti-inflammatory fats.

EXTRA TIPS

► If your symptoms appeared after you had started a course of medication then talk to your GP about changing what you are taking.

► Apply aloe vera gel to areas of the skin that are affected. Aloe vera has soothing and healing properties. Vitamin E can also be rubbed into affected areas to reduce scarring. Just pierce a vitamin E capsule and rub in the oil. Test a small patch first to check for reactions.

► Find out what you are intolerant to. Keeping a food and symptom diary may be useful or have a food intolerance test. Common culprits include wheat, gluten grains, dairy products, soya, eggs, yeast and chocolate.

► Lupus is often a sign of a toxic system. Do frequent one- or two-day detoxes so that the liver can get on top of its load and the body can eliminate inflammatory substances.

In 2000, I was poorly with a mystery virus. Medical professionals believe I may have suffered an attack of systemic lupus. Whatever it was it wasn't funny and whilst ill in bed I read your book. My family now live pretty much in line with the fruit, veg, superfoods, beans and lentils rules you set down. We eat in 'abundance' and none of us are overweight; nowadays we are all healthy. My kids don't eat sugary, processed food; they always head for the fruit bowl if snacking. I am back to being a healthy mum and wife; these days good sensible eating keeps me like that.

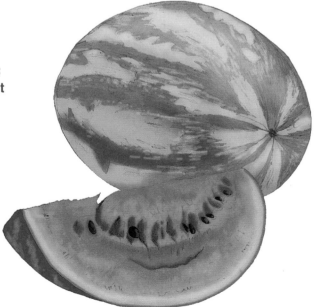

METABOLIC SYNDROME

Metabolic syndrome refers to a group of symptoms that are often found together in individuals. Common symptoms associated with the syndrome include weight gain around the middle, high blood pressure, high triglycerides, blood-sugar problems and imbalanced cholesterol levels. Those with these symptoms are at increased risk of heart attacks, strokes, diabetes, atherosclerosis, polycystic ovaries (in women) and prostate cancer (in men).

CAUSES

One of the most common causes of metabolic syndrome is a diet high in sugar, refined carbohydrates and alcohol. These foods all break down into glucose once digested. The glucose goes into the blood stream causing a rapid and dramatic rise in blood-sugar levels. As the body cannot survive if blood-sugar levels are high, insulin is secreted by the pancreas in order to carry the glucose from the blood into the cells. Once in the cells, glucose can be stored for later use as energy or converted to fat for long-term storage. As insulin very much favours storage of glucose rather than its release for energy, the more insulin you produce the more likely you are to convert glucose to fat.

Diets high in sugar, refined carbohydrates and alcohol mean that insulin is constantly being called upon to carry the glucose into the cells. This can lead to the cells becoming 'deaf' to insulin as they get so used to it being present. This can be likened to background noise which you notice when you first hear it but soon forget it is there. More insulin is secreted until the cells let the glucose enter. As, by now, insulin levels are higher than they should be, more glucose is stored as fat and less is available for energy. This often leads to the deposition of fat around the middle of the body, hence the characteristic apple shape that is so common nowadays. Other risk factors for developing metabolic syndrome include:

▶ A family history of type 2 diabetes.
▶ High blood pressure.
▶ High blood triglycerides.
▶ Polycystic ovaries.
▶ A sedentary lifestyle.
▶ Being overweight. Waist circumference measurements are one of the markers used to diagnose the condition; women with a waist measurement of more than 35 inches and men with a waist of more than 40 inches are at increased risk of developing metabolic syndrome and should get their blood pressure and blood triglycerides checked.
▶ The risk also increases as you get older.

Action plan

The key for treatment is to keep insulin levels as low as possible. This entails eliminating foods that raise blood glucose rapidly. It is also vital to take measures to protect the cardio-vascular system. Eating plenty of calcium-, magnesium- and potassium-rich foods is key.

✤ EAT/DRINK
▶ Protein, which slows down the breakdown of carbohydrates into glucose. Good combinations include chicken or fish

with vegetables (not potatoes) or lentils, beans, soya, nuts or seeds with whole grains such as brown rice, oats, quinoa, millet, buckwheat and amaranth.

► Fibre, which helps to keep insulin levels low and blood sugar stable. Make sure all your meals and snacks contain fibre from whole grains, nuts, seeds, fruit, vegetables, beans and pulses. Oats are particularly recommended as they contain a fibre called beta-glucans which can help with blood-sugar control after meals and reduces cholesterol.

► Garlic, which has protective effects on the cardio-vascular system, often a problem area for those with metabolic syndrome.

► Oily fish have protective and anti-inflammatory effects on the cardio-vascular system and can improve the cells' response to insulin. Other sources of omega-3 fats include flax seeds, hemp seeds, pumpkin seeds, walnuts and avocados. The cold-pressed oils of these seeds can also be used in salad dressings.

► Potassium-rich foods such as apricots, avocados, prunes, figs, green vegetables, peas, lentils and beans.

⠿ AVOID

► Sugar, refined carbohydrates and alcohol. All foods that break down into glucose rapidly need to be avoided as these increase insulin levels and the conversion of glucose to fat. Foods to avoid include sugar, soft drinks, alcohol, biscuits, cakes, pastries, chocolate, sweets, white pasta, white rice, white bread, white flour products, crisps and potatoes.

► Salt. Sodium raises blood pressure which is one of the risk factors for metabolic syndrome.

► Tea, coffee and caffeinated soft drinks. Caffeine indirectly raises blood-sugar levels and therefore insulin. Replace these with herbal teas and freshly pressed vegetable juices.

HERBS AND SUPPLEMENTS

► Take chromium picolinate. Chromium has been found to be one of the key nutrients for those with metabolic syndrome. Chromium has anti-diabetic and anti-obesity properties as well as blood-pressure-lowering and cholesterol-lowering properties.

► Supplement with alpha-lipoic. This can help to improve glucose uptake by muscle cells, meaning less glucose is stored as fat.

► Take co-enzyme Q10. This can improve the function of insulin-producing cells in the pancreas.

► Supplement with vitamin B complex daily. The B vitamins play a key role in blood-sugar control, energy production and cardio-vascular health.

► Supplement with magnesium citrate daily. Magnesium is also needed for blood-sugar control, energy and cardio-vascular health.

► Take glucomannan fibre. Research has shown that glucomannan from konjac can stabilize blood sugar in those with insulin resistance.

⠿ EXTRA TIPS

► Eat regularly spaced small meals and snacks. Large meals are always going to provoke a rise in blood glucose and insulin levels. Have six small meals and snacks a day rather than the traditional three. Remember, this does not necessarily mean you eat more over the day, but that you eat smaller meals plus snacks.

► If you are overweight, take dietary and lifestyle steps to lose weight. Being overweight puts you at increased risk of all the other risk factors associated with the syndrome.

► If you smoke, stop. Nicotine indirectly raises blood-sugar levels.

► Exercise daily. Exercise improves the cells' response to insulin, meaning less is produced. It also helps to normalize appetite and reduce cravings.

► Get outside in daylight every day. Vitamin D is manufactured in the skin in response to sunlight. Vitamin D has been shown to improve the cellular response to insulin by 60 per cent. Supplements may need to be taken in the winter months.

MIGRAINE

Migraines are severe headaches that are often preceded or accompanied by flashing lights, blurred vision, nausea, vomiting and sensitivity to light. Some people also suffer from strange tastes and smells. Sufferers tend to get them periodically. They can last from an hour to several days and can be severely debilitating. Migraines are thought to be linked to a constriction of blood vessels in the brain. The constriction may be followed by dilation of the blood vessels in which they fill with blood.

CAUSES MAY INCLUDE

► Stress.
► Liver imbalance.
► Lack of sleep.
► Food intolerances.
► Poor posture or previous neck injury.
► Blood-sugar imbalances.
► Constipation.
► Female hormonal fluctuations.
► Exhaustion.
► Toxicity.
► Teeth grinding.
► Dental problems.
► Medications.
► Dehydration.
► Bright or flashing lights.
► Smoking.
► Foods that are high in the amino acid tyramine.
► Sufferers of *Candida albicans* (see page 219) may find they have a sensitivity to weather changes that can bring on a migraine.

Action plan

Keep a diary that includes everything you eat and drink to help identify triggers.

⠿ EAT/DRINK

► Water. Migraines may be caused by simple dehydration. Drink at least 8 glasses of water throughout the day to help prevent migraines. If you feel one coming on then sip a large glass of warm water.
► Nettle, feverfew and camomile teas together.
► Magnesium-rich foods. Magnesium relaxes muscles and nerves and is often low in migraine sufferers. Good food sources include green vegetables,

avocados, alfalfa sprouts, millet, brown rice, quinoa, soya, sea vegetables, hazelnuts and watercress.

► Hemp and flax seeds. These are high in essential fats that have an anti-inflammatory effect. Oily fish and other nuts and seeds are also good sources.

► Rye broth. This can help to relieve a migraine once it has started and may also be useful as a preventative.

⠿ AVOID

► Tyramine-containing foods: chocolate, cheese, coffee, red wine, oranges, aged meats and foods containing MSG (monosodium glutamate).

► Other problem foods may include potatoes, tomatoes (especially if cooked), dairy products, salt, wheat, gluten, yeast, beer and preservatives and additives. These all contain tyramine, an amino acid that can trigger migraines in some people.

HERBS AND SUPPLEMENTS

► The herb feverfew can help in the long term. It will not help rescue a migraine once it hits but taken daily the effects are cumulative. Eat the leaves of the plant if possible for the best effect.

► Nettle tea can also be beneficial for its high mineral content.

► Extract of butterbur may help.

► Magnesium can help to relax the muscles and nerves.

► Vitamin B6 deficiency is common in those who suffer from migraines. If taking this long term, take a B complex vitamin as well.

⠿ EXTRA TIPS

► Keep a food and symptom diary to identify any other offending foods.

Bear in mind that a migraine may be caused by something eaten one or even two days before. The reaction is not necessarily immediate.

► Keep blood-sugar levels stable. Eat small meals and snacks regularly and avoid sugar, refined carbohydrates, caffeine and alcohol.

► Check your posture, especially if working at a computer all day. Try to keep the spine long and the shoulders down as this allows for good circulation to the head.

► See a chiropractor or osteopath. Straightening out areas of tightness or injury can improve circulation and reduce migraine attacks.

► If you get a migraine, put your feet in a basin of hot water and place a cold towel on your head.

MORNING SICKNESS

See pregnancy section in Food and the Stages of Life, page 112.

MULTIPLE SCLEROSIS

Multiple sclerosis (MS) is a disorder of the central nervous system. It is characterized by the destruction of the myelin sheaths that surround the nerves. The myelin sheaths are replaced by scar tissue. The condition tends to get worse over time with periods of remission alternating with flare-ups.

Symptoms include dizziness, poor co-ordination or balance, tingling and numbness in affected parts, stiffness, slurred speech, aches, pains, weakness, fatigue, impotence and difficulty in walking. As it progresses, all movements may become affected and even breathing may be difficult.

CAUSES

MS is thought to be an auto-immune condition, meaning that the immune system attacks the myelin sheaths as if they were a foreign body. Stress, poor diet and nutrient status, adrenal fatigue, dehydration, acidosis, excessive alcohol use, environmental toxins, candida, mercury poisoning, food intolerances and genetics may all play a part.

Action plan

The sooner after diagnosis that dietary and lifestyle changes are made, the more effective they are likely to be. However, it is never too late to make improvements.

⠿ EAT/DRINK

► Essential fats. These are important for the whole nervous system. Good sources of beneficial fats include oily fish, hemp seeds, flax seeds, pumpkin seeds, sesame seeds and sunflower seeds. The cold-pressed oils of these seeds can also be used in salad dressings.

► Green vegetables which are high in magnesium and folic acid. Magnesium is needed for the function of the nervous system and for energy within the cells. Folic acid is also needed for nervous system function and is often low in those with MS. Good vegetables to include are broccoli, Brussels sprouts, savoy cabbage, pak choi, cavolo nero and kale.

► Freshly pressed, organic vegetable juices. These are full of nutrients needed for detoxification and the immune system. Include carrots, apples, radishes, beetroot, celery, fennel, cabbage, kale, ginger and parsley.

► Berries, which are packed with antioxidants needed for cellular repair. Include raspberries, strawberries, blueberries, bilberries and blackberries.

► Water – at least 2 litres a day. Get into the habit of sipping water between meals and drink herbal teas instead of tea and coffee. Water is needed for all aspects of cleansing and repair. Get a water filter fitted if possible to ensure the purity of the water.

► Pumpkin seeds. These are a great source of zinc that tends to be low in those with MS. It is an important mineral for the nervous system and for healing. Other good sources of zinc include flax seeds, sunflower seeds, whole grains, fish and pulses.

► Fruit and vegetables. These foods are alkalizing. Other alkalizing foods include almonds, millet, Brazil nuts, quinoa, chestnuts and buckwheat.

⠿ AVOID

► Meat and eggs as they are particularly acid-forming.

► Margarine, heated fats, fried foods, crisps, pastries and processed meats as these contain fats that interfere with the function of the essential fats.

► Wheat and other gluten grains (rye, oats, kamut, spelt and barley), dairy products, yeast, eggs, soya, chocolate, tomatoes, potatoes and citrus fruits to which you may be intolerant.

► Sugar, refined carbohydrates, alcohol, caffeine, additives, salt and processed foods. All of these put a strain on the body, can deplete nutrients, create toxins and prevent healing.

HERBS AND SUPPLEMENTS

► Add a superfood powder to your fresh juices. These include barley grass, wheat grass, spirulina or my own living food energy powder.

► Take probiotics twice a day. Probiotics are beneficial bacteria that can improve gut function, reduce yeast and improve nutrient absorption. They also manufacture some B vitamins that are needed by the nervous system and for energy.

► Take vitamin B complex. The B vitamins are needed by the nervous system and for energy. Look for one containing choline and inositol as these can aid fat digestion and liver function. Folic acid and vitamin B12 are particularly important for the nervous system so make sure your supplement contains folic acid. Vitamin B12 is difficult to absorb so consider getting monthly B12 injections.

► The co-enzyme Q10 helps to improve circulation and oxygenation in the cells.

► Take an antioxidant supplement. The antioxidants include vitamins A, C, E, zinc, selenium and n-acetyl cysteine. Look for one containing a combination of these as they all work synergistically (i.e., they all increase each other's effectiveness).

⁞ EXTRA TIPS

► Avoid pesticides, chemicals and pollution. These can all create a further burden on the immune system and some are toxic to the nervous system.

► Eat organic foods and use only natural beauty and household products.

► Swimming is a good exercise for those with MS. Exercise that creates a lot of heat can aggravate the symptoms. Find a pool that uses non-chlorine methods of keeping the water clean, such as ozone. Yoga and walking may also be beneficial.

► Get outside every day. Vitamin D is needed for calcium utilization and calcium is needed for proper nerve function. Vitamin D is made by the action of sunlight on the skin. Make sure you have some skin exposed to daylight for at least 30 minutes a day.

► Massage sesame oil into your skin daily before you shower. This soothes the nervous system and helps to stimulate circulation and oxygenation to the tissues. The increased blood flow encourages cleansing and healing.

► Look into intravenous vitamin therapy.

MUSCLE CRAMPS

See Cramps, page 238.

N

NAUSEA AND TRAVEL SICKNESS

Nausea is a feeling of sickness that can debilitate, leaving you feeling drained of energy and wanting to vomit. The feeling can be mild to severe.

Symptoms of travel sickness may include headaches, dizziness, fatigue, loss of appetite and sleeplessness. This type of nausea is obviously caused by travelling, e.g., by ship. Other possible causes are lack of air, anxiety, and restricted vision or conflicting information going to the brain during motion which can upset the balance in the inner ear.

CAUSES OF NAUSEA MAY INCLUDE

- B vitamin deficiency.
- Lack of food.
- Malnutrition.
- Food poisoning.
- Infection.
- Stress.
- Digestive disturbances.
- Migraines.
- Anorexia.

Action plan

The following plan will help ease your nausea.

EAT/DRINK

- Plain wholemeal toast or dry crackers to help settle the stomach.
- Miso soup. It helps to neutralize stomach acid.
- Pumpkin seeds which can help to reduce nausea.
- Ginger tea or a cup of hot water and a slice of ginger. Ginger should not be boiled as this will destroy its volatile oil. Gallstone sufferers should not use ginger. Those suffering from travel sickness should drink ginger tea before and during the journey. Children can be given crystallized ginger at regular intervals on the journey to stave off sickness.
- If you suffer from travel sickness, eat fruit (especially papaya) or cooked whole grains, such as brown rice, before setting off.

AVOID

- If you suffer from travel sickness, avoid alcohol, spices and fatty foods before and during travel.

HERBS AND SUPPLEMENTS

- The Ayurvedic herb chiretta prior to meals can help nausea associated with stomach weaknesses and indigestion.
- Take a digestive enzyme supplement with meals to help with nutrient uptake from the foods you eat.
- Take ginger root in capsules. But not if you are pregnant. Ginger in mild form like ginger biscuits or tea is fine for morning sickness. In high doses, ginger acts as an emmenagogue (tones reproductive organs and menstrual flow) which means that it could trigger a miscarriage early in pregnancy.
- Drink some peppermint tea. This is especially helpful if your nausea is accompanied by a headache. If you suffer from travel sickness, put two drops of peppermint oil into warm water and sip before your journey. Peppermint oil can also be put on a handkerchief and inhaled during travel.
- Lemon balm tea is helpful for nausea related to stress and emotional upset.

▶ Essential oils of ginger and cardamom can help, too. All you have to do is place three drops on your wrist or a handkerchief and breathe in the aromas.

▶ Start taking a good multivitamin/mineral complex to cover any possible nutrient deficiencies.

▶ Take the supplement vitamin B6.

▶ If you suffer from travel sickness, take magnesium and vitamin B6 before the trip. These both have anti-nausea effects and can relax the nervous system.

⠿ EXTRA TIPS

▶ Make sure you are eating enough food. Lack of food can trigger nausea. Eat little and often.

▶ Acupressure can help. There is a pressure point which can help to stave off nausea.

Extra tips for those suffering from travel sickness

▶ Avoid strong smells such as engine oil, cleaning products and perfumes. These can all contribute to nausea.

▶ Look at a distant but stationary object such as the horizon. This prevents conflicting messages being sent from the eyes to the brain.

▶ Increase oxygen levels. Open the window if you are in a car or go out on deck if you are on a ship.

▶ Travel sickness is partly psychological so try not to focus on it. Use distractions such as conversation or relaxing music. Reading is not recommended.

▶ Nostril breathing has helped many of my clients. Close the right nostril with your thumb, then inhale fully and slowly through your left nostril. Alternate 10 times.

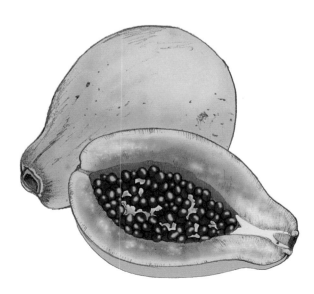

O

OEDEMA

Oedema basically means fluid retention in body tissues under the skin. The body can retain fluids anywhere but commonly affected areas include the abdomen, fingers, ankles, feet, breasts and under the eyes. The area affected generally looks swollen and puffy.

CAUSES

There are various underlying factors that are likely to be playing a part. They include:

► Hormonal imbalances – oedema is common pre-menstrually in women.
► Excess sodium relative to potassium – sodium encourages the retention of water by the body.
► B vitamin deficiency, especially B6.
► Liver congestion.
► Kidney or urinary system problems.
► Thyroid imbalance.
► Diabetes or blood-sugar imbalance.
► Abuse of laxatives or diuretics.
► Dehydration.
► Food intolerances.

Action plan

It is important to investigate and address possible underlying causes.

❖ EAT/DRINK

► Beans and lentils. These all contain potassium needed to counteract the effects of sodium. Fruit and vegetables are also excellent sources of potassium.
► Kale and savoy cabbage. These are dark green vegetables that are high in vitamin B6, potassium and magnesium – all needed for proper fluid balance in the body.
► Water – up to 2 litres a day. People with oedema often avoid drinking much as they think they will retain more water. However, you need to drink water in order to help the body let go of old fluids and sodium.
► Vegetable juices as they can help to replace the sodium with potassium.

⁘ AVOID

► Foods to which you are intolerant. Common culprits in oedema are wheat and the other gluten grains, yeast and dairy products.
► Salt, which is found in all processed and packaged foods. Flavour your foods with celery seeds, dill, parsley, kelp flakes and coriander instead.
► Alcohol, coffee, tea, soft drinks, pickles, refined carbohydrates and sugar. These can all affect fluid balance in the body and challenge the organs of detoxification.

HERBS AND SUPPLEMENTS

► Drink herbal diuretics to increase the flow of urine. Good ones to choose include nettle tea, dandelion tea, corn silk tea, yarrow tea and dandelion coffee.
► Take evening primrose oil, especially if you suffer from pre-menstrual water retention.
► Take blue-green algae and alfalfa sprouts. These can both aid cleansing and supply magnesium and potassium.
► Supplement with B complex plus extra B6. Vitamin B6 is especially important for normalizing body fluids and is best taken in conjunction with other B vitamins to avoid imbalances.

▶ Apply a lavender-oil-soaked cloth to the affected area. This can help to relieve the swelling. Raising the area above the hips is also useful.

▶ Dry skin brush daily. Use a natural bristle brush on dry skin and brush from the feet upwards. Always brush towards the heart. This helps to get the circulation and lymph moving, thus preventing stagnation.

▶ Exercise daily. Get moving as much as possible during the day to prevent the pooling of fluids.

OSTEOARTHRITIS

Sometimes called 'wear-and-tear arthritis', this tends to strike people in their fifties and above and affects more women than men. It refers to the erosion of cartilage that covers the ends of bones between joints. The usually smooth cartilage becomes rough and this results in friction, pain and inflammation. The changes in the cartilage stimulate the overgrowth of bone cells as the body tries to correct the imbalance. This overgrowth can lead to bony spurs that contribute to more pain.

Joints affected include those of the wrists, hands, knees, spine and hips. Symptoms include pain, stiffness, swelling, deformity and reduction in mobility of the affected joints. Cold, damp climates may aggravate symptoms with improvements being seen in warm, dry climates.

Conventional treatment usually involves the use of ibuprofen and other non-steroidal anti-inflammatory drugs (NSAIDs). These reduce pain and inflammation but do nothing to address the underlying causes. They can have a negative impact on gut health.

Action plan

The focus is on removing triggers and including foods that reduce inflammation.

⁞ EAT/DRINK

▶ Oily fish – salmon, mackerel, sardines, pilchards, herrings, trout and halibut. These contain the anti-inflammatory omega-3 essential fats EPA and DHA.

▶ Nuts and seeds – especially walnuts, pumpkin seeds, flax seeds, hemp seeds and their cold-pressed oils.

▶ Fruits – these are high in anti-inflammatory nutrients and can help to alkalize the body. Arthritis is often a sign of acidity in the tissues. Eat two to three pieces of fruit a day between meals on an empty stomach.

▶ Vegetables. These are also alkalizing and anti-inflammatory. Eat two to three portions of vegetables with lunch and dinner. Some should be eaten raw. If cooking them, try steaming, baking, roasting or stir frying rather than boiling.

▶ Alfalfa sprouts – these are high in minerals needed for healthy bones.

▶ Sulphur-rich foods. Sulphur is needed for the repair of cartilage and bone and aids in the absorption and utilization of calcium. Foods containing sulphur include asparagus, eggs, garlic and onions.

► Green vegetables, which contain vitamin K and folic acid needed for healthy bone and cartilage formation.

► Whole grains, such as brown rice, whole wheat and rye as these contain histidine which can remove excess metals from the body. Those with arthritis often have high levels of copper and iron.

► Fresh pineapple, which contains the enzyme bromelain that can help to reduce inflammation. Eat the core of the pineapple as this is where most of the enzymes lie.

► Fibre from whole grains, flax seeds and pulses as this removes wastes from the body.

► Kombucha tea which contains many important nutrients and enzymes that can improve connective tissue and mobility and reduce pain.

::: AVOID

► White potatoes, peppers, chillies, aubergines, tomatoes and tobacco. These members of the nightshade family contain solanine which can promote inflammation in some people.

► Wheat, dairy foods, eggs and chocolate to which you may be intolerant. Problem foods are often those eaten on a daily basis so look at your diet and see what crops up most frequently. Have a food intolerance test if you are not sure what to eliminate, www.gillianmckeith.info.

► Saturated fat from meat and dairy products which can have an inflammatory effect. Especially avoid processed meats such as ham, bacon, salami, sausages, burgers and pepperoni, etc.

► Margarines and hydrogenated fats which cause damage in the body and block the body's use of the anti-inflammatory essential fats (see above).

► Tea, coffee, wine and spinach which contain oxalic acid which can increase acidity and worsen inflammation.

► Salt, sugar, refined carbohydrates and processed foods which can all be detrimental to health and can increase weight and inflammation.

HERBS AND SUPPLEMENTS

► Cat's claw can reduce the pain of arthritis.

► White willow, black cohosh and meadowsweet all contain salicylic acid which is anti-inflammatory and can reduce pain.

► Burdock root, celery seed, devil's claw, horsetail, nettle, wild yam root, comfrey root, ginger and parsley may all be useful in the treatment of arthritis.

► GLA, EPA and DHA essential fatty acids supplements, which can all be anti-inflammatory.

► Bromelain which can be taken between meals to reduce inflammation and with meals to aid digestion of proteins.

► Magnesium, boron and vitamins K and D which can all aid the proper utilization of calcium and may prevent the build-up of bony spurs between joints.

► Co-enzyme Q-10 which can aid the repair of connective tissue and improve energy.

► Glucosamine and chondroitin sulphate are the two essential components of cartilage and in supplement form have been shown to slow the degenerative effects of osteoarthritis.

► Vitamins C and E for anti-inflammatory and protective effects.

► Zinc, which is often low in those with arthritis and needed for immune function and repair.

► Probiotics, hydrochloric acid and/ or digestive enzymes can all aid proper utilization of calcium and improve the absorption of other nutrients.

⁘ EXTRA TIPS

► Avoid iron supplementation (unless prescribed by your doctor) as iron may contribute to pain, swelling and joint destruction. Get your iron from foods such as molasses, broccoli, Brussels sprouts, fish, peas and beans instead.

► Physiotherapy, chiropractice and osteopathy may all be worth considering.

► Rub capsicum cream onto affected joints. This is derived from cayenne pepper which can reduce the sensation of pain in the body.

► Place cold packs on inflamed joints to reduce inflammation.

► Have hot then cold showers to promote circulation and healing.

► Spend time outside in the daylight. This promotes the formation of vitamin D in the skin which aids proper bone formation.

► Lose weight if you are overweight. Excess weight puts pressure on the joints and contributes to damage.

► Get regular, moderate exercise. Do not put pressure on affected joints but do try to strengthen surrounding muscles and ligaments. Walking and swimming are suitable for most people.

OSTEOPOROSIS

Osteoporosis – meaning, quite literally, 'porous bones' – occurs when the inner mesh of bone, which resembles a sort of honeycomb, develops larger and larger holes, making the bone fragile and prone to fracture. Osteoporosis affects one in three post-menopausal women and one in 12 men over the age of 50 in the UK. Commonly known as brittle bone disease, many people often are not even aware that they have the condition until a fracture occurs. Another indication is curvature of the spine, sometimes referred to as 'dowager's hump'.

The whole skeletal system may be affected, but it is the bones of the wrist, spine and hips which are most vulnerable. Bone is living tissue and its inner mesh, which consists primarily of protein, calcium and other minerals, is self-regenerating. Old bone is constantly being broken down by cells called

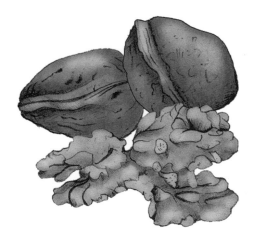

osteoclasts and replaced with new bone by osteoblasts. Bone density usually peaks at about the age of 35, after which time it starts to decline as part of the normal ageing process. It is crucial to build strong bones in adolescence and during your 20s.

CAUSES
► Lack of vitamin D.
► Lack of calcium.
► Lack of magnesium.
► Poor diet.
► Salty food.
► Too much coffee, fizzy drinks and alcohol.
► Malabsorption.
► Too much meat.
► Smoking.
► Sufferers of coeliac disease.
► Antidepressants.
► Antacids containing aluminium.
► Genetic disposition.
► Inflammatory bowel disease.
► Crohn's disease.
► Too much sugar.
► Lack of exercise.

Action plan

Increasing mineral assimilation is key to preventing an acceleration of the problem.

⣿ EAT/DRINK

► Fruit and vegetables. These aid mineralization of the bones. They are also rich in vitamin C and boron, a trace mineral also needed for healthy bones.
► Green vegetables for magnesium, the calcium mobilizer. It is more critical than even calcium for the bones. Green vegetables contain magnesium, calcium and vitamin K, all of which are needed for healthy bones. So you can go for watercress, cabbage, broccoli, lettuce, rocket, alfalfa sprouts, Brussels sprouts, dandelion leaves, green herbs, collard greens, seaweeds and kale which will give you a good dose of calcium as well as magnesium and vitamins K and C. Without magnesium, calcium cannot be absorbed into bone.
► Nuts and seeds, which are also excellent sources of calcium and other bone nutrients, particularly almonds, sesame seeds and raw shelled hemp seeds.
► Seaweeds: wakame, kombu, nori and agar for calcium. Wakame is known as the woman's seaweed because of its calcium content. Substitute fresh wakame for lettuce in sandwiches. You can mix any seaweed into soups, stews and casseroles. Seaweeds also nourish the thyroid gland. The thyroid gland, which governs metabolism, plays an essential role in controlling bone turnover. If it isn't working properly, the result could be bone loss.
► Foods high in essential fats which are vital for healthy bones. Good sources include oily fish, pumpkin seeds, raw shelled hemp seeds and sunflower seeds.
► Beans (try kidney beans) and a grain called quinoa which is not only rich in calcium but is also an excellent protein food.
► Phyto-oestrogen-rich foods which help to strengthen bones. Good sources include soya such as tofu, chick peas, lentils and linseeds, as well as fruit and vegetables generally.

► Figs as a source of magnesium, calcium and phosphoris for bones.

► Oats. Soak rolled oats overnight in water and eat raw in the morning or make porridge and add ground flax seeds. They contain silica, important for bones.

► Hazelnuts. These are good sources of calcium and magnesium as well as essential healthy omegas.

► Alfalfa meal which provides vitamin K and can be mixed into smoothies.

► Papayas and pineapples as good sources of food enzymes to help digestion, and therefore improve absorption of nutrients.

► Celeriac contains a good array of bone-friendly minerals and is a perfect alternative to potato mash.

► Silicon rich foods to improve availability of calcium and manganese. Horsetail tea, lettuce, buckwheat, millet, oats, brown rice, strawberries, celery, apricots, carrots and finally silica gel from health food stores.

AVOID

► Fizzy drinks. Many canned and bottled drinks contain phosphoric acid which can leach important bone-building minerals from your bones.

► I recommend limiting meat in your diet. Digestion of meats and meat proteins leaves acid residues in the body that need to be neutralized with alkalizing minerals. And these alkalizing minerals might be taken away from the bones, leading to a weakened bone structure.

► Caffeine and alcohol as they are considered to be anti-nutrients, which means they interfere with the absorption and utilization of nutrients, including calcium and magnesium, in the body.

Alcohol interferes with protein and calcium metabolism and affects bone-building cells.

► Salt and sugar. They can both increase the excretion of minerals and decrease the absorption of calcium. They are often found in breakfast cereals, processed foods, ham, bacon, sausages, some tinned and packaged foods and confectionery.

► Go easy on foods containing oxalic acid: rhubarb, cranberries, plums, spinach, chard and beet greens as this can bind to calcium.

HERBS AND SUPPLEMENTS

► The herb horsetail is a source of silica for calcium metabolism.

► Drink ginseng tea and nettle tea, too.

► Take magnesium supplements or magnesium/calcium supplements where the magnesium ratio to calcium is higher. Calcium citrate/malate is the preferred form of calcium.

► As well as calcium and magnesium, you need manganese, vitamin D, boron and silica. Manganese is critical for preventing the bone deformity scoliosis (see page 362).

► Take digestive enzymes to make sure that you are absorbing nutrients and breaking down food efficiently.

► Also take plant-based hydrochloric acid supplements before meals. Most post-menopausal women are low in stomach acid.

► For people who live in northern or southern latitudes and don't get enough sunlight during winter months, you must supplement every day during the winter months with vitamin D and boron which helps to convert vitamin D into active form.

► Good bone health also depends on vitamin B12.

► You also need vitamin K and folic acid for bone health.

⠿ EXTRA TIPS

► Do not smoke. Smoking prevents mineral absorption needed for healthy bones.

► If you are on anti-depressants or antacids, you must pay even more attention to your bones. Studies have found that the elderly who are on anti-depressants and other drugs are more likely to break a hip than those who don't take such drugs. So supplement with a good bone-building formula.

► Get outside for at least 30 minutes every day. Vitamin D is formed by the action of daylight on the skin and is vital for the retention of calcium as it stimulates calcium absorption from the gut.

► Do weight-bearing exercises. Exercise is one of the most effective ways of building bones. Good bone-building exercises include weight lifting, aerobics, walking, jogging, skipping, Pilates and yoga. Do not only do cardio-vascular activity at the expense of lifting weights. But be very careful with weight-bearing exercises if you already have osteoporosis. Seek the guidance of your GP.

► If you suffer from coeliac disease (see page 231), a condition in which gluten (a component of grains) reduces the small intestine's ability to absorb essential nutrients, such as calcium and magnesium, then you will need to supplement as you are at greater risk.

► Natural progesterone cream from wild yam can help to slow down bone loss.

► Presoak grains and legumes before cooking to minimise phytic acid content which can bind to zinc, calcium and magnesium.

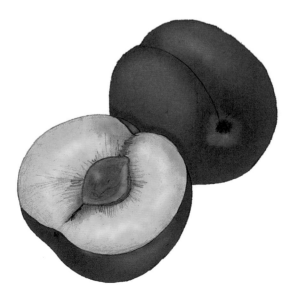

PANCREATITIS

Pancreatitis literally means inflammation of the pancreas. It occurs when the pancreatic duct is blocked by gallstones, scarring or tumours. The pancreas produces digestive enzymes that help to break down protein, fats and carbohydrates from food as well as insulin and glucagon that control blood-sugar levels.

Pancreatitis can be acute or chronic. Acute pancreatitis may only last a few days and may resolve completely. Some people suffer recurrences but others have just the one attack. Symptoms include sudden or gradual pain in the upper middle of the abdomen. The pain may radiate to the back of the body. The pain may come on after eating and last a few days. Nausea, vomiting, fever, chills, swollen, tender abdomen, low blood pressure, dehydration, jaundice, rapid heart beat, blood-sugar problems and lethargy may all result.

Chronic pancreatitis starts off as acute but if the pancreas becomes damaged and scarred it may not recover and the damage can worsen. Often there is no pain in chronic pancreatitis; this may be a sign that the pancreas has stopped working altogether. Inability to digest food, weight loss, anaemia, diabetes, osteoporosis and liver problems may all occur in those with chronic pancreatitis.

CAUSES

A range of factors can contribute to pancreatitis but the most common ones are alcohol abuse and gallstones.

▶ Alcohol abuse.
▶ Gallstones.
▶ Medications.
▶ Oxidative stress.
▶ Antioxidant deficiencies.
▶ Injury.
▶ Genetics.
▶ Surgery.
▶ High blood-calcium levels.
▶ Infections.
▶ High blood fats.

Action plan

If alcohol is a problem for you, see the entry on Alcoholism, page 175.

✛ EAT/DRINK

▶ Low-fat foods. People with pancreatitis do not digest fats well. However, make sure you eat some sources of essential fats daily as these are anti-inflammatory and needed for health. Good sources are oily fish, hemp seeds, sunflower seeds, linseeds, pumpkin seeds, walnuts, avocados and cold-pressed oils.
▶ Freshly pressed vegetable juices, broths, soups, herbal teas and water.
▶ Fruit and vegetables. There may be a link between oxidative stress and the development of pancreatitis, and research suggests that antioxidants may help to reduce pain and severity of pancreatitis. Raw or lightly cooked fruit and vegetables provide abundant antioxidants to combat this.
▶ Brazil nuts. These contain selenium, an antioxidant that can help to prevent oxidative damage and reduce pain and inflammation.
▶ Dandelion-root coffee which can stimulate bile flow. This aids fat digestion and elimination and can help pancreatic function.

P

► Give up alcohol. Alcohol puts a huge strain on the pancreas and is often a major cause of the condition.

► Sugar, refined carbohydrates, processed fats and saturated fats. These all put a strain on the pancreas and liver and can raise blood fats. High blood fats are found to be a factor for many people with pancreatitis.

HERBS AND SUPPLEMENTS

► Herbs that are rich sources of antioxidants include pycnogenol.

► Take digestive enzymes with meals. If the pancreas is struggling to do its work you may not produce sufficient digestive enzymes to break down food fully. Digestive enzymes can help with this.

► Supplement with a blood-sugar-balancing formula. The pancreas plays a key role in maintaining normal blood-sugar levels. Look for one containing chromium, B vitamins, zinc, magnesium, manganese and vitamin D.

► Supplement with antioxidants: vitamin C, vitamin E, betacarotene, selenium and methionine.

EXTRA TIPS

► Eat small, regular meals and snacks and avoid large, heavy meals. This will put less strain on the pancreas and digestive system and help to keep blood-sugar levels stable.

► Sprinkle a teaspoon of lecithin granules onto food daily. Lecithin is an emulsifier that can help with fat digestion.

► Don't smoke. There may be a link between smoking and chronic pancreatitis. Smoking creates free radical damage and uses up antioxidants.

PEPTIC ULCER DISORDER

A peptic ulcer is an open wound on the lining of the stomach (gastric ulcer) or small intestine (duodenal ulcer). There is usually much inflammation around the area. The pain of a peptic ulcer is caused by the acid that is usually in the stomach and is vital for the proper digestion of protein.

Stomach ulcers are caused when the lining that usually protects the stomach wall from stomach acid gets worn away or the mucous membranes in the stomach wall fail to secrete sufficient protective mucus.

Duodenal ulcers occur when acid from the stomach gets into the small intestine. This may be due to a fault in the valve that controls what passes from the stomach to the small intestine. Irritation and ulceration can occur in both these cases.

Symptoms include a burning pain an hour or so after eating or between meals. The pain may be reduced when food is eaten as the food effectively dilutes the acid in the stomach.

CAUSES

► Excess or insufficient stomach acid or an insufficient production of the protective lining of the digestive tract can all lead to the formation of an ulcer.

► One of the key factors leading to the development of peptic ulcers has been found to be the presence of the *Helicobacter pylori* bacterium in the stomach. This organism is found in 95 per cent of people with peptic ulcers. While many people believe that ulcers indicate excessive levels of stomach acid, H.pylori is more likely to thrive if there is insufficient acid in the stomach. H. pylori also, in turn, inhibits the production of stomach acid so interferes with proper digestion and absorption.

It is important that H.pylori is eradicated in order for proper healing to take place. Using antacids reduces stomach acid and creates an environment in which H.pylori can take hold, so these are not necessarily the answer.

Other causes and triggers include:

► Stress.
► Use of aspirin and other medications.
► Smoking.
► Excessive alcohol use.
► Missing meals.
► High meat diet.
► Chewing gum.

Action plan

The key aims in treating a peptic ulcer are to eradicate H. pylori, to heal the wound and to normalize stomach acid and digestion generally.

⠿ EAT/DRINK

► Cabbage juice. It has excellent gut-healing properties. Combine it with carrot juice to make it more palatable.
► Raw garlic.
► Soft, easily digested foods. Avocados, soft fruits, sweet potatoes, baked squash, soups and smoothies are ideal.
► Well-cooked whole grains. Millet is particularly beneficial to the stomach. Well-cooked quinoa and short-grain brown rice can also be soothing.
► Water, which can quickly dilute the stomach acid that may be causing pain and irritation. Do not drink water with

meals but have a large glass 30 minutes before meals and an hour after.
► Nut and seed butters and cold-pressed oils rather than nuts and seeds. The nut butters and oils are good ways of getting the anti-inflammatory essential fats without the danger of irritation.

⠿ AVOID

► Alcohol, tea, coffee, salt, chocolate, spices, sugar, fatty foods, fizzy drinks, processed foods, dairy products and red meat. High-protein foods such as red meat, dairy and eggs need a lot of acid to be broken down so can increase irritation and pain. Also avoid very hot or very cold foods as these can cause further irritation.

HERBS AND SUPPLEMENTS

► Slippery elm tea. Slippery elm can coat the lining of the digestive tract, thus protecting it from irritation. Arrowroot powder can also be used for the same effect.
► Drink camomile tea to soothe the digestive system. Stress is commonly implicated in ulcers so calming teas can be beneficial. Other useful herbs include meadowsweet, skullcap and marshmallow root.
► Take bromelain with meals. Bromelain is found in the core of fresh pineapples. It can be taken as a supplement with meals to aid digestion and reduce inflammation.
► Take mastic gum to clear H. pylori infection.
► Take deglycyrrhized liquorice. Liquorice has a long history of healing the digestive tract.
► Take L-glutamine powder. L-glutamine is a major source of fuel for the digestive tract and can help the healing of the

mucous membranes that line it.
► Take large doses of vitamin C. This
has been shown to eradicate H.pylori
in some patients.
► Supplement with acidophilus. This can
help to improve the balance of bacteria
in the gut and digestion generally.

⠿ EXTRA TIPS
► Sleep with the upper body slightly
raised to prevent acid rising up into the
oesophagus. This is useful if heartburn
at night is a problem.
► Antacids are not helpful in the long
term. These work by switching off the
body's production of stomach acid.
Stomach acid is a necessary part of
digestion and without sufficient
quantities of it food can sit in the
digestive tract fermenting and
putrefying. This can lead to all kinds
of digestive and absorption problems.
A stomach that is not sufficiently acidic
will allow bacteria and pathogens to get
into the digestive tract. Antacids do
nothing to heal the digestive tract or
to eradicate the causes of the problem,
they only provide symptomatic relief.
► If you smoke, give up. Smokers are more
likely to have peptic ulcers. Smoking
depletes the body of healing nutrients
and suppresses the immune system.
► Chew food thoroughly to reduce the
amount of work the stomach and intestines
need to do and improve nutrient absorption.
Chewing also mixes food with saliva
which is alkalizing. Relaxing when eating
helps to improve digestive function. Food
cannot be digested if you are eating while
feeling stressed.

PERIODONTAL DISEASE
Periodontal disease is a fairly wide term
referring to various disorders of the teeth
and gums. Problems often start with
inflammation around the teeth and gums,
known as gingivitis. This is caused by the
build-up of food and bacteria. This forms
plaque and the plaque leads to infection
and inflammation of the gums. The
inflammation causes the build-up of more
plaque as it is harder to clean between
the teeth and the swollen gums.

   As the condition progresses, the
infection causes the bone supporting
the teeth to break down. Abscesses, bad
breath and bleeding gums may all be
part of the picture. Ultimately there
may be loss of teeth.

CAUSES
Diets high in sugar and refined
carbohydrates, frequent snacking on
sugary food and drinks, improper tooth
brushing, teeth grinding, dry mouth,
smoking, alcohol use and nutrient
deficiencies can all predispose someone to
periodontal disease. Osteoporosis, diabetes
and heart disease may be underlying
conditions so these need to be checked out.

Action plan
Follow these tips to help strengthen your
teeth and gums.

⠿ EAT/DRINK
► Raw carrot and celery sticks. Chewing
on these can help to strengthen the teeth
and jaw.
► Vitamin C-rich fruit and vegetables.
Vitamin C is needed for healthy gums and
has anti-inflammatory effects. Good

sources include berries, green vegetables, currants, melons, peas, peppers, watercress and kiwi fruits. Avoid very acidic fruits such as citrus fruits and juices as these can cause further damage to the teeth.

► Almonds, figs, sesame seeds, green vegetables, quinoa, amaranth, chickpeas, oats and haricot beans which contain calcium and magnesium. These minerals are needed for healthy bones and teeth.

⠿ AVOID

► Sugar, refined carbohydrates, alcohol and cigarettes. These can all lead to the build-up of plaque and have a negative effect on nutrient status.

► Fizzy drinks. These are high in sugar and phosphoric acid, both of which have a negative effect on the teeth and gums.

SUPPLEMENTS

► My top supplement recommendation is co-enzyme Q10, which improves oxygenation of the tissues and aids healing. It is often low in those with gum disease.

► Supplement with vitamin C with bioflavanoids. These are needed for gum health and repair. Make sure you get a buffered vitamin C as other types can be acidic and this would be detrimental to tooth health.

► Take a bone-supporting formula. The teeth and bones are made of similar minerals so similar nutrients can support both. Look for one containing calcium, magnesium, vitamin D, boron, zinc and B vitamins.

⠿ EXTRA TIPS

► Apply clove oil to painful or infected areas. Clove oil is well known for providing relief from teeth and gum problems.

► Floss! Flossing removes food particles from between the teeth where brushing does not always reach. Floss at least twice a day.

► Use natural mouthwashes. These can help to remove plaque and plaque-forming bacteria. Tea tree oil, grapefruit seed extract, goldenseal, myrrh oil and sage are all good antibacterial oils to look for. A sea-salt water mouthwash can also be used to kill bacteria. Alternating between them may be even more effective.

► Visit your dentist and hygienist regularly. This can help to identify problems before they become advanced and harder to treat.

► Decaying teeth may need to be extracted or filled. Avoid mercury fillings where possible due to mercury's effect on the nervous system. Go for ceramic fillings.

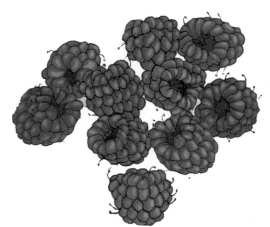

PNEUMONIA

Pneumonia refers to inflammation of the lungs usually caused by an infection. The infection causes the lungs to become congested with mucus and pus. Symptoms include fatigue, shivering, fever, chest pain, coughing up sputum, sweating, muscle aches, sore throat, swollen lymph glands, bluish tinge to the skin and difficulty breathing.

CAUSES

The initial infection may be viral, bacterial or fungal. Most at risk are the very young, older people and those with other disorders such as diabetes, HIV, cardio-vascular disease or a compromised immune system. Smokers are also at increased risk because of the damage done to their lungs and immune system by nicotine. Other factors that may be implicated include malnutrition, stress and pollution.

Action plan

Treatment for pneumonia should always be in conjunction with a medical practitioner.

⁚⁚ EAT/DRINK

► Fruit and vegetables. These are the most cleansing and easily digested foods. They provide an abundance of antioxidants needed by the immune system to fight the infection.

► Betacarotene-rich foods. Betacarotene is an antioxidant that can be made into vitamin A in the body. It is especially protective of the mucous membranes in the lungs and can aid healing. Carrots, pumpkins, squash, apricots, spinach and watercress are all good sources.

► Warm water – at least 2 litres a day. Fluids are necessary to clear thickened mucus and congestion from the lungs.

► Freshly pressed vegetable juices, herbal teas and broths. Fasting on freshly pressed juices for the first few days can help to shorten the suffering and reduce the fever.

⁚⁚ AVOID

► Dairy products. These can increase the amount of mucus the body produces and increase congestion in the lungs.

► Sugar, tea, coffee, refined carbohydrates, alcohol and additives. These can suppress the immune system, put a strain on the liver and digestive system and/or deplete the body of nutrients.

HERBS AND SUPPLEMENTS

► Useful herbs include aconite, green hellebore, gelsemium, belladonna, echinacea and elecampane root. However, these may all be indicated at different stages of the infection so advice should be sought from a medical herbalist before taking any.

► Astragalus may be helpful for recovery.

► Supplement with vitamin C with bioflavanoids. Vitamin C has antibacterial and anti-viral properties and is needed for healing the mucous membranes.

⁚⁚ EXTRA TIPS

► If you smoke, give up. Smoking damages the lungs, depletes the body of nutrients, interferes with proper breathing and compromises the immune system.

► Put a castor oil pack over the chest three times a week. Castor oil packs are useful for clearing congestion. Hold a hot-water bottle over the pack for the best effects.

PREMENSTRUAL SYNDROME OR TENSION (PMS OR PMT)

There are a number of types of PMS or PMT, and it is not uncommon for women to experience more than one type during each cycle:

► Anxiety – mood swings, irritability, anxiety and tension.

► Cravings – cravings for sweet foods, chocolate or carbohydrates in the few days leading up to the period in addition to possible increased appetite, fatigue and headaches.

► Depression – a group of symptoms that includes depression, crying, confusion, forgetfulness and poor coordination.

► Hyperhydration – water retention, breast tenderness and swelling, bloating and weight gain.

CAUSES MAY INCLUDE

► Liver stagnation.

► Blood deficiency.

► Hormonal imbalance (normal hormonal balance at menstruation depends on proper liver function).

► Too much red meat.

► Salty, sugary diet.

► Stress.

Action plan

Diet can make a huge difference, both in balancing your hormones and addressing nutrient deficiencies.

⠿ EAT/DRINK

► Fibre, which is found in whole grains, pulses, nuts, seeds, fruit and vegetables, helps to remove old oestrogens from the body.

► Magnesium-rich foods such as green vegetables, nuts, seeds, tofu and pulses.

It may be worth taking a supplement before the symptoms start each month. Magnesium can help to reduce water retention, balance blood sugar and ease menstrual headaches.

► Essential fatty acids as these are needed for the entire hormonal and nervous systems. Sources include flax, sunflower, pumpkin and sesame seeds and their cold-pressed oils, nuts and oily fish such as mackerel, sardines, salmon, trout and herring.

► Foods that contain the B vitamins, needed for hormone and blood-sugar balance. Sources include whole grains such as millet, quinoa, brown rice and buckwheat as well as nutritional yeast flakes, which can be sprinkled on food.

► Yams, brown rice, sunflower seeds, buckwheat, avocados, legumes – all of which are good sources of vitamin B6, which has been shown to reduce the symptoms of PMT.

► Collard greens, which are a good source of calcium. Apart from building bones, calcium helps to reduce PMS symptoms during the luteal phase (the second half) of the menstrual cycle.

► Sunflower oil which is rich in vitamin E. Vitamin E has been shown to be helpful for tender breasts associated with PMS and also for mood swings.

► Hemp and pumpkin seeds which are an excellent source of zinc. Zinc is an important mineral for the conversion of essential fatty acids. It also plays a major part in balancing hormones.

► Asparagus, which is an excellent source of potassium and quite low in sodium.

It also has a strong diuretic effect. It may therefore be useful for PMS-related water retention.

► Okra for its potent mix of vitamins and minerals, including B6.

⁖ AVOID

► Alcohol, tea, coffee, chocolate and fizzy drinks as these tend to disrupt hormone levels.

► Red meat and dairy products which contain saturated fats that can disrupt hormones so should be cut down for two weeks before and during your period.

► Sugar and refined foods to keep blood-sugar levels stable as this affects mood and energy. Eat small, frequent meals and snacks and take regular moderate exercise to improve blood-sugar control.

HERBS AND SUPPLEMENTS

► Use a complete superfood such as spirulina, wild blue-green algae or chlorella. Blend it into a smoothie. You should increase the intake of these superfoods as your period approaches.

► Take the herb milk thistle before and during menstruation. Silymarin contains some of the most potent liver-protecting and liver-stimulating substances known.

► PMS has been linked to faulty liver fat metabolism. So, sprinkling a tablespoon of lecithin granules onto salads or putting some into a smoothie a few days each week until you see a difference in symptoms is well worth the effort.

► The following herbs may be helpful if taken a couple of days before and during menstruation: agnus castus for breast pain; angelica cong quai for cramps; cramp bark for abdominal discomfort; liquorice for water retention; black cohosh for fibroids.

► Decongest your liver with lipotropic agents. A good lipotropic formula should consist of choline, methionine and/or cysteine.

► Take zinc citrate and magnesium. Zinc is important because it helps to normalize hormones, especially prolactin.

► Increase your intake of B vitamins, including B6 (a magnesium deficiency can lead to decreased B vitamin activity). They are important for energy, mood, digestion and water balance. Do not use isolated B6; take it with a B complex or with botanical royal jelly.

► Vitamin A has been shown to reduce PMS symptoms. Take it in betacarotene form.

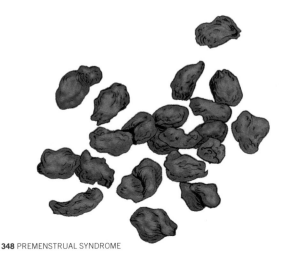

► Vitamin E helps to regulate hormone levels.

► Take flax oil, primrose oil or borage oil daily. Women with menstrual problems have been shown to exhibit essential fatty acid abnormalities.

⁙ EXTRA TIPS

► Regular moderate exercise throughout the month helps to regulate hormones, remove toxins, enhance nutrient absorption, strengthen the organs and ultimately to lessen PMS symptoms.

► Stress also plays a huge role in hormonal balance as the adrenal glands (responsible for our stress response) also produce some oestrogen and progesterone. Relaxation techniques such as yoga, tai chi, deep breathing and meditation can all help.

NOTE ON SUPPLEMENTS

These should be taken every day approximately four days before the period and during the period. After menstruation, you can stop taking them until the following month. Eventually, once your liver is strengthened and your body more balanced, you may find that you don't need all these nutrients and herbs.

PROSTATE CANCER

The prostate gland is a small gland found at the base of the bladder. It secretes prostatic fluid – the fluid in which sperm is carried. Prostate cancer develops when cells in the prostate start to grow in an uncontrolled way. They can then invade surrounding tissues and may spread to other body parts via the lymph.

Prostate cancer is becoming increasingly common. It tends to be a slow-growing cancer and may be asymptomatic. Autopsies show that many men who die of other causes actually have cancer of the prostate gland without being aware of it.

Symptoms include pain or burning during urination, a need to urinate frequently, poor urine flow or an inability to urinate, blood in the urine or semen, impotence, lower back pain or pelvic pain. There may, however, be no symptoms. Many of these symptoms may be due to benign prostatic hyperplasia (BPH) so a correct diagnosis is important.

Diagnosis is often by measuring levels of prostate specific antigen (PSA). Otherwise, rectal examination and ultra-sound scans can also be carried out. Ultimately a biopsy is needed to confirm the diagnosis.

CAUSES MAY INCLUDE

► A history of venereal disease.

► A high-fat diet.

► High testosterone levels.

► A family history of prostate cancer.

► Nutrient deficiencies.

► Exposure to environmental chemicals.

► Pollution.

Action plan

Any changes you make must be sanctioned by your GP, but the following may be of help.

⣿ EAT/DRINK

▶ Fruit, vegetables, nuts, seeds, whole grains and pulses which have been shown to slow the growth of prostate cancer as measured by PSA levels.

▶ Tomatoes which are one of the best sources of lycopene. Lycopene is a plant chemical that can reduce the chances of developing prostate cancer and can slow its progression. Maximum lycopene can be derived from tomatoes that have been puréed. Watermelons and pink grapefruits also supply some lycopene.

▶ Olive oil and avocados. These are high in mono-unsaturated fats that have favourable effects on slowing the development of prostate cancer. They are also good sources of vitamin E, deficient levels of which are linked to the development of cancer.

▶ Soy products. These contain isoflavones which can reduce testosterone levels. This may be useful if the prostate cancer is linked to high testosterone levels. Good soy foods to include are tempeh, tofu, natural soya yoghurt, edamame, miso, natto and tamari. Soy isolates such as textured vegetable protein tend not to have the same beneficial effects.

▶ Brazil nuts, which are one of the best sources of selenium, an important anti-cancer nutrient that is particularly important for prostate health. Make sure they are organic as their nutrient content is likely to be higher than conventionally grown nuts.

▶ Cruciferous vegetables (broccoli, Brussels sprouts, cauliflower and kale) contain potent anti-cancer chemicals. These are also found in pomegranate juice which contains antioxidants that can slow the progression of prostate cancer.

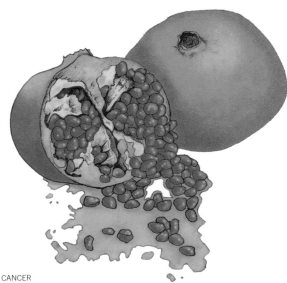

▶ Oily fish, hemp seeds, flax seeds and walnuts. These are all sources of the essential omega-3 fats which are often low in those with prostate cancer.

▶ Soluble fibre. Men with diets high in soluble fibre have been found to have lower levels of PSA than those who do not eat much fibre. Good sources of soluble fibre include oats, barley, lentils, peas, beans, fruit and vegetables.

▶ Organic foods in general which are higher in nutrients and lower in potentially damaging chemicals.

⠿ **AVOID**

▶ Meat and meat cooked at high temperatures (such as chargrilled, barbecued or fried meats). Cooking meat at high temperatures leads to the formation of heterocyclic aromatic amines which are carcinogenic (cancer forming).

▶ Salt, alcohol, caffeine, sugar, fatty meats, fried foods and dairy products. These can potentially challenge the immune system, deplete the body of nutrients and increase the risk and progression of cancer. Fats to avoid include saturated fats from fatty meats and dairy products and processed or heated fats such as those in margarines, pastries, crisps, burnt or fried foods.

EXTRA TIP

▶ Spend time outside in daylight every day. Prostate cancer is more likely to develop in men with low levels of vitamin D. The best source of vitamin D is from the action of sunlight on the skin. Aim for at least 30 minutes a day.

PROSTATE ENLARGEMENT

This is also called benign prostatic hyperplasia (BPH) and is characterized by an enlarged prostate gland. This is extremely common in men over the age of 40.

Symptoms include frequent urination, hesitancy, and intermittent flow with reduced force. There may also be pain on urination and pain in the lower stomach area. If left untreated the retained urine can flow back into the bloodstream and cause dangerous complications. If left untreated the prostate can become cancerous.

UNDERLYING CAUSES

▶ Hormonal imbalances – testosterone levels in men tend to decrease with age while other hormones, such as prolactin and oestrogen, increase. Often there is an increase in the level of dihydrotestosterone (DHT) in the prostate. DHT stimulates the production of prostate cells leading to enlargement.

▶ High cholesterol levels – cholesterol metabolites can cause damage to cells in the prostate.

Action plan

While surgery is often thought to be the only option, BPH responds well to nutritional and herbal interventions. Men over the age of 55 are advised to have a medical examination to ascertain whether there is any enlargement of the prostate.

⠿ **EAT/DRINK**

▶ Pumpkin seeds – these are a great source of zinc. Zinc has been found to reduce the size of the prostate. Other good sources include flax seeds, whole grains, pulses, fish, eggs and lean meats.

► Barley water. This is cleansing for the kidneys and bladder. Grated ginger or lemon juice can be added for extra flavour.

► Seeds and cold-pressed oils. Try hemp, flax, sunflower and sesame seed oils for their anti-inflammatory effects.

► Oily fish, such as salmon and mackerel.

► Organic foods – pesticides can increase levels of DHT in the prostate.

► Whole grains – these are high in vitamin B6 and other B vitamins needed for normal prostate function and hormone balance. Brown rice, millet, quinoa and oats are all good sources.

► Kelp, which is high in nutrients needed for a healthy hormonal system.

► Water – at least 8 large glasses a day – for the prevention of infections in the urinary system and for good urine flow.

⠿ AVOID
► Saturated animal fats in fatty meats and dairy products as these can increase inflammation.

► Sugar, caffeine, alcohol and refined foods – these are low in nutrients and can also deplete the body of nutrients. They also stimulate insulin, high levels of which may be implicated in BPH. Alcohol, in particular, is implicated in BPH so should be avoided completely.

HERBS AND SUPPLEMENTS
► Pygeum is a herb that is being increasingly used in BPH with good results.

► Support the urinary tract with herbs – nettle, parsley, dandelion leaf, slippery elm bark and uva ursi can all be beneficial.

► Supplement with zinc citrate, chelate or gluconate and EFAs. After this, take saw palmetto.

⠿ EXTRA TIPS
► Engage in regular exercise – exercise increases oxygen and nutrient flow to the area. Avoid cycling as this can put pressure on the prostate.

► Have hot then cold showers – start with a normal hot shower, then switch to cold for 30–60 seconds directing the water to the abdomen. Then switch back to hot for two to three minutes. Repeat two or three times, This improves circulation and lymph flow to the area.

PSORIASIS

Psoriasis is a distressing, common skin disorder that first appears in the late teens to thirties. It manifests as reddish, silvery, raised, scaled lesions. Once you have it, it is very hard to get it into remission. However, there are occasionally spontaneous remissions and it never appears again. It can manifest as thick scalp dandruff or scalp lesions that spread mainly over the middle torso, back, elbows, knees, groin, genitals, anus and very occasionally the face and neck. It tends not to itch although it might, and it looks unsightly. The nails can be affected too, taking on a mottled appearance and even falling off. It can cause sufferers to cover up even in the summer, hide away, avoid the beach and feel embarrassed, miserable and depressed.

With psoriasis, the skin cells are multiplying at a much higher rate than with normal skin, causing a pile-up of skin as new cells come in too fast before the old cells have had time to shed. There is an imbalance between what's called AMP (cyclic adenosine monophosphate) and GMP (cyclic guanidine monophosphate). Increased GMP results in rapid skin cell development and increased AMP results in decreased cell replication.

It takes perseverance to deal with this condition and you have to be really determined to stick at it.

CAUSES MAY INCLUDE
► Hereditary condition.
► Inherited fault in antibody-antigen response to foreign organisms like *Candida albicans*.
► Toxin overload.
► Sluggish bowels.
► Emotional stress.
► Liver imbalance and impaired liver function.
► *Candida albicans* yeast overgrowth.
► Nutrient deficiencies.
► Incomplete protein digestion.
► Bowel toxaemia.
► Overeating of animal fats.
► Alcohol.
► Bad illness, infection.
► Pregnancy and hormonal changes.
► Sunburn.

Action plan
You need to do everything possible to nourish the liver and improve fat metabolism.

EAT/DRINK MORE
► Fibre.
► Raw food. That means raw salads, smoothies, juices, soups (yes, raw soups), seeds.
► Fish, for the anti-inflammatory omega-3s. Eskimos generally don't seem to get psoriasis.
► Liver-friendly foods such as artichoke, cauliflower, cabbage and kale.
► Foods high in B vitamins, including brown rice, as many sufferers are deficient.
► Yarrow tea.

AVOID
► Sugar, alcohol, caffeine and refined grains. Remove pork from the diet. The nitrates that are added to this meat are often a trigger.

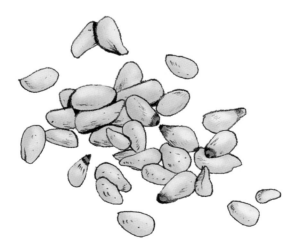

▶ Red meat and milk. They both contain arachidonic acid which for some is difficult to absorb and could exacerbate inflammation.

▶ Dairy products, eggs, wheat, corn and citrus as these are the most common causes of food sensitivities.

▶ Nightshades such as tomatoes, peppers, potatoes and paprika. They could be triggers.

▶ Gluten, which may be a trigger, so do not eat too much wheat. Vary your diet. Go to www.gillianmckeith.info.

HERBS AND SUPPLEMENTS

▶ Take milk thistle to improve liver function. I have seen the best results with this herb as it helps to filter blood toxins, inhibit inflammation and correct rapid cell growth. Also use the herb glutathione to slow down the underlying skin cell growth.

▶ Other herbs: cleavers, dandelion, yarrow and burdock in tea form and

tincture to help detoxify. Coptis may help to prevent new outbreaks. Sarsaparilla. Goldenseal may help indirectly to lower the proliferation of skin-cell development. Ayurvedic herb coleus forskolhli may slow down fast cell growth. Oregon Grape, or *Mahonia aquifolium*, has been lauded as an anti-psoriasis herb.

▶ Take glutamine powder before meals.

▶ Sprinkle lecithin granules on salads. Lecithin is helpful for fat metabolism and liver health.

▶ Improving digestion overall is critica. The herb gentiana in liquid form may be useful for this.

▶ A supplement of starflower oil is beneficial.

▶ Use green superfoods like spirulina, algae and chlorella.

▶ Incomplete protein digestion resulting in high levels of toxic metabolites in the bowel and a lack of stomach acid may be a link. So add betaine with HCL before all meals.

▶ Fish oils may well help.

▶ Take vitamin A supplements. But vitamin A therapy is best done under the watchful eye of a health practitioner. Do not take vitamin A supplements if you are pregnant.

▶ Take vitamin B complex.

▶ Zinc has a remarkable effect on the skin. When it is low, yeast levels can flourish and a lack of zinc may be a psoriasis trigger. You need zinc to absorb alpha-linoleic acid.

▶ Vitamin D supplements in liquid form may be helpful, too.

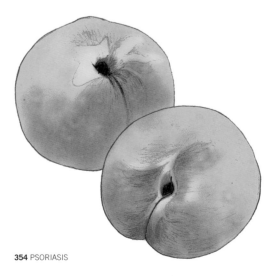

▶ Hypnosis can work wonders. See a therapist for best results.

▶ Watch out for soaps and detergents that dry out the skin.

▶ Sometimes exposing the skin to direct sunlight can help but in some cases it can actually make it worse. So it's an experiment really.

▶ Steroidal creams seem to be fairly effective for most sufferers. They dissolve the scales. However, they can cause thinning of the skin. And as soon as you stop using the steroidal cream, the scales return. So it's a sticking plaster effect, not a cure.

▶ Define the trigger. From my own clinical experience with clients, emotional stress seems to be the biggest trigger. Suppressed emotions can trigger skin problems.

▶ Check for the gluten sensitivity, which might be a trigger. If you are sensitive to gluten, replace oats, wheat, rye, barley, kamut and spelt with brown rice, wild rice, red rice, quinoa, buckwheat and millet.

▶ Investigate the link between overgrowth of the intestinal yeast, *Candida albicans* and psoriasis. You must get tested for this and if the test is positive, you need to follow the protocol for candida recovery (see page 219).

About 24 years ago I suffered a slipped disc. At the same time, psoriasis appeared as a line down my spine, and from there it spread across my body down my arms and legs. I read that psoriasis had always been mistakenly treated as a skin complaint but it was more to do with toxins in the body. So I went on a strict detox. I had only water for the first day, then water and one fruit the second day gradually adding foods over a period of a month. By this time I was on a completely whole food diet that did not include meat. During this month the psoriasis gradually disappeared up my arms and legs, across my body until I was left with a line down my spine which completely disappeared by the end of the 4th week. I had not used any creams and now I can completely control the return of psoriasis through diet alone.

R

RAYNAUD'S DISEASE

Raynaud's disease, also known as Raynaud's phenomenon, refers to constricted circulation to the extremities. The arteries of the hands, feet, nose and ears go into spasm when exposed to cold temperatures. The extremities go white or blue and numb in response to cold. They may also become swollen. Women are more likely to be affected than men and winter is the time when symptoms are most apparent.

CAUSES MAY INCLUDE
- Arteriosclerosis.
- Migraines (see page 328).
- Smoking.
- Use of calcium channel blockers.
- Medications.
- Poor circulation.

Action plan

The aim here is to improve circulation.

EAT/DRINK
- Buckwheat as a cereal or grain. Buckwheat contains rutin which can help to strengthen capillary walls.
- Foods that can help to improve blood circulation, such as beetroot, rye, soya beans and sardines. These are used traditionally in Chinese medicine for disorders of the circulatory system such as Raynaud's.
- Warming spices such as ginger, cinnamon, cloves, cumin and turmeric. A pinch of cayenne pepper added to stews and casseroles can also be warming.
- Oily fish, nuts, seeds and cold-pressed oils benefit the circulatory system.
- Hawthorn tea.

AVOID
- Cold foods and drinks.
- Saturated fats from fatty meats and dairy products.
- Alcohol, which lowers your body temperature.
- Sugar and refined carbohydrates.
- Caffeine and nicotine. These both constrict the blood vessels and reduce circulation.

HERBS AND SUPPLEMENTS
- Take ginkgo biloba as tea, capsules or tincture during autumn and winter. Ginkgo is well known for its benefits to circulation.
- Take co-enzyme Q10. This can improve oxygenation in the tissues.
- Vitamin B complex will help to improve circulation and nerve transmission. Additional vitamin B3 is helpful, too.
- Green superfood powder supplements are a great source of bioavailable nutrients.

EXTRA TIPS
- Dry skin brush daily to get the lymphatic and circulatory systems moving. Follow this with a hot then cold shower to further improve circulation. Switch from hot to cold twice to three times for even greater effects.
- Avoid getting cold. Wrap up warmly, wear gloves and warm socks if the weather is cold.
- Massage the arms, legs, hands and feet with a few drops of rosemary oil in a tablespoon of olive oil. Rosemary is warming and massaging can improve circulation.

RHEUMATOID ARTHRITIS

Rheumatoid arthritis (RA) is a chronic, inflammatory condition and what is called an auto-immune disease where the body is actually attacking its own tissues and cells.

Symptoms include swelling and joint pain which seems to start gradually in the small joints of the hands, wrists, feet, elbows, hips, knees or shoulders. One or more of these areas may disfigure and end up deformed. The skin turns ruddy and purple in colour over the swollen areas too. Most sufferers also complain of general malaise, fever, tiredness and lack of appetite.

CAUSES
► Hereditary predisposition.
► Low stomach acid.
► Food allergies.
► Abnormal gut and bowel permeability.
► Liver link.
► Deficiencies of B vitamins, especially pantothenic acid and zinc.
► Essential fatty acid and gamma-linolenic acid deficiency.
► Smoking.
► Chronic stress.
► Adrenal weakness.
► Constipation.
► Toxaemia.
► Vitamin D deficiency.
► Parasitic infection (blastocystis homenis).

Action plan

You need to change your diet to get on top of this condition. The more vegetarian based, the better. My clients respond best when they are on a vegan diet (no dairy, meat or fish) or almost vegan diet with the exception of including some fish.

⠿ EAT/DRINK
► Fruit and vegetables for antioxidants.
► Get more oils into your body, so eat oily fish like salmon, herring, mackerel and sardines. These contain anti-inflammatory omega-3 fats.
► Eat from all the different berries for their flavanoids which may help in reducing swellings. Papaya is a wonderful food which contains anti-inflammatory properties.
► Eat the yellow foods such as squash, carrots and yams. These contain betacarotene needed for a healthy immune system.
► Add turmeric to your stews. Turmeric contains the flavanoid curcumin which has anti-inflammatory properties.
► Use olive oil and gold of pleasure seed oil liberally on your salads.
► Eat foods rich in molybdenum, such as aduki beans. This compound helps liver detox, and a healthy liver affects the health of every cell in the body. Try aduki bean soup, salads, bakes and stews.
► Go for the cruciferous vegetables such as kale, cabbage, collards and Brussels sprouts.
► Drink celery juice for its diuretic effect, but, if you find that hard going on its own, just make sure that you add celery to your veggie juices. Mix it with carrot, kale or cabbage.
► Chomp on celery stalks, too. You can dip the stalks in mustard or hummous.
► Sprinkle ground flax seeds on your porridge for their anti-inflammatory effect.

► Eat raw shelled hemp seeds for snacks and mash them into avocados.

► Add ginger to your meals, too. You can grate it finely. It is thought that it may block the prostoglandins that cause inflammation.

⁚⁚⁚ AVOID

► Researchers have identified various foods as being the most likely triggers of rheumatoid arthritis. These include corn, wheat, cow's milk, pork, oranges, oats, rye, eggs, beef, coffee, malt, cheese, grapefruit, lemons, tomatoes and soya.

► Oranges and orange juice can be mucus forming and irritating to the digestive tract.

► Take out the nightshades and see if it makes a difference. Nightshades include white potatoes, tomatoes, paprika, aubergines, bell peppers and, of course, tobacco. Some people are sensitive to the solanine in these foods. It is thought that the solanine interferes with the enzymes in the muscles, often causing pain and discomfort. In sensitive individuals, it could create arthritic-like symptoms. This nightshade rule of mine is the same for osteoarthritic sufferers, too. Solanine is also a calcium inhibitor and arthritic sufferers may be deficient in calcium.

► I have found in my practice that arthritics tend to do best when I take gluten out of the diet. There are some studies on arthritics which have revealed elevated levels of the gliadin antibodies. Arthritic-like symptoms have diminished in coeliac sufferers on a gluten-free diet. So even though you may not have coeliac disease but you do have arthritis, you could benefit greatly from a gluten-free diet.

► Get totally rid of junk foods, food with chemicals and colourings, fizzy drinks, pies, pastries, cakes and biscuits as you don't know what's in them. If you want a treat, make your own.

HERBS

► The herb yucca in extract form or capsule form can be very helpful for this condition. It's best to take yucca in combination with the herb devil's claw. Take 2 capsules 3 times daily.

► Astragalus extract is good source of the B vitamins, for the release of energy from food.

► The Ayurvedic herb boswella has been found to be useful with this condition.

► Take celery seed extract. It has been found to have anti-inflammatory properties.

► Take capsules of cayenne containing capsaicin which is thought to block pain.

SUPPLEMENTS

► The supplement quercetin also has anti-inflammatory properties. Take it between meals.

► Alternatively, take bromelain in between meals.

► Take borage oil capsules 3 times daily.

► Take betaine hydrochloric acid tablets with pepsin before meals. But speak to your GP about this first. In all the cases of RA that I have come across, every person has exhibited very low stomach acid. This supplement may help to reduce food allergy symptoms by helping to break down proteins.

► Ask your GP about the possibility of vitamin B12 injections.

► Vitamin B complex with extra B5, 3 times a day, is a must. 1,500–2,000mg is what's needed to make a difference.

► Use royal jelly paste as another way of getting the B vitamins, especially vitamin B5.

► Take vitamin E daily in capsule form.

► If your arthritis gets worse in winter, there could be a vitamin D deficiency. It's not a bad idea to supplement with D in the winter, especially if you have little exposure to sun at other times of the year.

► Also add a beneficial bacteria to your daily regime to improve gut function and nutrient absorption.

► Two tablespoons of flax oil daily would be of enormous benefit. You can alternate with fish oils.

► Take glutamine powder before meals for gut health.

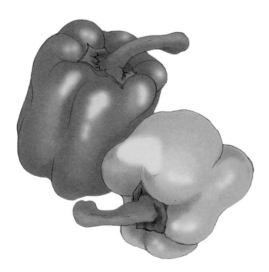

▦ EXTRA TIPS

► Keep a food diary and see just how much wheat, corn, red meats, dairy, white potatoes, peppers, paprika, tomatoes and caffeine you are consuming.

► For a month or so, adopt my food-combining principles to maximize digestion. That means fruit by itself, never for dessert, and not mixing dense proteins such as chicken or fish with dense carbohydrates such as potatoes or rice at the same meal.

► Get tested for food allergies. Food allergies and intolerances have been strongly implicated with this condition. Go to www.gillianmckeith.info for details on food sensitivity testing. See your GP about allergies.

► Get tested for parasites. There are certain parasitic infections, one being blastocystis homenis, that can cause arthritic-like symptoms. A stool test is needed for this. Go to www. gillianmckeith.info for details.

► As daft as it may sound, if the pain is in the wrist area, you may want to look into the wearing of magnet bracelets. Some people have reported to me an improvement. It's worth a try.

► Creams containing the ingredient capsaicin (from chillies) may help to soothe pain and reduce inflammation.

► Get regular body massages with oils. But even more important, have regular head massages with oils. This may improve circulation in the brain influencing the pituitary gland and hormonal release. The hormonal system has an effect on auto-immune reactions.

► When you have a bath, put a couple of tablespoons of apple cider vinegar in the water. This is a traditional soothing remedy going back donkey's years.

I'm 17; soon to be 18. When I was 14, I developed a life-threatening thrombosis after a netballing injury and ever since have been in and out of hospital fighting rheumatoid arthritis as well as recurring clots. After feeling sorry for myself for so long I decided that what I made of my life was up to me. After watching your show I realized my diet was playing a large role in my overall health. After turning to healthier alternatives I now have a much better appetite and enjoy food more. My condition physically has improved and I no longer require intravenous medications for pain control! I'll still have these conditions for the rest of my life, but I know for a fact that my quality of life is so much better.

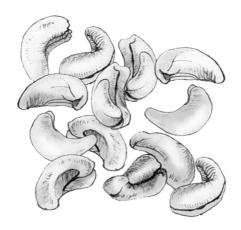

ROSACEA

It's not exactly acne but it looks a little like that. A chronic redness and red flushed look appears on the cheeks and also around the nose and chin. The skin becomes thickened, feels rough and may come out in red welts and red spots. It tends not to affect teenagers and is more common in fair-skinned women.

CAUSES MAY INCLUDE

► Parasites, organisms.
► Alcohol.
► Caffeine.
► Some dairy products.
► Pork.
► Spicy foods.
► Poor digestion.
► Hormonal imbalance.
► Stress.
► Sluggish liver and lymphatic function.
► Lack of digestive enzymes.
► Hereditary predisposition.
► Bright sunlight.
► Food intolerances.

Action plan

Try to find the root cause by systematically working through the potential trigger areas.

⁚⁚ EAT/DRINK

► Cabbages, cauliflower, sprouted broccoli seeds, celery, kale, seaweeds. Rosacea is often a sign of liver toxicity and these foods are all helpful to the liver.
► Fibre and raw foods and vegetable juices to prevent constipation.
► Pineapples and papayas as a good source of food enzymes that aid digestion.

▶ Brown rice and lentils, beans, dates, wheat germ, beets, green vegetables like spinach, almonds and sunflower seeds which are all sources of vitamin B, as in my experience most people with this condition are deficient.

▶ Drink a cup of warm water with a squeeze of lemon first thing in the morning and last thing at night to alkalize your system.

▶ Take two teaspoons of apple cider vinegar before main meals to aid digestion.

▦ AVOID

▶ Dairy products. They simply make the condition worse.

▶ Pastries, pies, cakes, sugary biscuits, margarine, shortening, fried foods and foods containing the dangerous form of fat, trans-fatty acids.

▶ Vitamin B3, niacin, on its own as this may cause you to flush. Instead, take as part of a B complex.

HERBS AND SUPPLEMENTS

▶ Take the herbal extract milk thistle. This helps liver function.

▶ Drink nettle tea at room temperature which is a good source of the Bs.

▶ Herbal tinctures of red clover and astragalus can help. Make sure they are alcohol-free, though.

▶ The herb burdock root has traditionally been used for this condition. It works on the liver which is often sluggish.

▶ Agnus castus may help to regulate any underlying hormonal imbalance exacerbating the problem.

▶ Go on a 24-hour detox and take the herb cleavers to help to get the lymph moving to carry the toxins more efficiently out of the body. Follow this with a couple of days of just broths, raw foods and veggie juices.

▶ In every case of rosacea that I have ever seen, the person has always tested deficient in the B vitamins, in particular riboflavin, vitamin B2, which is essential for carbohydrate metabolism, vitality, energy and the clarity of the skin. So take vitamin B complex.

▶ Low levels of stomach acid are one of the main causes of rosacea. Take betaine with HCL before meals and a digestive enzyme supplement such as pancreatin with or at the end of meals.

▶ Vitamin C and bioflavanoids are anti-inflammatory.

▶ Avoid vitamin B3, niacin, on its own as this may cause you to flush.

▦ EXTRA TIPS

▶ Get tested for food intolerances. Go to www.gillianmckeith.info for a home-test kit. There is often a connection, especially with those rosacea sufferers who get lots of headaches.

▶ I have also found a connection between parasites, organisms, amoebas and unbalanced bacterias with this condition. So please do a digestion test (www.gillianmckeith.info).

▶ Avoid facials with steaming. It sometimes makes things worse.

▶ Take up yoga or meditation to aid relaxation and deal with stress (see page 373).

▶ If you have been taking antibiotics to help with this condition see page 188.

SCABIES

Scabies is a skin disease caused by infection from the acarus scabei mite. The mite burrows into the top layer of the skin and lays its eggs. Initially, the mites cause small, red lumps on the skin. Other symptoms include intense heat, itching, irritation and red, scabby, dry skin. The infection usually starts on the hands and can spread from there often affecting the arms, toes and buttocks. The itching may last for a couple of weeks.

Scabies is diagnosed by inspecting a skin scraping under a microscope for evidence of the mites or eggs. Scabies is highly contagious. It is spread by skin-to-skin contact so outbreaks can occur in schools and institutions.

Action plan

Increase your immunity so that you are less likely to succumb to infection.

❖ EAT/DRINK

▶ Vegetable juices contain nutrients needed for healing.

▶ Garlic. It is anti-parasitic and antibacterial. It can be eaten and applied topically. Rub cut cloves of garlic onto the affected areas but be careful as garlic is quite powerful and can make the skin sore.

▶ Zinc-rich foods including pumpkin, sunflower and sesame seeds.

▶ Shitake mushrooms and pau d'arco tea for immune-boosting properties.

▶ Sprouted seeds for antioxidants.

⋯ AVOID

▶ Sugar, refined carbohydrates and processed foods. These all suppress the immune system and slow healing.

⁖ EXTRA TIPS

▶ Tea tree can be applied to the affected areas of skin to destroy the mites.

▶ Apply sulphur as a dusting powder to destroy the mites.

▶ To aid healing, apply aloe vera gel or calendula cream to the affected areas.

▶ Avoid contact with infested people and their clothing where possible.

▶ Keep nails short and clean; the mites can get under the fingernails if you have been scratching your skin.

▶ Clothing and bedding that is in contact with the skin should be boiled to destroy mites and eggs.

▶ Where possible, remove the mites from their burrows with a sterilized needle.

SCOLIOSIS

This is a condition that I have lived with since the age of 14. I have a theory that my body was not metabolizing enough vitamin D and the mineral manganese in my formative years when my bones were developing. Now as a practitioner, I always recommend to young teenagers that they take extra supplements of bone building minerals to enhance skeletal growth.

The spine is twisted sideways creating a lateral curve and can also come outwardly creating a humped appearance. Scoliosis is usually diagnosed as being thoracic or lumbar or both depending where the curving is on the spine. As the spine twists, it pulls the ribs out of normal position, too. Single and double curves can occur creating a C shape or a sort of S shape. Often the hip will be affected, too. Although it can be apparent at birth, it more often occurs during the growth spurt years in childhood. The teenage years are the ones to watch for the development of this condition but it can occur earlier.

In addition, the muscles around the spine become overly tense often resulting in low-grade to excruciating pain. Not everyone experiences the pain as a symptom, although many do. Traditional treatment involves wearing a brace and more radically, surgery where a metal rod is inserted into the back. Girls are affected more by this condition than boys.

UNDERLYING CAUSES AND RISK FACTORS

► Vitamin D deficiency.
► Manganese deficiency.
► General mineral deficiencies.
► Hereditary.
► Hormonal influences during growth spurt years.
► Carrying heavy bags on one shoulder for prolonged periods of time.
► Playing musical instruments that require a lopsided position like the violin.
► A diet high in sugar and simple. carbohydrates during vital development years.
► Dormant virus that attacks the spine.

Action plan

It is the type of condition that tends to get worse over the years for all kinds of reasons. As the years have gone on, my pain has worsened. I have gone through long periods of excruciating agony. But there is hope. There are ways to mitigate the pain.

⊞ EAT/DRINK
► Start each day with a cup of warm water or a cup of warm water and lemon.
► Eat foods to feed the kidneys. The kidneys suffer a great deal with this condition. Include kidney beans, onions, fennel, spring onions, chives, beetroots, parsley and celery, quinoa, black sesame seeds, walnuts, aduki beans and black beans in your diet.
► Almonds are a good source of magnesium. It is important to eat magnesium rich foods which can help to mobilize calcium into the bones.
► Eat kale and other dark green leafy vegetables for their bone building minerals.
► Once every month, have a juice, soup and broth detox day.
► Hazelnuts contain vitamin E, which can help prevent tissue degradation in the muscle support, important with scoliosis. Other vitamin E foods include avocados, almonds, asparagus, cabbage, whole grains, edamames and leafy greens.

⊞ AVOID
Challenging foods that will stress the kidneys and liver, particularly sugar and alcohol.

HERBS AND SUPPLEMENTS
► Take the herb cleavers one week a month. 30 drops in water twice daily.
► Drink goldenrod or oatstraw tea to nourish the kidneys. You can find this in a specialist herbal shop or health-food store. Alternate with dandelion tea.

► A good multivitamin should be taken daily.

► B complex, 50mg twice daily, to help nourish the central nervous system.

► Magnesium citrate is essential to mobilize calcium into the bones.

► It is thought that a vitamin D deficiency or a manganese deficiency could be a trigger. So even although you may have the scoliosis now, it is still prudent to take supplements as a preventative for a worsening curve. Take vitamin D in liquid form for easy assimilation.

► Look out for white spots on the nails especially in teenagers during their growth years. They may indicate a zinc deficiency. Take zinc citrate. It will take a while to correct this deficiency but it is essential to do so.

⠿ EXTRA TIPS

► A hot-water bottle can help to relax the back area. Place the bottle at the back area when you are about to go to sleep or rest.

► Learn deep breathing techniques.

► Do not carry heavy bags. Children should not lug around heavy school bags. If your child must have a bag, make it a backpack rather than a one-shouldered bag.

► Create a Positive Appreciation book that you write in every day. This will keep you focused on the positive aspects of life and not dwelling on yourself, your condition or any pain. Find one thing each day that you appreciate and write it down.

► Check out the Katharina Schroth method for scoliosis. This treatment involves a set series of prescribed exercises that do seem to make a difference for the better. You can find out about this by contacting www.gillianmckeith.info/scoliosis.

► Rolfing technique. I urge anyone with this condition to try this. Japanese acupuncture can help a great deal in relieving pain.

Tuina massage can help to relieve painful pressure points. This type of massage is usually performed by an acupuncturist.

► Alexander Technique teaches lengthening and body posture. I highly recommend you investigate this technique.

► Pilates is a form of exercise that works amazingly for me. From the first day I started I was in less pain and I now do it every day. Pilates works on strengthening your core muscles and this is of enormous benefit to a scoliosis sufferer. If the muscles around the spinal area are stronger, they are more supportive and can keep the spine from moving so much. An added plus is a nice, flat toned stomach, so you can't beat that!

► Exercise. You can't afford to sit in a chair all day typing on a computer. Find something that you love, from walking to swimming to yoga or Pilates.

► Have regular reflexology treatments. Ask the reflexologist to focus on the liver, kidneys and back area.

SCHIZOPHRENIA

Schizophrenia is characterized by symptoms such as hallucinations, voices that talk to or about the patient, paranoia, violent outbursts, delusions, loss of zest for life, social withdrawal and feeling flat. Schizophrenia is debilitating for both the patient and their family. It affects about 1 per cent of the population.

CAUSES MAY INCLUDE

► A family history of mental-health problems.

► Biochemical abnormalities.

► Stress.

► Damage during birth.

► Environmental toxins.

► Head injuries.

► High histamine levels.

► Some medications.

► High copper: zinc ratios.

► Nutrient deficiencies, particularly magnesium, zinc, folic acid, B vitamins and essential fats.

Action plan

Getting a handle on nutritional deficiencies can help alongside treatment.

⠿ EAT/DRINK

► Whole natural foods. This is the best way to ensure that you get the necessary nutrients and avoid toxins and dietary challenges. A diet of fruit, vegetables, nuts, seeds, pulses, whole grains, fish and lean meats is the way to go. Eat food that has been cooked or prepared from scratch wherever possible.

► Green vegetables, whole grains, beans and lentils. These are high in folic acid, B vitamins and magnesium which have been found to be low in those with depressive disorders.

► Oily fish, such as salmon, trout, herring, sardines and mackerel. These contain omega-3 fatty acids that have been shown to be low in those with schizophrenia.

► Ground flax seeds, hulled hemp seeds and their cold-pressed oils. These contain essential fats needed for neurotransmitters in the brain, as well as the antioxidant vitamin E needed to protect the brain.

► Pumpkin seeds, fish, lean white meats, eggs, pulses, peas and sunflower seeds for their zinc content.

⠿ AVOID

► Sugar, refined carbohydrates (white flour products, white rice, white pasta, etc.), alcohol, caffeine, drugs, nicotine and additives. It is vital to keep blood-sugar levels stable as swings in blood sugar can affect mood and brain chemistry.

► Potential food sensitivities or allergens.

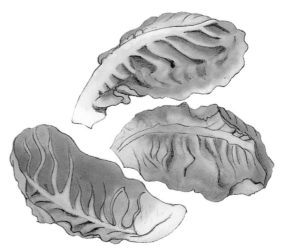

Eating foods to which you are intolerant can alter brain chemistry and create mood swings and addictions. Gluten (from wheat, rye, oats and barley) and dairy products are common culprits. Others may include chocolate, peanuts, eggs, soya and corn.

▶ Artificial sweeteners and additives. These can upset brain chemistry so avoid all processed foods.

▶ Saturated fat from fatty meats and dairy products. Diets high in saturated fats have been found to be detrimental to the symptoms of schizophrenia.

HERBS AND SUPPLEMENTS

▶ Supplement with fish oils containing EPA. EPA is an oil found in fatty fish that has been shown to be deficient in many people with schizophrenia.

⠿ EXTRA TIPS

▶ Do aerobic exercise daily for at least 20 minutes. Exercise is great for improving blood-sugar control, improving brain chemistry, dissipating stress hormones and improving mood generally. Jogging, brisk walking, swimming, cycling, skipping, dancing and rebounding can all make you feel better and improve overall health.

▶ Get outside every day in daylight. Daylight is vital for normalizing body rhythms and moods. Aim for at least 30 minutes a day.

▶ Deal with stress. Schizophrenia may be linked to chronic and acute stress. If stress is a problem for you then consider talking therapies, yoga, tai chi and visualizations. Support groups can also be helpful.

▶ Insulin resistance (see page 326)

has been found to be common in those diagnosed with schizophrenia. This is particularly important if you are on anti-psychotic medication as there is some research that suggests that schizophrenics who take anti-psychotic medication may be at increased risk of developing diabetes.

▶ Avoid toxic metals such as lead, aluminium, cadmium and mercury. These can interfere with brain chemistry and nutrient absorption. Sources include pollution, amalgam fillings, deodorants, cigarette smoke, some paint, lead water pipes, aluminium cooking utensils and some fish such as tuna, swordfish and shark.

▶ Reduce copper intake and exposure and increase zinc intake. Those with schizophrenia tend to have high copper relative to zinc. Use a water filter and avoid copper cookware.

SEASONAL AFFECTIVE DISORDER

Seasonal Affective Disorder (SAD) is a condition in which sufferers become depressed and lethargic during the winter months. Symptoms include fatigue, apathy, weight gain, craving comfort foods, overeating and anxiety.

CAUSES

The production of melatonin by the pineal gland in the brain is triggered by daylight. Melatonin helps to set the daily rhythm and impacts on mood. Serotonin, known as a feel-good chemical, is a precursor to melatonin. During the winter the pineal may not be exposed to enough daylight for it to have the full effect. Serotonin and melatonin levels are likely to be reduced due to shorter days, increased cloud cover and little time spent outside with subsequent effects on mood and energy.

Action plan

There are many nutritional ways to help, through boosting your energy levels and mood.

⸬ EAT/DRINK

▶ Whole grains. Complex carbohydrates, such as those found in brown rice, quinoa, millet, oats and rye, improve the transport of tryptophan into the brain. Here, tryptophan is converted to serotonin, the feel-good chemical.
▶ Other tryptophan-rich foods include bananas, chicken, salmon, turkey, oats, brown rice and soya products, such as tempeh and tofu.
▶ Brewer's yeast flakes. These are high in the B vitamins, which are needed for normal brain chemistry. Avoid these if you are intolerant to yeast.
▶ Pumpkin, hemp, sunflower and flax seeds. These contain zinc and essential fats, both vital for brain function and hormonal balance.

⸬ AVOID

▶ Wheat, as this is linked to depression and lack of energy.
▶ Foods that cause slumps in energy and mood. Sugar, alcohol, caffeine, refined carbohydrates and processed foods all cause highs followed by lows. You may crave these comfort foods but they will perpetuate feelings of sluggishness and depression in the long term.

HERBS AND SUPPLEMENTS

▶ Supplement with St John's wort. This can keep levels of serotonin up and has been found to be as effective as anti-depressant medications but with fewer side effects. Do not take this if you are on other medications.
▶ Drink lemon balm, peppermint and camomile teas. These all have anti-depressive and calming properties.
▶ Supplement with fish oils. These are important for normalizing brain chemistry and are often deficient in those with depressive disorders.

⸬ EXTRA TIPS

▶ Get outside in daylight every morning. This is important for setting the body's rhythms and moods.
▶ Exercise every day, preferably outside. Aim for at least 20 minutes daily. Do anything you enjoy: cycling, walking, jogging, rollerblading, skipping and re-bounding are all good for getting the heart rate up and triggering the release of endorphins in the brain. These are feel-good chemicals released during exercise.
▶ Use full-spectrum light bulbs. Light is measured in lux; a normal light bulb will light a room to up to about 800 lux. A room lit with full spectrum lighting will have about 10,000 lux. You can also help to maximize your light intake by keeping curtains and blinds open and by working near a window.
▶ Investigate light boxes and light therapy.

SEBORRHOEA OR SEBORRHOEIC DERMATITIS

Seborrhoea refers to red, inflamed, scaly patches on the skin and scalp caused by overactive sebaceous glands (oil-secreting glands). Areas most commonly affected are the scalp, face and chest. In babies it often appears as cradle cap.

CAUSES

► Nutrient deficiencies, particularly vitamin A, B vitamins, essential fats and biotin, may be a factor.

► Yeast overgrowth and lack of stomach acid are both common in those with seborrhoea. It may also indicate that the body is trying to eliminate wastes through the skin so colon and liver cleansing would be indicated.

► Food intolerances may also be a problem.

Action plan

Great nutrition can really help with this condition.

⠿ EAT/DRINK

► Vegetables and veggie juices. These are cleansing and nourishing. Include green vegetables for their chlorophyll content and orange vegetables for their beta-carotene, which can be converted to vitamin A in the body.

► Oily fish and seeds. These have anti-inflammatory effects. Aim for oily fish two to three times a week and 2 tbsp of seeds daily. Hemp and linseed oils can be used in salad dressings.

► Whole grains for their B vitamins. B vitamin deficiency is often part of the problem. Brown rice, millet, quinoa and buckwheat are all good sources.

► Pau d'arco tea for its anti-fungal properties.

⠿ AVOID

► Sugar, refined carbohydrates, alcohol and yeast. These may all exacerbate symptoms of a yeast overgrowth.

► Saturated and processed fats. These are found in dairy products, chocolate, fatty and processed meats, such as ham, bacon and sausages, crisps, pastries, biscuits, cakes and many processed and packaged foods.

► Gluten grains. These have been linked to cases of seborrhoeic dermatitis. They include wheat, rye, oats, barley, spelt and kamut. Other food intolerances may also exacerbate the symptoms so a food intolerance test may prove useful, see www.gillianmckeith.info.

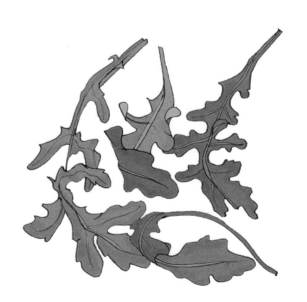

HERBS AND SUPPLEMENTS

▶ Drink burdock-root coffee. Other useful drinks include dandelion coffee and nettle tea for the liver.

▶ Borage oil capsules and evening primrose oil capsules for anti-inflammatory properties.

▶ Supplement with probiotics. These can help to crowd out yeasts and improve absorption of B vitamins.

▶ B complex twice daily.

▶ Vitamin B12 sublingual or liquid drops.

▶ Vitamin A for a short time (not when pregnant) to help improve immunity.

▶ Betaine or digestive enzyme for digestive support.

⠿ EXTRA TIPS

▶ Use neem shampoo and conditioner if the scalp is affected and neem cream on the skin. Neem has anti-fungal and anti-inflammatory properties. Tea tree oil shampoo also has anti-fungal properties and can be alternated with neem shampoo.

▶ Rub the scalp with flax oil and vitamin E oil. Leave on for a little while.

SHINGLES

Shingles is caused by the *Herpes zoster* virus that is also responsible for chickenpox. Once the virus has entered the body it is always present. Therefore, anyone who has had chickenpox will be harbouring the virus in a dormant state in the nerves around the spine. If the immune system becomes weakened the virus may be reactivated.

Shingles affects the nerve endings causing a blistering rash, pain, itching and tenderness. The rash usually affects the skin of the abdomen but may also affect other body parts.

The rash may be preceded by a few days of feeling feverish and achy. Once the rash starts, the blistering usually lasts a week or two, sometimes longer. The pain may continue after the blisters have scabbed over and dropped off, sometimes for several months. This is known as post-herpetic neuralgia.

Shingles can cause serious damage such as blindness, paralysis and secondary infections in those with weakened immune systems.

CAUSES

Shingles generally occurs when the immune system is weakened from stress, chemotherapy, radiotherapy, contact with an open blister or nutrient deficiencies. About 20 per cent of people who get shingles suffer a recurrent attack.

Action plan

Improving the nervous system is important for the long term.

⠿ EAT/DRINK

▶ Foods rich in lysine may be effective in reducing severity. These include chicken, fish, beans, mung beans, srouts and most fruit and vegetables, with the exception of peas.

▶ Fruit and vegetables to support immune function and alkalize the body. Viruses thrive in an acidic environment.

▶ Mixed vegetable juice. For extra benefits add a few drops of a green superfood such as wheat grass, barley grass, spirulina or blue-green algae. This will support the liver and the immune system.

::: AVOID
► Foods high in arginine: chocolate, gelatin, wheat, carob, coconut, oats, peanuts, soya beans, sesame seeds and wheat germ.

HERBS AND SUPPLEMENTS
► Aloe vera juice before meals.
► Drink calming teas before bed to aid sleep: camomile, St John's wort, valerian, lemon balm and lime flowers can all be helpful.
► Make a paste out of slippery elm powder and water and apply this to the blisters to soothe and speed healing. Aloe vera gel is also calming and soothing.
► If you have pain, at the onset take echinacea regularly.
► Astragalus, skullcap and lobelia are all good nerve tonic herbs.
► L-lysine for its antiviral effects.
► Vitamin C for its immune supportive effects.
► Sublingual vitamin B12 to support the nervous system.
► Vitamin B complex twice daily.
► Zinc citrate daily.

::: EXTRA TIPS
► Do not touch the sores unless applying an ointment or poultice to aid healing. This can increase irritation and spread the infection.
► Relax and get as much rest as possible.
► Take care with personal hygiene; do not share towels, etc.

► Mix a few drops of eucalyptus, lavender or bergamot oils to a tablespoon of almond oil and apply to the lesions as soon as they appear. This reduces the time it takes for them to dry out and fall off.
► A cloth bag of oats can be put under the tap when running a bath to help soothe the skin.
► Topical ointment with capsaicin powder (from cayenne peppers).

SINUSITIS

Sinusitis is inflammation of the sinus cavities. The lining of the sinuses swell up and block the nasal passages. It can make you feel miserable, grumpy, tired out, and is painful, too. Headaches, coughs, runny nose, nasal discharge, congested nose and fever are the usual symptoms. Sinusitis can be acute due to bacterial, viral or fungal infections and also chronic where there is usually an allergy or immune trigger.

CAUSES MAY INCLUDE
► Poor immunity.
► Allergies.
► Swimming in chlorine.
► Passive smoking.
► Environmental pollution.
► Dairy products.
► Food intolerances.
► Constant colds and flus.
► Zinc deficiency.
► Central heating.
► Lung weakness.

Action plan

Decreasing the mucus secretions
is helpful in the short term, while the
plan for the long term is to improve
your immunity.

EAT/DRINK

► Up to 2 litres a day of water, but not ice
cold. Water makes the nasal secretions
thinner and easier to get out of your nose.

► Brown rice, peas, black-eyed beans.

► Veggie juices, soups, broths, salads,
and other raw fruit and veg.

► Cayenne, ginger, garlic, fenugreek
seeds, turmeric and horseradish in your
cooking may improve elimination.

► Raw garlic and freshly grated
horseradish may help shift mucus.

► Get daikon root from the health-food
store and make a daikon miso soup.
Daikon is a fantastic mucus resolver.

AVOID

► Dairy products such as eggs, cow's
milk and cheese.

► Alcohol.

► Corn, peanuts, aubergines and wheat.

► Sugar.

► Baked flour goods.

HERBS AND SUPPLEMENTS

► Use sage, thyme and basil herbs for
antibacterial properties.

► Drink elderflower tea.

► Take vitamin A. Often sufferers of
sinusitis have weakened immune systems
and vitamin A helps to strengthen
immunity.

► Vitamin C with bioflavanoids and
quercetin can help too.

► Take n-acetylcysteine supplement for
draining out the nose.

► Bromelain in between meals can help
to reduce inflammation. If you take
bromelain with meals, it will act as a
digestive enzyme. If taken in between
meals, it has anti-inflammatory
properties.

► Echinacea extract and the herbal
extract goldenseal should help to reduce
mucus build up.

► After a course of echinacea, switch
to astragalus.

EXTRA TIPS

► Try a steam inhalation with oil of
eucalyptus and tea tree oil together. You
can also try peppermint oil. Essential oil of
pine in a bowl of hot water brings relief, too.

► To give yourself a right good clear out,
make a lemon juice and horseradish
drink. This is an age-old remedy for
clearing the sinuses.

► A hot facial compress or hot, damp face
cloth can bring relief. Some people prefer
ice-cold compresses but the hot one is
more soothing, I think. You could
alternate hot with cold.

► Acupressure which you can do yourself
helps. Press with your index and middle
fingers on each side of your nose; hold the
pressure for a couple of minutes. It should
bring some relief.

► If your GP has you on medication,
make sure you take probiotics to keep the
level of good bacterias high in your gut.

► Pull and massage your toes daily as
the sinus nerve endings are on the toes.

► Have regular reflexology sessions.

► Avoid really dry rooms. Get a humidifier
if it's winter and you have the central
heating on. Try to keep rooms well

ventilated and windows open to let
fresh air circulate.

► Learn how to deep-breathe and take
up a gentle, breathing type of yoga.

► Take regular baths with lavender
and frankincense oils. These oils are
strengthening to the immune system.

► Keep a food diary for a week noting
how you feel after each food or beverage.

► Be careful not to eat the same foods
every day. Best advice is a four-day
rotation.

► Avoid swimming in chlorinated pools.

► Adding colloidal silver to your nasal
spray is also beneficial. You can get
colloidal silver in health-food stores.

SORE THROAT

This inflamed feeling and pain in the
tonsil area or back of the throat may
sometimes be accompanied by a slight
fever.

It is possible you may have a
streptococcal infection so don't wait on
this one. Severe sore throats should not
be left unchecked as they can be serious,
affecting the heart and triggering
rheumatic fever. And you may need
antibiotics. So see your GP.

CAUSES MAY INCLUDE

► Toxicity.

► Colds.

► Low immunity.

► Shouting and over-using the voice.

► Chronic stress.

► Glandular fever.

► Zinc deficiency.

► Streptococcal infection.

► Viral infection.

► Allergies.

Action plan

This plan will help boost your immunity.

EAT/DRINK

► Lots of liquids (not alcohol). But make
sure they are not ice cold or they will
make your throat worse.

► Herbal teas, veggie juices, warm broths,
and blended soups.

► Pineapple juice.

AVOID

► Dairy products and sugars. They are
potentially mucus-producing and won't
help.

► Gargle with warm salt water. Make
it sea salt, though. For extra relief, you
can also add a few drops of tea tree oil
and thyme.

► Gargle with apple cider vinegar mixed
with sea salt and warm water.

HERBS AND SUPPLEMENTS

► Drink sage tea. Sage is known to soothe
a sore throat.

► Get a high-powered beneficial bacteria
from the health-food store.

► Take vitamin C supplements. Those
with poor, sugar-laden diets tend to be
low in vitamin C.

► Take vitamin A but not if pregnant. But
instead of pre-formed vitamin A, I would
prefer you to take betacarotene. This
converts into vitamin A once in the body.

► Suck on zinc gluconate lozenges. They
dissolve naturally. You can get them from
health-food stores.

▶ Take goldenseal tincture. Keep doing this until you get some relief and then follow with echinacea. There's nothing to stop you gargling with this, too.

▶ Once you have recovered from the sore throat, go on a six-month course of the herb astragalus to help to raise immunity. Also take spirulina, the green superfood.

⠿ EXTRA TIPS

▶ Make sure that you floss and clean your teeth regulary to prevent infections in the mouth and throat.

▶ Chronic sore throats are a common side effect of glandular fever. You also sometimes have a sensation of a ball or marble in your throat. Get it checked by your GP. You may need a blood test.

STRESS

Stress is the manifestation of how you respond to and handle stressors in your daily life. Some people are better at dealing with stressors than others as they are less reactive. This is important as stress causes a pumping out of toxic substances into the blood stream which can leave you tired, irritable and angry. Stress can also play havoc with your digestion and weight balance, impede your organ function, and raise blood-sugar levels to an unnaturally high level. Poor response to stress causes a damaging, excessive secretion of the hormones adrenalin and cortisol. These hormones, produced by the adrenal glands, are designed to help your body

respond to emergency situations such as running for your life or fighting. If they stay in your system for a long time, they will give your brain a toxic bath. At the same time, your heart rate will increase, blood-sugar levels will elevate, blood vessels will constrict, breathing will get heavy. All of this is fine if it is only temporary and the situation warrants such a physical response.

Your ability to keep your weight balanced depends on the adrenal glands producing balanced levels of hormones 24 hours a day. When your body is continuously pumping out excess hormones at inappropriate times and for prolonged periods, eventually these critical glands are unable to perform at all.

Weight problems, canker sores, blood pressure problems, stomach ulcers, gastrointestinal disorders, muscle weakness, clogged arteries, impaired memory, colds, flus, skin disorders, even repetitive strain injuries have all been connected with high levels of the stress hormone cortisol over a prolonged period. Stress places unnecessary pressure on your entire endocrine system. Stress impairs this system's immune function and can thus trigger illness.

CAUSES

Nowadays, the slightest non-physical problems are causing this 'fight or flee' reaction in our bodies. Ordinary stressors like a baby crying, arguments, unhappiness, relationship issues, sexual performance worries, marriage, the workplace, upsetting phone calls, traffic jams, frustration, anger, fear, isolation are triggering an unnatural, prolonged surge of these hormones. If you don't indulge in a form of physical exercise at that moment to 'burn off' these excess hormones caused by your negative stress response, your brain ends up getting fried, adrenal glands get wasted, and you feel totally wiped out. The body is not designed to neutralize excess hormones when no physical action is called for.

Action plan

You can teach yourself to be less reactive and the right food choices can dramatically assist the body to handle stress.

⁙ EAT/DRINK

► Green asparagus, which helps in the formation of red blood capsules. Asparagus is also high in the antioxidant enzyme glutathione which helps the liver to function at optimum levels and anything that has a positive effect on your liver has a positive effect on your mood and your ability to deal with stress.

► Garlic, which contains a detoxifying chemical called allicin, a powerful antibiotic with both antiviral and anti-fungal powers as well as cholesterol-lowering, blood-pressure-lowering and mood-boosting effects.

► Avocados, which contain 14 minerals, all of which regulate body functions and stimulate growth. Especially noteworthy are its iron and copper contents which aid in red-blood regeneration and the prevention of nutritional anaemia, one very common cause of fatigue and inability to cope effectively with stress. It also contains sodium and potassium and

there may be links between potassium deficiency and susceptibility to stress.

► Brown rice, legumes, parsley and green vegetables, which are high in vitamin B. The B vitamins are needed for your nervous system to function and cope with the effects of stress.

► Sprouts, green vegetables and unrefined cereals containing magnesium which appears to be depleted when there are high levels of stress in the blood stream.

► Sunflower and sesame seeds. Not only are sunflower seeds a rich source of potassium, they are also rich in B vitamins (in particular B6 and pantothenic acid) and zinc, which play a critical role in the health of the adrenal glands. Evidence suggests that during times of stress the levels of these nutrients can plummet.

► Cabbage, which is a good stress-busting source of the antioxidant vitamins A, C and E, betacarotene and the mineral selenium. Antioxidants fight the damaging effect of free radicals in your body, released in response to stress, and they also help the conversion of tryptophan to serotonin and thus play their part in boosting mood.

► Almonds, which are rich in magnesium which is especially important for supporting adrenal function as well as in the metabolism of essential fatty acids. Low levels of magnesium can be associated with nervous tension, anxiety, irritability and insomnia. Soak them overnight for easy digestion.

► Berries. Blackberries, strawberries

and raspberries are rich in manganese and vitamin C. Insufficient vitamin C can weaken your immune system and make you feel generally stressed and run down.

► Cucumbers are wonderful digestive aids and have a purifying effect on the bowel and the liver. They are packed with nutrients, vitamins (vitamins A, B and C) and minerals (calcium, phosphoros and iron) that have a marvellous effect on the skin. When the liver is properly nourished it can help to balance hormones, boost mood, beat stress and deliver vibrant health.

⁞⁞⁞ AVOID

► Caffeine. This is found in coffee, tea, chocolate, colas, etc. It causes the release of adrenalin, thus increasing the level of stress. Caffeine addicts wear out the stress hormone-producing adrenal glands. These stress hormones interfere with metabolism. It is suggested that there is a link between caffeine intake and high blood pressure and high cholesterol levels. Furthermore, both tea and coffee act as diuretics so flush out many vital nutrients and trace elements.

► Alcohol, which is a major cause of stress. Alcohol and stress, in combination, are quite deadly. Alcohol stimulates the secretion of adrenalin resulting in problems such as nervous tension, irritability and insomnia. Excess alcohol will increase the fat deposits in the heart and decrease the immune function. Alcohol also limits the ability of the liver to remove toxins from the body. During stress, the body produces several toxins. In the absence of its filtering by the liver, these toxins continue to circulate through the body, resulting in serious damage.

► Sweets. Sugar has no essential nutrients. It provides a short-term boost of energy through the body, resulting possibly in the exhaustion of the adrenal glands. This can result in irritability, poor concentration, and depression.

► Salty foods. Salt increases the blood pressure, depletes the adrenal glands, and causes emotional instability. Use a salt substitute that has potassium rather than sodium.

► Fatty foods. Avoid the consumption of foods rich in saturated fats, such as animal foods, dairy products, fried foods and common junk foods. Margarines and other processed vegetable oils are high in trans-fatty acids, which can hinder the body's assimilation of health-boosting essential fatty acids.

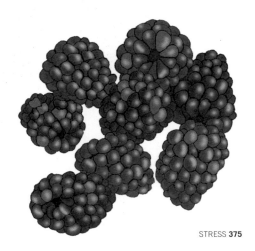

► Cow's milk and other dairy products may stress the body because they contain substances such as the protein casein, which are difficult and unsuitable for humans to digest and can also trigger allergic responses.

► Too much red meat can overwork the kidneys and liver, deplete calcium and stagnate digestion. This can lead to kidney stones and liver disease and colon and bowel disorders. High-protein red meat also elevates brain levels of dopamine and norepinephrine, both of which are associated with higher levels of anxiety and stress.

► Refined, white processed bread, flour and rice which stress the body because they are low in nutrients and high in empty calories. In order to digest refined foods your body has to use its own vitamins and minerals, so depleting its stores.

► Spicy foods. Spices contain volatile oils which are capable of physically irritating the lining of the stomach.

HERBS

► The herbs astragalus and Siberian ginseng should be taken together to help the adrenal glands to adapt and cope better. Note: If you have high blood pressure, do not use extracts of panax (Chinese) or American ginseng. Siberian ginseng increases the tone and function of the adrenal glands, helping to balance the hormonal excretions. Ginseng has been shown in studies to protect against the effects of physical and mental stress. Astragalus helps the body to cope with stress.

► Liquorice root is most beneficial for correcting low cortisol output. The adrenal glands get a chance to rest and recover.

► Avena sateeva from oats can help bring about a sense of calm.

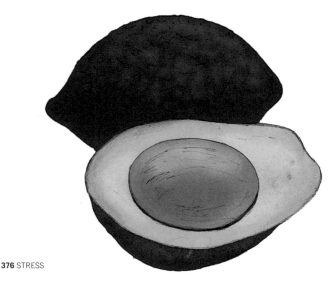

► Rhodiola is an adaptogenic herb that increases the body's natural resistance to stressors. It increases beta-endorphins in the blood stream thus inhibiting stress-induced hormonal changes.

► Evening primrose. When stressed, the body saps up huge quantities of vitamins, in particular pantothenic acid, vitamin B5, vitamins E and C. Your body also finds it difficult even to absorb the nutrients that you so desperately need. Evening primrose supports the adrenals by aiding in the assimilation of these vitamins, particularly pantothenic acid.

► Herbal teas can be very effective at relieving many stress symptoms. These teas are derived from the flowers, leaves, seeds, stalks, stems and roots of plants. They contain natural substances that nourish the central nervous and glandular systems. Find which of the following work best for you: lemon balm, hops, oatstraw, kava, ginseng, camomile, passionflower, skullcap, liquorice, valerian.

► The body's feel-good hormones, serotonin and norepinephrine, can also be made from trytophan and L-phenyl alanine, amino acids present in certain protein foods. Algae contains approximately 60 per cent protein and is derived from all 8 essential amino acids. Studies have shown improved academic results and coping skills when children take algae.

SUPPLEMENTS

► Take B5 pantothenic acid, vitamin B12, folic acid, magnesium, zinc and essential fatty acids to aid adrenal function.

► The following vitamins are critical in the support of your adrenal glands. There's plenty of evidence to show that levels of these key nutrients plummet during times of stress. And these nutrients are also needed for the enjoyment of sex: vitamin C, panthenic acid, vitamin B5, vitamin B6, zinc, magnesium, vitamin B12 and folic acid.

► Take the amino acid tyrosine when under prolonged significant stress.

EXTRA TIPS

► Avoid foods containing additives, preservatives and other chemicals. Additives place a huge stress on your body because it has to work harder to deal with them, with the result that energy and valuable nutrients are spent when they could be used for more profitably, for example, in boosting the immune system.

► Get plenty of exercise.

► Yoga, visualization and meditation can all be beneficial for stress relief. Check out the Oriental exercise regimens of tai chi and chi gung.

T

TONSILLITIS

(see Sore Throat, page 372)

Tonsillitis literally means inflammation of the tonsils. There is usually a streptococcal infection present, though sometimes there may be a viral infection. Symptoms include sore throat, inflamed tonsils, fever and pain on swallowing. You may have bad breath, too.

Children's tonsils used to be whipped out at the first signs of throat problems but that is no longer the case. Once you have lost your tonsils, you are without a piece of your anatomy that is an immunity defender. Tonsils filter bacteria thus supporting the immune system.

If your child is always getting sore throats, take a look at how much milk he or she is drinking. There may well be a connection.

CAUSES

Chronic tonsillitis may indicate that the organs of elimination (bowel, liver, kidneys and lungs) are clogged up. This can lead the lymphatic system, including the tonsils, to become overloaded.

Action plan

You need to boost your immunity.

❖ EAT/DRINK

▶ Organic vegetable juices. These are packed full of nutrients needed by the immune system to fight infections. They will also aid cleansing of the system.

▶ Soups and fruits to allow the body to cleanse and heal without being challenged further.

▶ Garlic.

⁞ AVOID

▶ Dairy products, sugar, refined foods, salt and saturated fats. These can all create mucus and can clog up the system, thus preventing healing from taking place.

HERBS AND SUPPLEMENTS

▶ Drink slippery elm tea to soothe the throat.

▶ Gargle with sage tincture to fight the infection locally.

▶ To prevent recurrence, take three drops of thuja tincture in warm water every evening.

▶ Camomile tea and cleavers tea help to reduce inflammation.

▶ Drink cups of warm water with half a teaspoon of vitamin C powder, 20 drops of echinacea tincture and 10 drops of astragalus tinctures every three hours.

▶ Take vitamin C with bioflavanoids. Vitamin C has antibacterial and antiviral effects.

▶ Take zinc to help the immune system to fight infections and aid healing.

▶ If you are taking antiobiotics make sure you also supplement with probiotics.

⁞ EXTRA TIPS

▶ Wrap a witch hazel cold compress around your neck.

▶ Get a reflexology session.

TOOTH DECAY

(see Periodontal Disease, page 344)

TRAVEL SICKNESS

See Nausea (page 332)

ULCERATIVE COLITIS

See Crohn's Disease (page 239).
See Peptic Ulcer (page 392).
See Irritable Bowel Syndrome (page 314).
This is another inflammatory bowel condition which causes chronic inflammation of the large intestine and rectum. It is thought to be an auto-immune condition. The side effects are extreme pain, fever, anaemia, fierce bowel movements, gas, bloating, stomach distension, alternating bouts of explosive, bloodied diarrhoea with periods of constipation. The rectum may have fissures and haemorrhoids or even abscesses. This condition often results in rapid weight loss due to the fact that nutrients from foods are not being absorbed effectively. Acids and by-products have eaten away at the intestinal lining resulting in serious inflammation and ulcering.

Make sure you get a proper diagnosis. Sometimes colitis symptoms can mimic appendicitis. If you have rectal bleeding, please see your GP as this could also be a sign of colon cancer.

CAUSES MAY INCLUDE
► Food allergies.
► Food sensitivities.
► Dairy intolerances.
► Intestinal parasites or protozoa disease.
► Bad bacterias.
► Excessive arachidonic acid.
► Liver stagnation.
► Emotional problems, stress.
► Poor immunity, auto-immune disease.
► High sugar intake.

Action plan

Diet plays a crucial part both in causing and helping to alleviate this condition.

⣿ EAT/DRINK
► Oats, peeled fruits and cooked leafy greens which seem to be tolerated.
► Puréed vegetables and fruits. Just remember to remove the seeds and skin.
► Veggie juices and broths which are safe bets. Cabbage juice is a well-known remedy for ulcers.
► Chicken, fish and turkey which seem to be fine with this condition.
► Fresh figs (every other day). If you can't find fresh figs, then get dried ones and soak them in water overnight.

⣿ AVOID
► Dairy, yeast and wheat which have been shown to cause varying levels of inflammation in the bowel. So avoid cheese, milk and even yoghurts for now.
► Junk food, fast food such as hamburgers, greasy chips, deep-fried fish or kebab.
► Raw food; that means food that is not cooked. It will irritate the already inflamed colon.
► White flour, white pasta and sugar.
► Caffeine as that can be a trigger. The same goes for colas, fizzy drinks and alcohol.

HERBS AND SUPPLEMENTS
With supplements that I recommend, you can open up capsules and mix them into juice or a smoothie. I do not expect you to take them all at once.
► Take a powdered probiotic to help to keep levels of good bacterias high.
► Take slippery elm powder or tea.

► Drink flax-seed tea. Place 1 tablespoon of flax seeds in a large mug of hot water. Leave to cool overnight. Strain and drink the broth in the morning.

► Silica gel will also help to reduce inflammation in the gut.

► The herb boswellia has been reported to help with ulcerative colitis.

► The following herbs are suggested for this condition but please see a herbalist who can make up the right formula for you. I have used the herb poke root (phytolacca) to help in the healing of ulcerations caused by this condition. The following are also helpful: marshmallow root (soothing to gut), goldenseal (helps to stop bleeding in times of flare-up), comfrey (muscle calming) and echinacea (helps to fight infection and to create a good bacteria count).

► You will need to supplement to make up for the lack of nutrient assimilation which is a problem with this condition. Take multivitamins daily. Also, a yeast-free liquid iron is helpful in addition to a multiple vitamin to make up for blood loss.

► Zinc levels tend to be very low so supplement with zinc citrate.

► A deficiency of magnesium is also very common. Magnesium citrate is needed. You really need a complete mineral supplement as many other minerals are usually low.

► Vitamin B complex is important too. And make sure you get enough folic acid, especially if you have been on medications.

► Fish oils which are high in omega-3s can help to diminish the symptoms.

► Take L-glutamine powder before meals.

► The bioflavanoid quercetin may help with smoother muscle contractions and to limit inflammation. You need to take it before meals.

► Liquid chlorophyll before meals can help a lot in healing the intestines.

► Sialic acid concentrate or n-neuraminic acid can help to heal the intestinal mucosa.

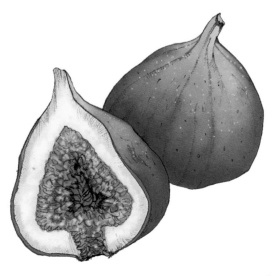

► You absolutely must get the help of a nutritionist. Do not struggle on your own.

► Get tested for parasites. Parasites can be the cause of many gastrointestinal problems. You need to look for the following: blastocystis hominis, entamoeba histolytica and giardia lamblia.

► Read food labels carefully and avoid any products that state 'carrageenan' as an ingredient. Carrageenan is used in some of the following: milk products, ice creams, cottage cheese, milk chocolate drinks. People with ulcerative colitis tend to have high levels of the bacteria bacteriodes vulgatas which helps carageenan to cause damage in the gut. So watch out.

► I always tell my clients with this type of problem to keep a seven-day food and beverage intake form. This way you will get an idea of the triggers.

► Avoid aspirin and conventional laxatives.

► If you are female and on the pill, I strongly suggest that you find another means of birth control as the pill causes liver stagnation which is not helpful for this condition.

► Really chew your food properly. Most people with ulcerative colitis have been vacuuming up their food. You have to chew the food until it becomes liquid.

► Have a course of acupuncture. Look into Japanese acupuncture. This may help to reduce attacks.

UNDERWEIGHT

It is hard to define what underweight is as some people are naturally thin and perfectly healthy. Others have underlying health problems associated with their weight. There are obviously many different reasons for being underweight and it is important to address the underlying causes.

POSSIBLE CAUSES

► Eating disorders such as anorexia nervosa generally involve psychological and emotional issues that need to be dealt with.

► Stress, which can affect appetite, digestion and metabolism (the rate at which we burn up calories). It can have a huge impact on what we are able to eat in terms of time and appetite.

► Malabsorption, which can occur if we lack sufficient digestive juices to fully break down and absorb all nutrients. This can obviously affect weight. Where digestive symptoms are present, bowel disorders should be ruled out or dealt with (e.g., Crohn's (see page 239), diverticulitis (see page 252) and colitis (see page 379)).

► Parasites. An imbalance in the gut bacteria can affect digestion and absorption and lead to weight loss.

► Compromised liver function. The liver plays a big role in the digestion of protein, carbohydrates and fats. If the liver is struggling with its load, the digestion and absorption of these macronutrients will be compromised.

► Overactive thyroid. The thyroid controls our metabolic rate. If it is overactive, calories will be burnt up faster than normal and weight loss is likely. Other symptoms include feeling hot, insomnia, irritability, nervousness, increased bowel movements and fewer or lighter periods.

► Food allergies (see page 178), intolerances and coeliac disease (see page 231). These can all affect digestion and absorption and should be investigated.

► Serious illness. Any sudden or dramatic weight loss should prompt investigation into potential underlying causes. Diabetes, AIDS, cancer and trauma can all cause dramatic weight loss.

► Medical treatments. Chemotherapy, radiotherapy and surgery may all cause weight loss and loss of appetite.

Action plan

Obviously, action taken should be dictated by the underlying causes. These will all need to be addressed in order to achieve a healthy weight.

⠿ EAT/DRINK

► Alfalfa sprouts – these are incredibly high in bio-available vitamins and minerals. A good all-round tonic.

► Whole grains. Include brown rice, oats, millet, quinoa, rye and buckwheat. These are a great source of B vitamins needed for proper metabolism. To increase nutrition, stir a teaspoon of olive, hemp or flax seed oil into the grains after cooking.

► Freshly pressed fruit and vegetable juices – these are especially good where absorption is poor or in illness or recuperation. They are great for increasing nutrient levels without putting a strain on the digestive system.

► Essential fats. These are found in oily fish, nuts, seeds, avocados and cold pressed oils. Eat foods from this list daily. They are needed for energy, metabolism, nutrient absorption and hormone balance.

⠿ AVOID

► Caffeine from chocolate, coffee, tea and colas. Coffee can speed up the metabolic rate and deplete nutrient levels.

HERBS AND SUPPLEMENTS

► Take digestive enzymes with meals to aid absorption of nutrients from food. These would particularly be recommended where digestive symptoms are present.

► Sprinkle lecithin granules onto food – lecithin aids fat digestion.

► Drink fenugreek seed tea daily – this is traditionally used to help with digestion, absorption and weight gain.

► Drink slippery elm bark tea – this is traditionally used to build up thin and undernourished people. Just mix 1 teaspoon of powder with some warm water and sip.

► Include herbs and mild spices in your diet – these aid digestion and absorption and can improve the appetite; caraway, cayenne, celery seed, dill, fennel, fenugreek and ginger are all useful.

► Supplement with zinc to improve sense of taste and smell and appetite.

► Take magnesium supplements daily – particularly if stress is an issue. Magnesium gets used up in stress and is needed for energy and relaxation.

► Take a free form of amino acid complex – particularly where absorption is poor. This provides a readily available source of protein needed for building up body tissue.

⁞⁞ EXTRA TIPS

► Get tested for parasites, yeasts and bacteria – where there are symptoms of bloating, flatulence, diarrhoea and/or constipation there is a possibility of undesirable entities in the gut. Ask your GP about testing or see a nutritional therapist who can arrange for the appropriate tests to be done. In the meantime, take probiotic supplements to help to re-establish healthy gut bacteria.

► Eat six small meals and snacks over the day and chew thoroughly. This will put less strain on your digestive system and make absorption easier. Always eat in a relaxed atmosphere.

► Stop smoking and drug use.

► Have regular olive-oil massages – rubbing oils into the skin can 'feed' and nourish the body where absorption is poor.

► Take moderate exercise such as walking and yoga – gentle exercise can improve appetite and assimilation of nutrients. Aim for 20 minutes a day. Stretching and taking some deep breaths before meals can improve digestion.

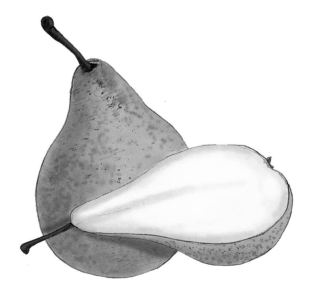

V

VARICOSE VEINS

Varicose veins are weak or broken spots in surface blood vessels that most commonly occur in the rectum, anus (haemorrhoids) or legs. They develop due to the improper functioning of the tiny one-way valves located in venous walls which help to transport the circulating blood back to the heart. If the valves are not working efficiently, blood collects in localized areas, causing veins to stretch and swell. Varicose veins all too frequently form during or just after pregnancy. Besides being unattractive, they might be accompanied by a dull ache, and in more severe cases, leg sores may even develop.

CAUSES MAY INCLUDE
► Prolonged standing or sitting.
► Lack of exercise.
► Diet low in antioxidants.
► Obesity.
► Pregnancy.
► Heredity.
► Poor circulation.
► Poor nutrition and weakened digestion.
► Liver weakness.

Action plan

There is much you can do to help prevent more varicose veins developing or the ones you have from worsening. Keep a food diary and have a look at ways you can make improvements. The following foods combine to help improve healthy veins, bowel and liver function.

❖ EAT/DRINK
► Fibre and antioxidant-rich plant foods, which help to keep tissues strong.

► Foods high in vitamin C and P (bioflavanoids) for healthy capillary walls. Good food sources of both vitamins (C and P are usually found together) include blackcurrants, grapes, cherries, plums, apricots, rose hips, green peppers, tomatoes, dates and buckwheat groats.
► Sprinkle wheat germ on your porridge.
► Leafy greens for their chlorophyll content.
► Include more seaweeds in your diet.
► Parsley is packed with nutrients so include in your cooking, not just as a garnish.
► Place 1 tablespoon of flax seeds in a mug of warm water overnight and drink the broth in the morning.
► Drink grapefruit juice to help keep you regular.
► Include onions, garlic and shallots in your cooking.

••• AVOID
► Processed foods.
► Foods that have an expansive or tiring effect on the cells, such as dairy products, sugar, alcohol, conventional tea and coffee.

HERBS AND SUPPLEMENTS
► Bilberry herb is the best herb to help varicose veins as it strengthens vein walls and capillaries.
► Nettle tea promotes venous elasticity. Alternate with dandelion tea for a change. Also try ginkgo biloba tea.
► Use tinctures of horsetail, which is a rich source of bioflavanoids.
► Pine bark extract or grape seeds extract is thought to help.
► If your bowels are not moving try the Ayurvedic fruit powder triphala for a few months. Milk thistle tincture can also help with constipation.

► Two nutrients that are particularly important for strengthening blood vessels are vitamin C and its mutual companion – bioflavanoids. Also known as vitamin P, bioflavanoids have the ability to regulate the permeability of blood capillaries. They stick to the collagen fibres in blood vessels, which restores the integrity of capillary walls.

► Become aware of other nutrients that might help to improve circulation to the veins. In addition to the vitamin C with bioflavanoids, I always recommend to my patients vitamin E, which improves blood circulation and reduces pain and swelling, vitamin B complex, lecithin and co-enzyme Q10. A general antioxidant formula that contains betacarotene, selenium and zinc will also be beneficial.

⁞⁞ EXTRA TIPS

► To help ease varicose discomfort, a compress infused with horsechestnut herb can be placed over the affected areas. To prepare the compress, mix half a teaspoon of horsechestnut powder with two cups of water and use it to soak a sterile cotton cloth.

► Witch hazel herb is another remedy that can be applied to the skin; a natural astringent, it tightens tissues and reduces pain.

► Treat yourself to a warm bath infused with essential oils. Try rosemary or frankincense in the mornings or lavender, camomile or rose at night.

► Don't stand or sit in the same position for long periods of time.

► Don't sit with your legs crossed.

► Avoid baths that are too hot.

► Try to maintain your ideal weight.

► Engage in regular exercise such as walking, swimming or cycling.

► Massage the legs regularly on a daily basis.

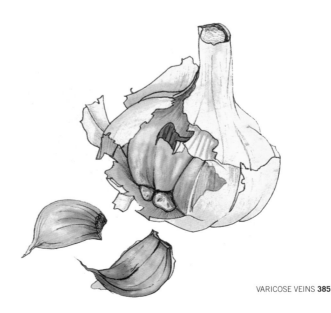

▶ Avoid wearing tight clothing that restricts circulation.

▶ Do leg inversions as follows: Lie on the floor on your back, placing your feet up onto a chair or couch. Relax in this position for about 15 minutes until the blood has a chance to move in a different direction, improving circulation in your legs.

▶ A weekly soak in a sea-salt bath is also an excellent way to relax and unwind, promoting detoxification and a soft, silky skin. Whichever way you choose to wash, round off with a do-it-yourself massage with either peach kernel or sweet almond oil.

▶ Skin brush. To improve the skin's job of getting rid of internal rubbish, you can help it by regular body brushing. Brushing the skin not only removes dead skin cells, it stimulates circulation and the lymph glands which flush out toxins. To skin brush effectively, you need a small, firm natural bristle brush. Brushing is best undertaken just before you bath or shower – on a dry body. Start at the soles of the feet and work your way up the legs in long, brisk strokes; then up the arms and down the back. Always brush upwards towards the chest and avoid sensitive spots such as moles, warts and broken veins. Never use the brush on your face.

▶ Aromatherapy vein massage. Add five drops of lavender oil and five drops of cypress oil to 20mls of carrier oil such as sweet almond or grapeseed. Gently massage into the legs, massaging upwards, towards the heart.

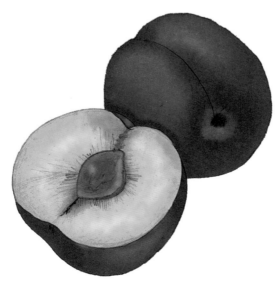

WEAKENED IMMUNE SYSTEM

The immune system specifically refers to the thymus, spleen, lymph, bone marrow and red blood cells. Obviously, other organs assist in the immune process as well, but these body parts technically establish the 'immune system'. A weakened immune system is when you have a poor response to illness, getting one cold after another, always feeling below par. It can be accompanied by apathy and lack of vitality and energy.

Concerns about the immune system are widespread, and rightly so. Poor diet, computer and mobile phone radiations, chemical pollutants, pesticides, extermination fluids, microwaves, ozone depletion, sun-bathing, stress – all these take a toll on our immune functions. The end result: more frequent and more severe colds, flu, allergies, mucus congestion and the fear of serious disease.

SYMPTOMS
▶ Allergies or food sensitivities.
▶ Feeling very tired all the time.
▶ Frequent colds or flus, more than three a year.
▶ Teethmarks or scalloped edging on the sides of your tongue.
▶ Swollen glands.
▶ Sore throats.
▶ Unexplained weight loss.
▶ Headaches.
▶ Pain under the right rib.

CAUSES MAY INCLUDE
▶ Nutrient deficiencies.
▶ Amalgam dental fillings.
▶ High, sugary diet.
▶ Processed foods.
▶ Smoking.
▶ Too much alcohol.
▶ Zinc assimilation.
▶ Regular consumption of tap water, fizzy drinks and sodas.
▶ Stress.
▶ Cold and damp.
▶ Gastrointestinal problems.
▶ Lack of exercise.
▶ Lack of sleep.
▶ Excessive use of computers and mobiles.
▶ Close family members with degenerative illnesses.
▶ Poor diet.
▶ Dehydration.
▶ High homocysteine levels (see page 296).
▶ *Candida albicans* (see page 219).
▶ Sluggish spleen and digestive function.

Action plan
Once you get some strength into the immune system, you will feel the difference.

EAT/DRINK
▶ Fruit and vegetables daily. They provide large amounts of antioxidants; these are our best defence against illness and can help to speed recovery from infections. Berries are a fantastic defender.
▶ Vegetable juices. These are one of the best ways of supporting the immune system and nourishing and cleansing the body. Try apple, carrot, beetroot, celery, ginger, radish and spinach.
▶ Water and herbal teas (see below). Dehydration creates lethargy, headaches and increases susceptibility to illness.

Drink your water warm as cold drinks can create stress if the weather is also cold.

► Chestnuts for vitamin C, riboflavin and easy-to-digest protein.

► Collard greens for immune-enhancing phytochemicals.

► Whole grains. These provide the comfort factor and help to raise serotonin levels in the brain without leaving you feeling stodged out. Brown rice, oats, quinoa, buckwheat and millet are all good grains to include.

► Sprouted broccoli seeds. When broccoli seeds are sprouted, they are at their highest level of life force and thus high in a compound called sulphorophane, a powerful antioxidant. They spark the most long-lasting immune support.

► The regular broccoli veggie which is still really good for the liver and you need good liver function for strong immunity.

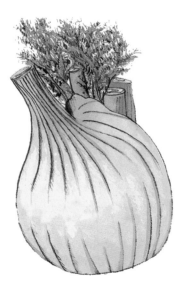

► Reishi and shitake mushrooms. Shitake mushrooms are easier to find. These incredible mushrooms are a natural source of a protein which induces immune response. They contain a compound called lebtinal which mobilizes our natural defences. They also protect the body by lowering heat toxins created from overly acid diets. An acidic body can weaken your immune system. They are also an excellent source of the antoxidant germanium which supports your immune system.

► Sea vegetables, aduki beans, kidney beans, black beans, the grain quinoa (use as porridge or in salads and soups) and fish. These are nourishing to the kidneys.

⦙⦙⦙ AVOID

► Heavy, fatty and stodgy foods. These foods feel comforting but ultimately deplete you of energy and leave you feeling lethargic and literally fed up.

► Sugar, refined carbohydrates, alcohol and caffeine. These suppress the immune system and provide empty calories without supplying the essential nutrients you need for health.

HERBS AND SUPPLEMENTS

► Astragalus is a superior immune tonic which maintains our defences. This super herbal food raises the body's resistance to external pathogens and strengthens the body's effectiveness in fighting viruses and infections.

► Echinacea has long been used to support the immune system when it has been compromised.

► Take a vitamin B complex, too, as you need B vitamins for antibody production and for immune-building white cells.

► Ginseng root. Siberian ginseng is a nutritive tonic. It neutralizes the effects of free radicals (destructive molecules) during periods of stress. It also helps the body adapt to stressors. It sends messages through the body's immune system, acting as a catalyst for the release of certain hormones essential for immune defence.

► Oregon grape contains a compound called berberine which supports the fight against nasty bacterias.

► Olive leaf. This immune herb contains effective natural antiobiotic support against dozens of bacteria strains.

► Ginger root nurtures the regulation of compounds important for immunity. It has a soothing, antiseptic support action on the body's ability to handle external wind and cold.

► Liquorice root. This herb and tea helps to counteract the immune suppressive effects of stress. It also moisturizes and soothes immune organ membranes.

► Lemon peel tea. Place the peel of a lemon in a cup and squeeze a little of the juice into a cup of warm water.

► Pau d'arco tea. This tea contains a strong anti-fungal, anti-parasitic, anti-microbial compound. It also helps to maintain the integrity of red-blood cells and other immune-supporting organs.

► Other teas to include are nettle, fennel, ginger, rose hip, liquorice and dandelion.

► Take the lymphatic herbal extract, cleavers.

⠿ EXTRA TIPS

► Get outside in fresh air and daylight every day. Daylight re-sets our daily rhythms by its action on the pineal gland. Fresh air is great for increasing oxygen levels to the brain and other organs. Have a brisk walk and swing your arms to get your circulation going. Cycling, jogging and skating are also great for circulation and improving mood.

► Turn down the heating. Central heating creates an environment in which bugs can thrive. Put on a jumper and move around at regular intervals to keep the circulation going.

► Go on a winter course of good bacteria. Viruses thrive in yeasty guts, so take care of your internal garden by replenishing it with good bacteria. People tend to get ill more easily when there is an imbalance between good and bad bacterias. Try to get high-potency powdered versions that require refrigeration. You could try Biocare's Replete.

► Always have some raw food with every cooked meal as the food enzymes from raw foods will help to keep you strong. Eating too much cooked food can compromise your immune system as research has shown that it puts white blood cells on constant alert which is weakening to immunity.

► Get a lymphatic drainage massage to help to move lymph through your lymphatic system, the body's drainage network.

► Dry skin brush daily before taking a shower.

► Practise thymus thumping. Make a fist and tap below the neck area 20 times. This will give a bit of a wake-up call to your thymus gland. If the thymus is weak, the body becomes more susceptible to immune-related problems. By getting the lymph moving through the thymus gland, the lymph fluid will make contact with immune-building white cells which are there to seek out foreign invaders before it is returned to the blood for circulation. Just give it a helping hand.

▶ Learn stress-relieving techniques. For example, if the thymus is subjected to undue stress, it then becomes more vulnerable to oxidative injury caused by free radicals. In effect, the thymus contracts. This creates a domino-effect, whereby the thymus is hampered or unable to properly provide many of the lymphocytes to fight infection in the blood. The person is then a victim of constant problems. This is a critical point, because if we nourish those key immune organs and body parts, we strengthen immune response.

▶ Buy a trampette and jump up and down daily for 20 minutes to get that lymph moving.

WORMS

Worms are a type of parasite that live in the gastrointestinal tract. And more people have them than you might think. They include round worms, pin worms and tapeworms. They are incredibly common due to foreign travel, poor quality factory-produced meats and the use of antibiotics and vaccinations that compromise the immune system. Diets high in sugar, refined foods and dairy products also provide the ideal environment in which worms can thrive.

Symptoms of an infestation include loss of or excessive appetite, cravings for sweets, weakness, abdominal pains, diarrhoea, anaemia, rectal itching and weight loss. Sometimes the larvae can be seen in the stool. Sometimes there are no symptoms at all.

Worms can lead to nutrient deficiencies and therefore a whole array of symptoms including growth problems, susceptibility to other infections and anaemia. Always get iron levels checked if worms or parasites are a problem.

CAUSES MAY INCLUDE

▶ Eating undercooked meat or fish.
▶ Sometimes raw vegetables.
▶ Walking barefoot in warm, moist climates.
▶ Poor hygiene.
▶ Contamination from pets.

Action plan

Worms need immediate attention as the effects can be far reaching. So see your GP, the following may also help.

⣿ **EAT/DRINK**

▶ Sesame seeds, pumpkin seeds and figs which have anti-worm effects.
▶ Pineapple, which is particularly useful against tapeworms as the bromelain in fresh pineapple destroys tapeworms. Make sure you eat the core of the pineapple as this is where most of the bromelain is found.
▶ Raw onions and garlic.
▶ Veggie juices. If you can stand it juice some raw garlic with your veggies, too.

AVOID

► Sugar, refined carbohydrates, processed foods, alcohol and sweet fruits (apart from figs and pineapples) as the sugars in these foods are what worms like best.

► Meat, fish or poultry that is not fully cooked or that has been left out at room temperature. Avoid pork and all pork products completely.

► Dairy products as these can be mucus-forming and worms thrive in a mucus-laden digestive tract. Other foods that can contribute to mucus build-up include wheat and other gluten grains (rye, oats and barley), soya, citrus fruits, meat and eggs.

HERBS AND SUPPLEMENTS

Follow a herbal protocol for 10 days, stop for a week and then resume for another 10 days to remove any that may have hatched since the initial 10 days.

► Dandelion juice.

► Drink aloe vera juice twice daily before meals to aid gut cleansing and healing.

► Black walnut extract three times a day on an empty stomach.

► This can be combined with a small handful of pumpkin seeds and/or a clove of garlic for an enhanced effect. The garlic can be minced and combined with miso and water if necessary. Freshly crushed cloves can kill the eggs.

► Other useful herbs include artemesia (mugwort), rhubarb root, gentiana root, cloves and wormwood. It is beneficial to drink a cup of artemesia tea before going to bed during treatment.

► Grapefruit seed extract can be taken internally – 20 drops in water three times a day. It can be used for washing vegetables if there is a risk that they contain bacteria or parasites – mix 10 drops of grapefruit seed extract in 4 pints of water.

► Culinary herbs that can help to support the immune system and are colon cleansing include fenugreek, flax seeds, fennel seeds, thyme, cayenne and turmeric.

► Drink slippery elm tea three times a day to aid colon cleansing and healing.

EXTRA TIPS

► Be scrupulous about hand washing and scrub under the fingernails daily.

► Wash underwear, bed linen and towels in very hot water after each use.

► It may be necessary to treat all members of the family and others who have been in close contact.

► Calendula cream or witch hazel can be applied topically to relieve anal itching.

► Put a clove of garlic inside your socks or shoes. The garlic will get absorbed into the skin and into the bloodstream. You may end up smelling of garlic but it will be worth it for a few days!

► Take probiotic capsules such as acidophilus to restore normal gut bacteria.

► Get home tested for parasites at my online clinic www.gillianmckeith.info

Index

Also available

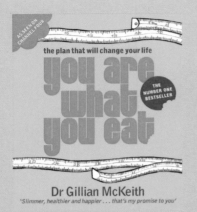

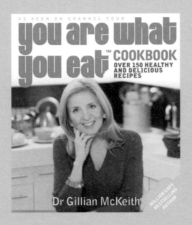

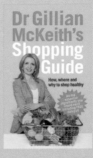

You Are What You Eat
The original nutrition sensation that will transform the way you approach your diet and your health.

You Are What You Eat Cookbook
With over 200 recipes to choose from, this is the perfect companion to the bestselling You Are What You Eat.

Dr Gillian McKeith's Shopping Guide
A brilliant guide to food shopping that includes what to buy and where to shop.

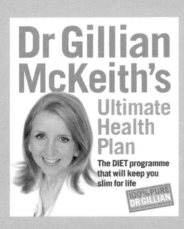

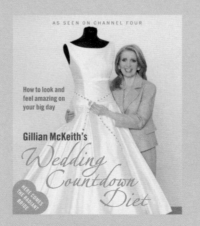

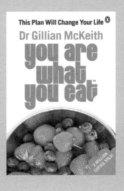

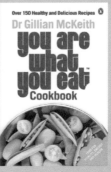

Dr Gillian McKeith's Ultimate Health Plan
The simple diet programme that will help you shed those pounds and reach the pinnacle of wellness.

Gillian McKeith's Wedding Countdown Diet
For every bride-to-be, Gillian's plan will help you look and feel fabulous on your big day.

Visit www.gillianmckeith.info

Empowering people to improve their lives through information, food and lifestyle

Join the club at www.gillianmckeithclub.com

As a member, you will have access to a wide range of tools, resources and features that will help to empower you further. With these tools you can begin to improve your health and well being, through quality information, great food, and a fulfilling lifestyle.

- ► Create your Personal Health Profile
- ► Take part in Gillian's Boot Camp
- ► Keep up to date with the latest Club News
- ► Chat in the Club Forum
- ► Find answers in the Research Centre
- ► Visit the Nutrition Clinic
- ► Join Live Chats with Gillian
- ► Receive weekly Top Tips
- ► Receive weekly Meal Plans
- ► Pick up new meal ideas in the recipe resources
- ► Receive the Newsletter

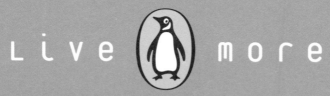

If you would like to receive more information on Healthy Penguin titles, authors, special offers, events and giveaways, please email HealthyPenguin@uk.penguingroup.com

Acknowledgements

Thank you to everyone at Penguin, especially Kate Adams for your dedication.

And to Sarah Rollason who will go to the ends of the earth and over mountains to help deliver my good food message. Fancy another cacao bar?

Appreciation to Nicola, Jo and Luigi. Let's meet up for one of my famous mango smoothies.

Thanks to Paula and Vicky. And Hannah too.

Warm thoughts to all my clients over the years; to all my website club members, congratulations on your commitment to the Mission. And big hugs to the many millions of viewers who watch and support my television programmes around the world.

Gigantic thank you to Josie. Let's have yet another spoonful of raw shelled hemp seeds to keep us going strong.

To Relton, Martin and Ilona who help to advance the mission.

Deepest gratitude and love to Howard. Your wisdom and passion is inspiring.

In memory of Oscar who brought so much enlightenment and love into my life.

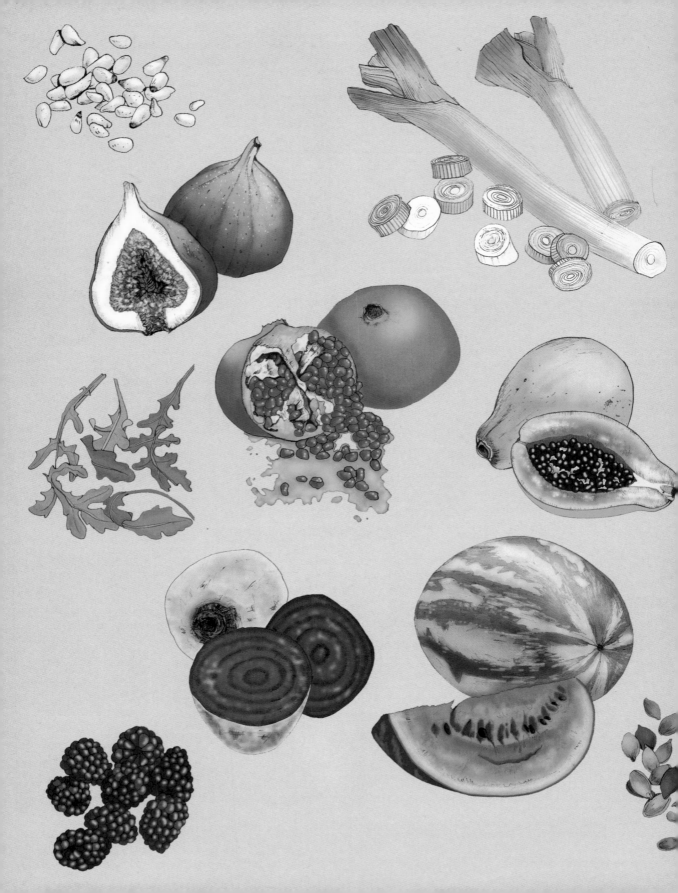